A Colour Atlas of

Paediatric Infectious Diseases

A Colour Atlas of
Paediatric Infectious Diseases

C.A. Hart
MB, BS, BSc, PhD, MRCPath
Professor of Medical Microbiology
University of Liverpool
Honorary Consultant Microbiologist
Alder Hey Children's Hospital
Liverpool

R.L. Broadhead
MB, BS, FRCP, DCH, DTMH
Professor of Paediatrics
University of Malawi
Senior Lecturer in Tropical Paediatrics
Liverpool School of Tropical Medicine
Liverpool

Wolfe Publishing Limited

Published by Wolfe Publishing Ltd, 1992.
Printed by BPCC Hazell Books Ltd, Aylesbury, England
ISBN 0 7234 1650 8

A CIP catalogue record for this book is available from the British Library.

Contents

Preface

Infectious disease is an ever expanding and exciting area of medicine as year by year new infectious agents are identified and old clinical syndromes are matched with new causative organisms.

In children's medicine, as in no other, infection presents a major part of clinical practice and there is a great need to provide an illustrated text to facilitate the diagnosis and understanding of infections.

Our aim in producing this Atlas is to provide an accessible guide to paediatric infections. With the clinician in mind, the book has been structured to present infections in the context of the organ systems that they affect, rather than in terms of aetiological agents. Inevitably this leads to a degree of overlap but it serves to reinforce the varied clinical picture of infectious disease in children.

Although we suggest certain general principles in the management of infection, this Atlas is in no way intended as a definitive guide to therapy. We provide a concise guide to specific infections and their aetiology, pathogenesis and diagnosis.

It is hoped that the reader will not only find this Atlas helpful in clinical practice but will also enjoy it. We enjoyed producing it.

C.A. Hart
R.L. Broadhead

Acknowledgements

We would like to thank Mrs B. Kitchen, Miss L. Woodyer and Miss C. Byrne for their secretarial help, and Mr B. Getty, Mr C. Fitzsimons and Mr K. Jones for photographic assistance. We are particularly grateful to those colleagues who generously provided some of the photographs reproduced in this Atlas:

Dr R. Arnold
Dr O. Arya
Dr R. Ashford
Dr D. Baxby
Dr N. Beeching
Dr D. Bell
Mr N. Blundell
Dr B. Brabin
Dr A. D. Bryceson
Dr H. Carty
Dr M. Chan
Dr Y. Chan
Dr J. Cheesbrough
Mr J. Cooper
Dr B. Coulter
Mr R. Cudmore
Mr W. Dinning
Dr S. Edwards
Dr A. Ellis
Dr M. Ellis
Mr R. Franks
Mr G. Friend
Miss A. Garden
Professor H. Gilles
Dr S. Gillespie
Dr S. Green
Mr M. Guy
Professor A. Harries
Professor R. Hendrickse
Dr D. Hobson
Mr S. Kaye
Professor D. Kelly
Mr R. Llewellyn
Professor D. Lloyd
Dr G. Lloyd
Mr B. Low
Professor M. Marcus
Dr J. Martin
Dr O. Marzouk
Professor K. McCarthy
Mr I. McFadyen
Dr T. McKendrick
Dr S. Mendelsson
Dr E. Molyneux
Professor G. Nelson
Dr I. Peart
Professor A. Percival
Professor W. Peters
Dr D. Pilling
Dr B. Pratt
Professor Radomyos
Dr J. Rhodes
Miss J. Robson
Dr T. Rogers
Dr A. Scott
Dr P. Shears
Dr J. Sills
Dr A. Spriggs
Mr J. Taylor
Dr A. Thomson
Professor D. van Velzen
Dr J. Verbov
Professor C. Vickers
Dr S. Walkinshaw
Dr P. Watt
Ms K. Weeks
Professor A. Wright
Dr G. Wyatt

Dedication

To David Thomas Hart

1 Neonatal infections

As improvements in neonatal intensive care have occurred, the degree of immaturity at which babies have a chance of survival has increased. These babies are not just immature in terms of lung function or gastrointestinal function, but also in terms of their immunity to infection. The neonate, and especially the premature neonate, is at high risk of developing infection. The neonate has difficulty in localizing such infections, which often disseminate to cause septicaemia (sepsis neonatorum).

Rates of infection vary from 1.8 cases of septicaemia and 0.2 cases of meningitis per 1,000 live births overall, to 74.5 cases of septicaemia and 18.6 cases of meningitis per 1,000 extremely low birthweight (<1,000 g) babies. The mortality rates from such infections can be high: for example, case fatality rates for neonatal meningitis can be as high as 50%.

All of this points to the fact that the neonate is an immune-compromised host. However, unlike most other immune-compromised hosts, the neonate's immunity will gradually improve to become fully competent.

The neonate as an immune-compromised host

Defects in the neonate's immunity are present in both the non-specific and specific immune systems.

Non-specific immune system

Defects occur both at body surfaces and within tissues (**Table 1**). The neonate in intensive care is the focus of a large paraphernalia of equipment (**1**), some of which involves breaches in body surfaces. Umbilical artery catheters can act as a direct connection between the external environment and the neonate's bloodstream (**2**); micro-organisms may gain access either through the lumen or on the outside of the catheter. Insertion of endotracheal tubes to ventilate a neonate (**3**) can either cause bacteraemia at the time of insertion, or act to deliver micro-organisms directly into the trachea, which should normally be sterile.

Table 1. Defects in Neonatal Non-Specific Immunity.

At body surfaces
Skin
Umbilical stump
Lack of normal flora
Intravenous and intra-arterial lines
Delicate, thin skin
Mucous membranes
Endotracheal tubes
Urinary catheters
High gastric pH and poor intestinal motility
Intestinal permeability
Poor normal flora
In tissues
Decreased complement levels
Poor temperature control
Diminished inflammatory response
Diminished phagocytic activity
Poor NK (natural killer) cell activity
Prosthetic implants (e.g. ventriculoperitoneal shunts)

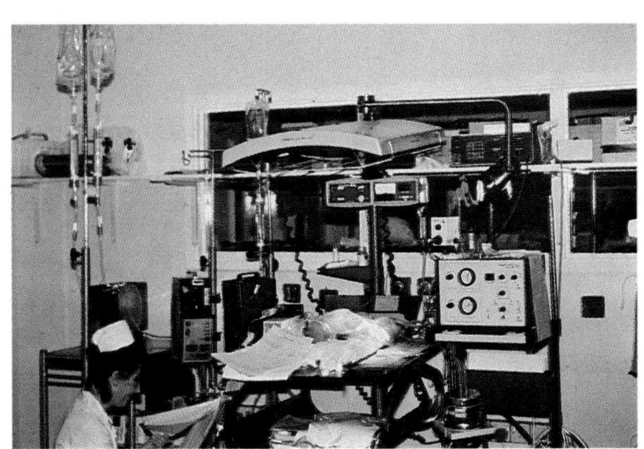

1 A premature neonate being managed in a neonatal intensive care unit.

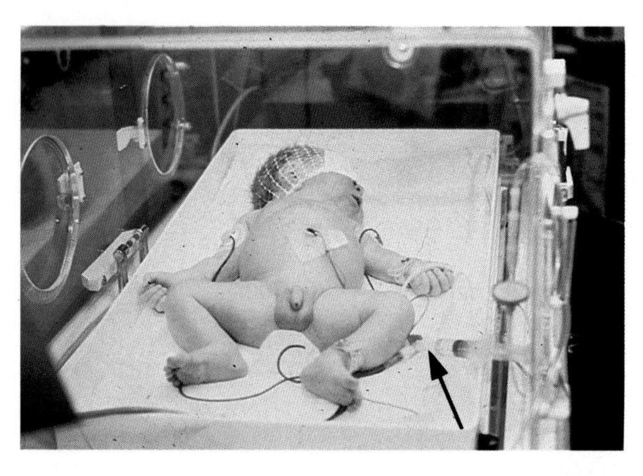

2 A neonate with an umbilical artery catheter *in situ*. The umbilicus is clean, but note the position of the 3-way tap.

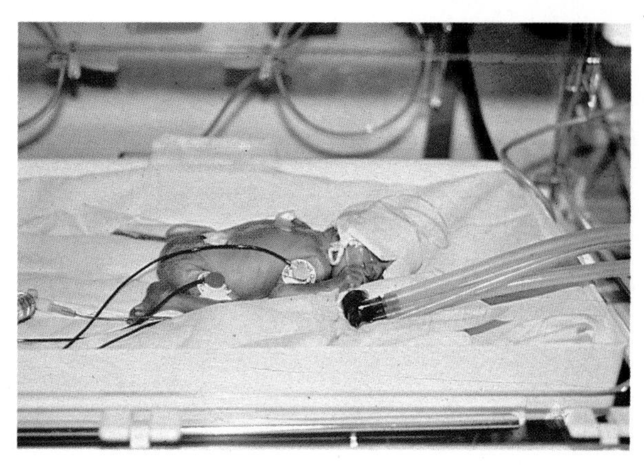

3 A premature neonate undergoing artificial ventilation.

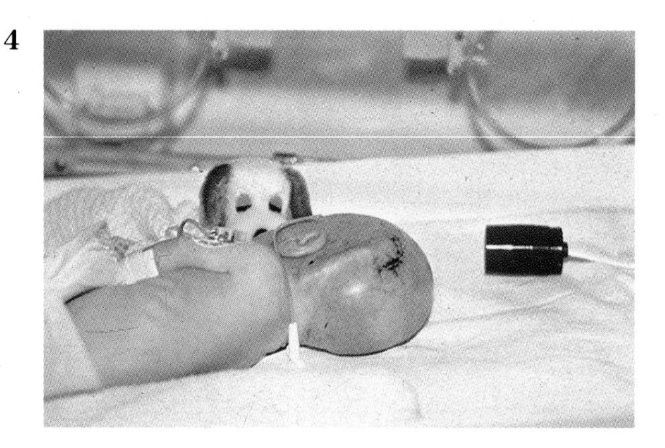

4 A neonate with a ventriculoperitoneal catheter inserted to relieve hydrocephalus.

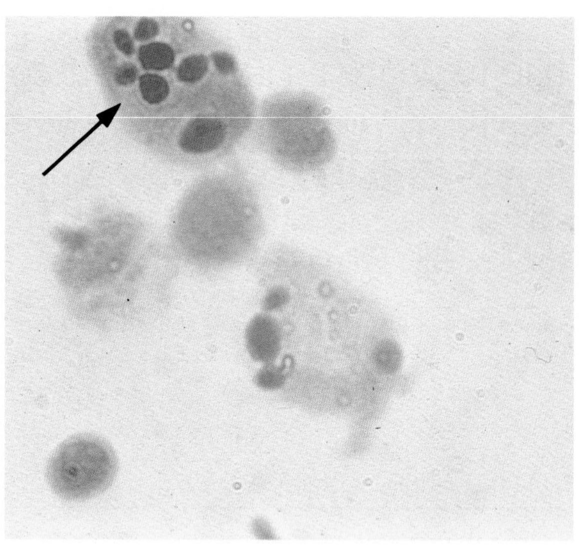

5 Gram-stained film of a peritoneal exudate from a neonate with *C. parapsilosis* peritonitis. Macrophages containing microcolonies of the yeast are visible (× *1,000*).

Insertion of ventricular shunts to relieve hydrocephalus might be supposed to pose little risk of infection (**4**) since the shunts are entirely sited beneath the skin. However, there is a risk of infection with bacteria gaining access at the time of insertion.

Such defects would be less important if the tissue defences were intact; unfortunately, they are not. Total complement activity in neonatal blood is about 50% that of adults, thus the natural bactericidal effect of a neonate's serum is impaired. The premature neonate has poor temperature control and thus has difficulty producing a febrile response to limit microbial replication. Although neonatal neutrophils are as efficient as adult neutrophils at ingesting and killing microorganisms, their response to chemotactic attractants is suboptimal. Consequently, mobilization of neutrophils from the blood to sites of bacterial invasion in tissues is suboptimal and accounts, in part, for the inability of premature neonates to localize infection. The ability of phagocytic cells to kill *Candida* spp. is also less than optimal especially in stressed neonates. **5** shows a gram-stained film of peritoneal exudate from a neonate with *C. parapsilosis* peritonitis. Microcolonies of the yeast are apparent growing within the macrophages.

Specific immune system

Most of a neonate's circulating antibody is derived transplacentally from the mother. It is only of IgG class (each subclass IgG_1–IgG_4 is transferred) and although transfer begins as early as 38 days post-conception, it is not maximal until 33 weeks. The fetus can produce antibody and has circulating B lymphocytes expressing IgG, IgM or IgA on their surfaces. However, antibody production is low, perhaps due to an excessive T8-suppressor cell activity. Fetal IgM production begins as early as week 17, and at term is 20% of adult levels; IgG production starts at week 28, and at term is 5% of adult levels; and IgA production begins at birth.

It appears that T-lymphocyte function in neonates approaches that of adults, apart from the apparent increase in T8 activity.

Neonatal infections

Infections in neonates may be conveniently divided into those acquired transplacentally, those acquired following rupture of the amniotic membranes and during delivery, and those acquired postnatally.

In general the signs of infection in neonates, and especially in premature neonates, are non-specific and include apnoeic attacks, grunting, fisting, alterations in acid–base balance and increased ventilatory requirements. Because neonates have poor temperature control, pyrexia is not a cardinal feature of infection. For example, out of 151 episodes of bacteraemia in a series of neonates studied by the authors, only seven (5%) were accompanied by pyrexia.

Intrauterine infections

Although women are exposed to a large variety of pathogenic micro-organisms during pregnancy, the development of infection is no more common than that outside pregnancy. Furthermore, it is the exception rather than the rule for the fetus to become infected. However, certain micro-organisms have a particular propensity to cause intrauterine infection. Most often, infection of the fetus follows infection of the placental syncytiotrophoblasts. These cells do not express class I transplantation antigens (HLA, A,B), and effective killing of virally infected cells depends upon the recognition by cytotoxic T cells of both viral antigens and major histocompatibility antigens.

Although there are specific syndromes associated with specific intrauterine pathogens, many infections present non-specifically with hepatosplenomegaly and a petechial rash (**6**). Specific diagnosis of intrauterine infection depends upon detection of an IgM-antibody response in fetal or umbilical cord blood (IgG could be of maternal origin) and detection of the pathogen, its antigen or its genome in the fetus or neonate.

6

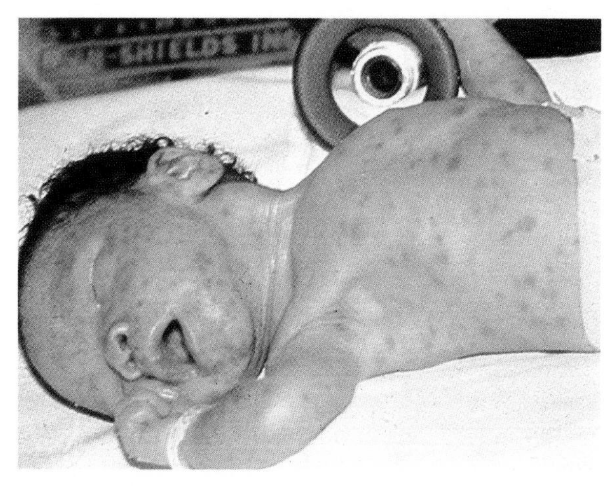

6 A neonate with a petechial rash due to intrauterine infection with rubella virus.

Some micro-organisms are well-established as intrauterine pathogens (**Table 2**); others are less well-established or occur infrequently (**Table 3**).

Table 2. Well-Established Transplacental Pathogens.

Microbe	*Incidence of Fetal Infection* (per 1,000 live births)	*Incidence of Congenital Damage* (% of infected)
Cytomegalovirus (CMV)	2–22	10
Herpes simplex virus Varicella–zoster virus	Unknown	Rare
Rubella virus	1	Up to 90
Parvovirus (B19)	1–10	<5
Human immunodeficiency virus (HIV)	0–80[a]	<1
Treponema pallidum	<1	40–90
Listeria monocytogenes	0.1	90–95
Toxoplasma gondii	0.5	10–30

[a]Varies according to local incidence of HIV infection.

Table 3. Less Well-Established or Rare Transplacental Pathogens.

Viruses	*Bacteria*	*Parasites*
Epstein–Barr virus	*Chlamydia psittaci*	Plasmodium
Enteroviruses	*Borrelia burgdorferi*	Trypanosomes
Poliovirus	*Mycobacterium tuberculosis*	Filaria
Vaccinia virus	*Leptospira* spp.	
Mumps virus		
Measles virus		
Influenza virus		

Rubella

Congenital rubella is the prototype for intrauterine infection. Rubella is a togavirus and is spread by droplet from the upper respiratory tract. Placental infection follows maternal viraemia and it is thought that infection reaches the fetus via emboli of infected vascular endothelium. Infection of the mother and placenta does not necessarily lead to fetal infection.

The results of fetal infection depend upon the stage of gestation. In the first trimester spontaneous abortion occurs in 20% of cases (**7**) and there is a risk of major malformation in 10–52% of cases. Congenital damage includes congenital heart disease (75%), intrauterine growth retardation (60%), thrombocytopenic purpura (55%), cataracts (50%) (**8**), microphthalmia (18%), and bony lesions (22%) including 'celery-stick' osteitis of the long bones (**9**). It should be remembered that intrauterine infection results in persistently infected clones of cells in the neonate, who will continue to excrete large amounts of rubella virus for a long time after birth (6–12 months). Infection in the second trimester is less often associated with congenital defects but profound sensorineural deafness occurs in a proportion of children, and is often not apparent for months or years after birth.

Great advances in the prevention of congenital rubella have been made following the introduction of live attenuated rubella vaccine. The current strategy aims to achieve eradication through the administration of vaccine to everyone at about 12 months of age. However, until full eradication of the disease has occurred, it may be necessary to revaccinate 11–14-year-old females in order to completely eliminate the risk of congenital disease. The vaccine should not be given to pregnant women even though there is a very low risk of congenital infection. Fetal infection after maternal reinfection with rubella does occur, although very rarely.

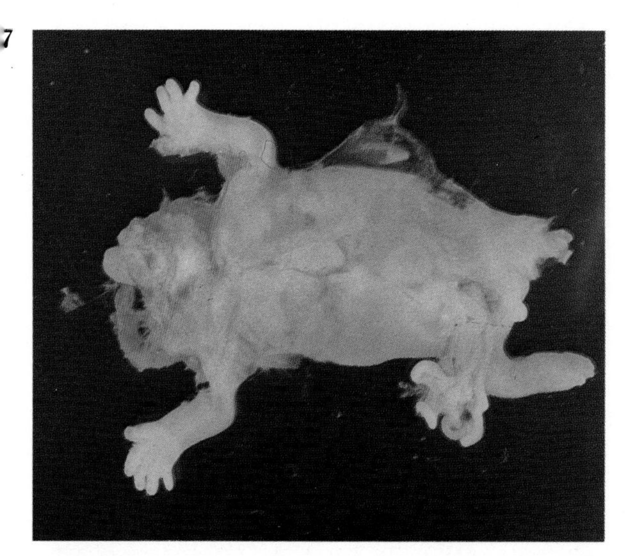

7 An embryo infected *in utero* by rubella virus.

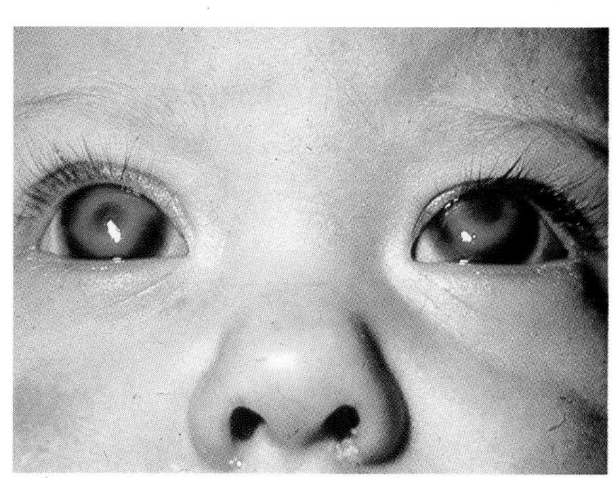

8 An infant with cataracts following *in utero* infection with rubella virus.

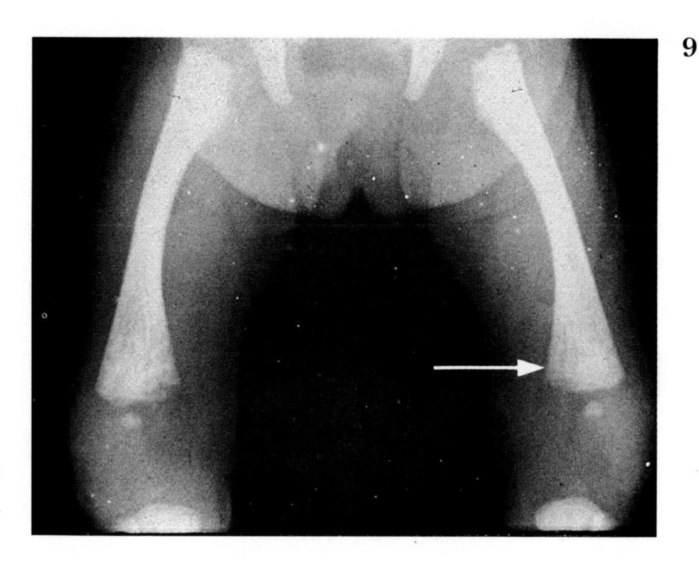

9 X-ray of the femurs of a child with congenital rubella osteitis demonstrating the typical longitudinal striae or 'celery-stick' appearance.

Cytomegalovirus

Cytomegalovirus (CMV) is a β-herpesvirus and has a close association with man. Infection is rarely symptomatic and infection persists for life. CMV does cross the placenta and is the most common infective cause of mental retardation. Fetal infection and congenital damage are more likely to occur if the mother experiences a primary infection during pregnancy. However, they can occur, albeit rarely, with secondary infections (recrudescence or reinfection). Between 0.2% and 2.2% of pregnancies are complicated by CMV infection. The risk of infection varies with social conditions, women in higher social classes being more likely to develop infection, since fewer reach child-bearing age having been infected. Although it is not so clearly demarcated as in rubella, infection with CMV early in pregnancy is more likely to result in congenital damage. However, the risk of congenital damage following fetal infection is low, being about 10%. The damage ranges from hepatosplenomegaly with a petechial rash to hearing loss, chorioretinitis, and severe mental retardation with gross intracranial damage. **10** and **11** show a lateral skull X-ray and ultrasound scans of a neonate with congenital CMV infection. These reveal hydrancephaly with enlarged ventricles and extensive periventricular calcification. Direct electron microscopy demonstrated typical herpesvirus particles (**12**), which on culture proved to be CMV. The virus is excreted for many months by congenitally infected babies. There is no safe and effective vaccine for the prevention of CMV infection.

10

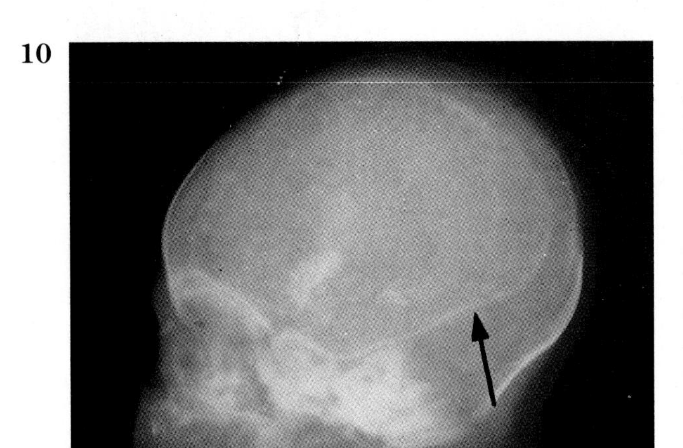

10 Lateral skull X-ray of a neonate with congenital CMV infection. An enlarged lateral ventricle with a calcified periphery is apparent.

12

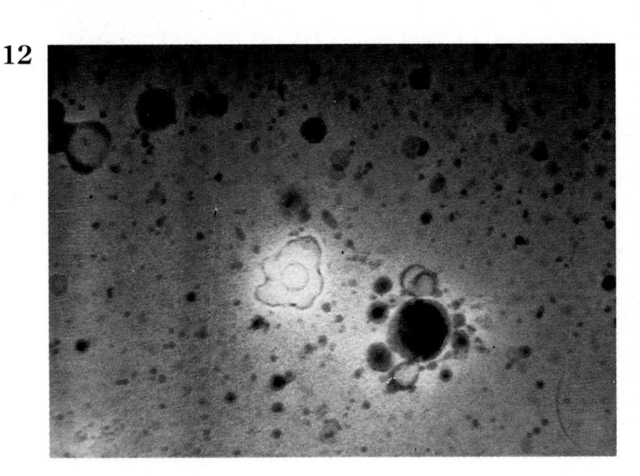

12 Negative-stain electron micrograph of urine from the child shown in **10** & **11**. An enveloped virus particle, typical of CMV, is visible (× *15,000*).

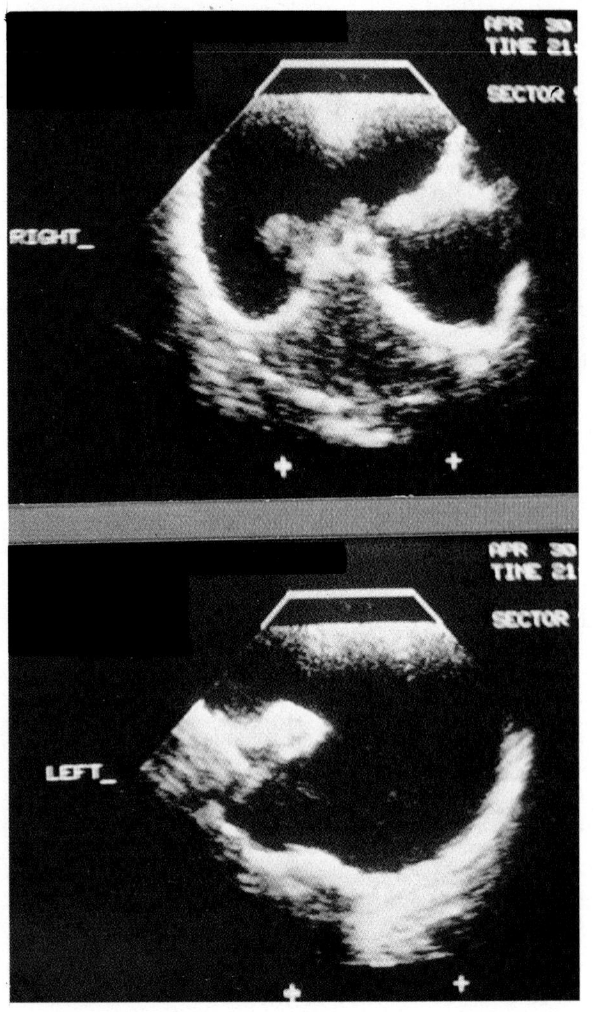

11 Ultrasound scan of the head of a child with congenital CMV. Hydrancephaly of the lateral ventricles with their calcified margins is clearly visible.

Herpes simplex and varicella–zoster viruses

Although both of these viruses can cross the placenta, and this is more likely to occur in primary than in recurrent infections, how often such infections occur in pregnancy is unknown. The incidence of congenital damage appears to be very low, with approximately 50 cases of each viral type reported in the world literature. Features associated with herpes simplex virus (HSV) include low birth weight, chorioretinitis and microcephaly. Those associated with varicella–zoster virus (VZV) include microcephaly, limb hypoplasia, chorioretinitis and mental retardation. In addition, VZV poses specific problems, especially if the mother develops chickenpox within the 7 days prior to delivery and the fourteenth day after delivery. Neonates born under such circumstances are at risk of developing life-threatening fulminant chickenpox (mortality up to 30%). Consequently, passive immunization with zoster immune globulin (ZIG) or plasma (ZIP) should be considered. Maternal chickenpox in the last trimester is associated with a higher risk to the mother of developing varicella pneumonia; it may also result in the development of shingles in the baby 3–6 months after delivery (**13** and **14**).

13

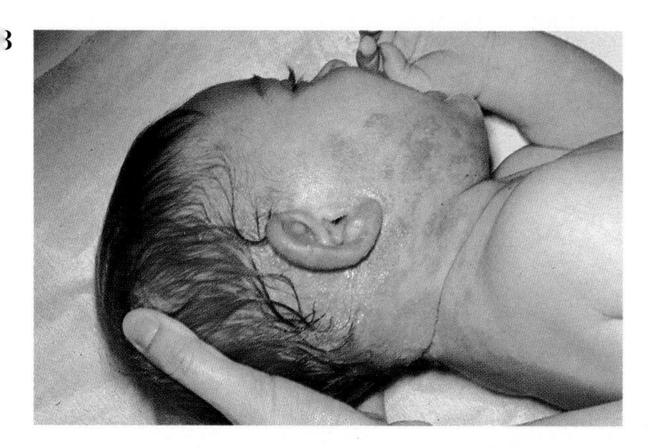

13 A 4-month-old child who was infected *in utero* with varicella–zoster virus. With waning maternal antibody, the virus has re-emerged to produce shingles.

14

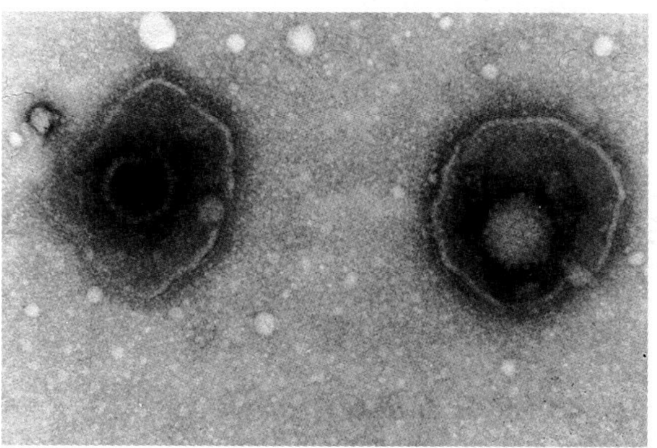

14 Negative-stain electron micrograph of fluid taken from one of the shingles vesicles that developed on the child shown in **13**. Typical enveloped herpesvirus particles are present (× *40,000*).

Human immunodeficiency virus

HIV is an enveloped (100–150 nm) RNA virus in the Lentivirinae subfamily of the family Retroviridae (**15**). It is the causative agent of acquired immunodeficiency syndrome (AIDS). Initial infection with HIV is followed by a long asymptomatic period during which the virus remains latent, predominantly in T4 lymphocytes. Infection can occur either transplacentally or intrapartum, and the relative importance of each is unclear. Transplacental infection early in pregnancy can be associated with intrauterine death. However, in most cases, infection is silent.

Diagnosis of intrauterine infection with HIV is problematic. Unlike other transplacental infections, it is not usually associated with a specific IgM response, and any IgG anti-HIV detected could be of maternal origin. Recent work indicates that measurement of neonatal IgA anti-HIV might be a better marker for infection. Between 25% and 50% of babies born to HIV-infected mothers will themselves be infected.

15

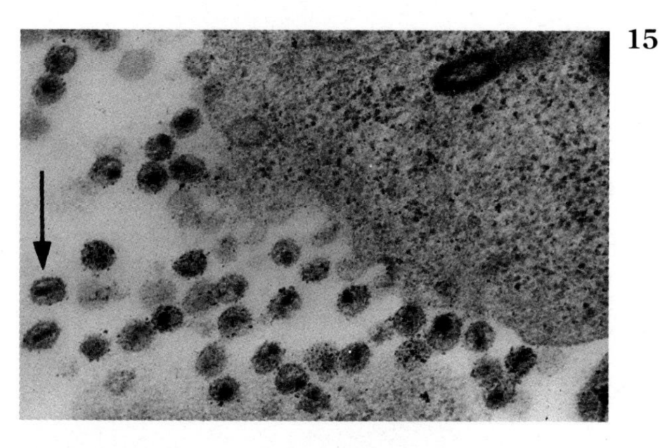

15 Thin-section electron micrograph of a lymphocyte infected with HIV. Extracellular enveloped virus particles with eccentric nucleocapsids are visible (× *15,000*).

Parvovirus

Human parvovirus B19 is a small (18–25nm) unenveloped DNA virus (**16**) that causes 'slapped-cheek' disease in children, a rubelliform rash with occasional arthropathy in adults, and aplastic crises in patients with sickle-cell or other haemolytic anaemias. It is also known to cross the placenta to infect the fetus. Although the most likely eventuality is delivery of a healthy baby at term, in a small number of cases (<5%) infection results in intrauterine death, stillbirth or hydrops fetalis (**17**). There is no vaccine to prevent infection.

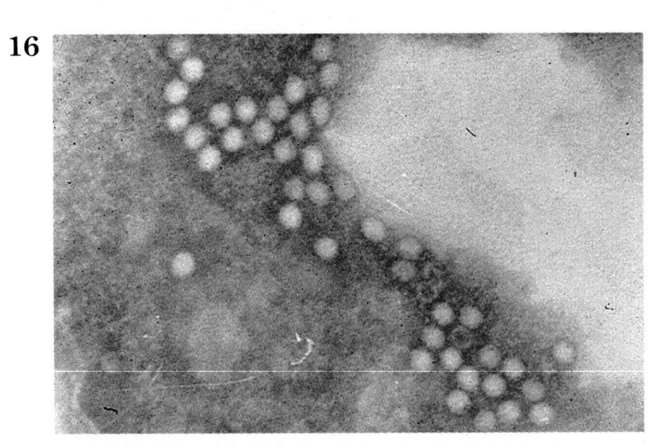

16 Negative-stain electron micrograph of human parvovirus (× *40,000*).

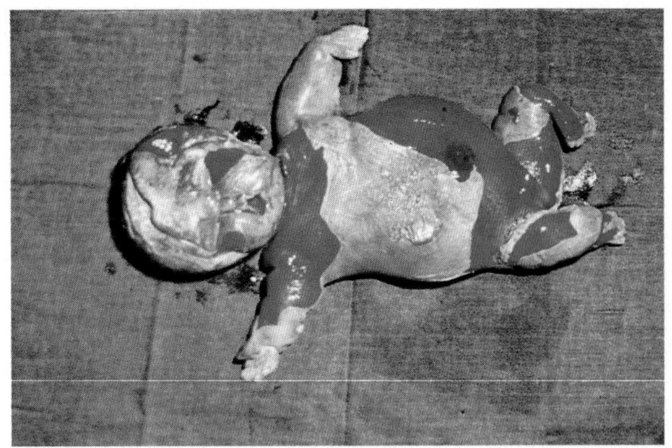

17 A hydropic fetus infected *in utero* by human parvovirus.

Treponema pallidum

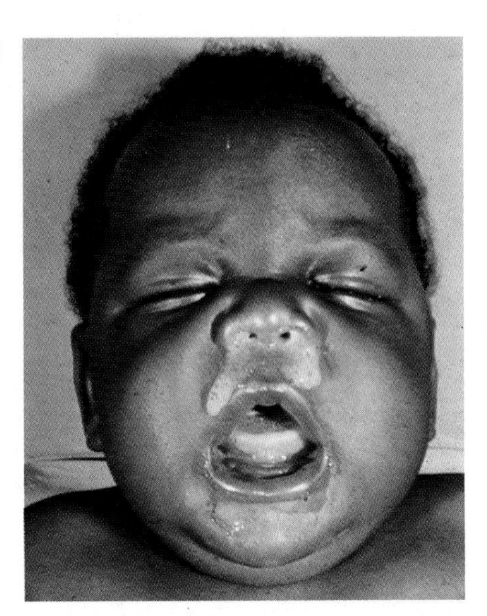

Although congenital syphilis is preventable, it still occurs. It causes fetal or perinatal death in 40% of affected neonates and is associated with congenital damage in a large proportion of survivors. Stigmata of congenital infection include snuffles (**18**), skin rashes including petechiae and, rarely, bullae (**19**), osteitis, periostitis (**20** and **21**), and dactylitis involving the proximal joints (**22**). The neonate excretes infective *T.pallidum* for some time after delivery. *T.pallidum* is still exquisitely sensitive to penicillin, which crosses the placenta to achieve therapeutic levels in the fetal circulation.

18 A neonate with a nasal discharge due to intrauterine infection with *T. pallidum*. This material contained large amounts of viable bacteria.

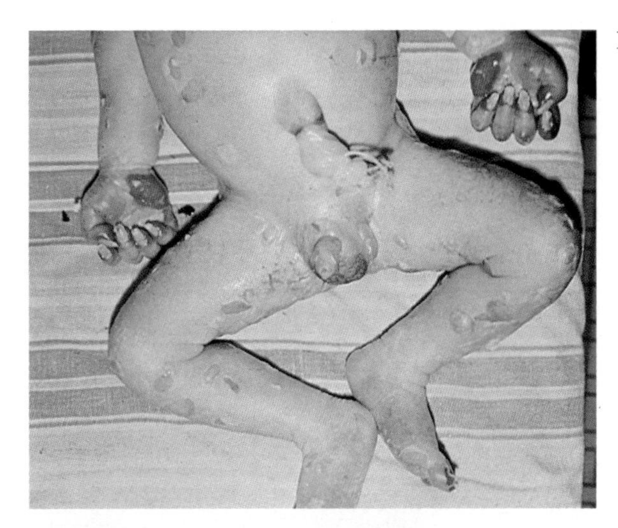

19 A neonate with congenital syphilis. Large bullae containing *T. pallidum* are visible.

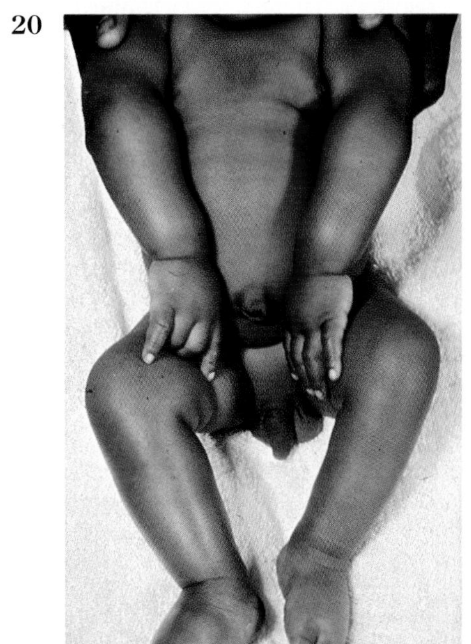

20 A neonate with osteitis due to congenital syphilis.

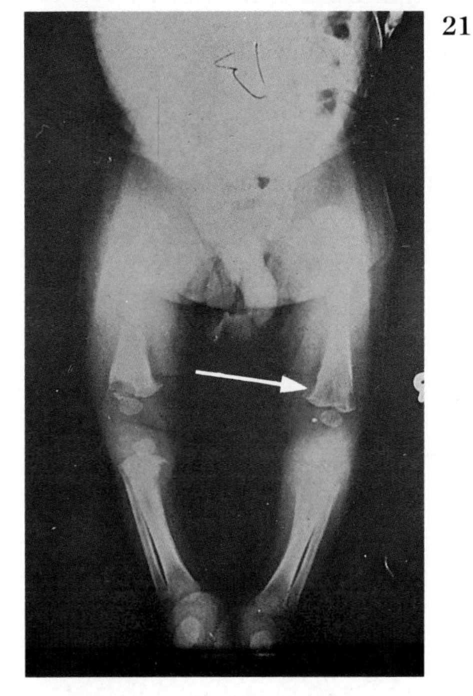

21 X-ray of the child shown in **20**, demonstrating areas of periostitis.

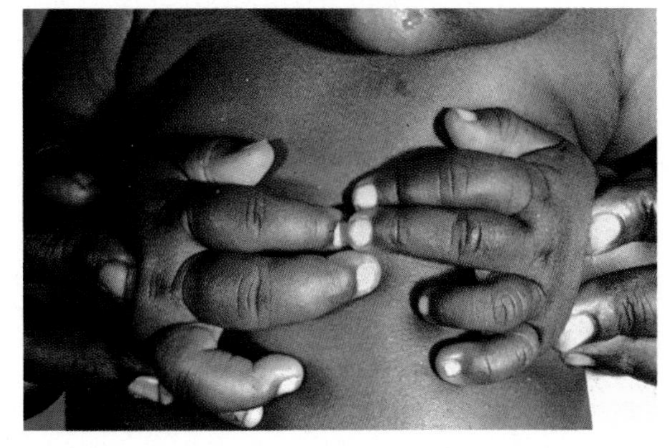

22 A neonate with dactylitis following an *in utero* infection with *T. pallidum*. Typically, this involves the proximal interphalangeal joint, but spares the distal joints.

Listeria monocytogenes

Maternal infection occurs following ingestion of contaminated foodstuffs including dairy products, such as cheese, cream and milk, salads, vegetables and cooked-chilled chicken. Maternal illness is often absent, but it may present with 'flu-like' symptoms. Spontaneous abortion, intrauterine death and stillbirth may result. If infection occurs late in pregnancy, it may lead to premature delivery of a neonate with infection of multiple organ systems, including meningitis. Ampicillin or penicillin is the treatment of choice; *L. monocytogenes* is resistant to the cephalosporins.

Toxoplasma gondii

23

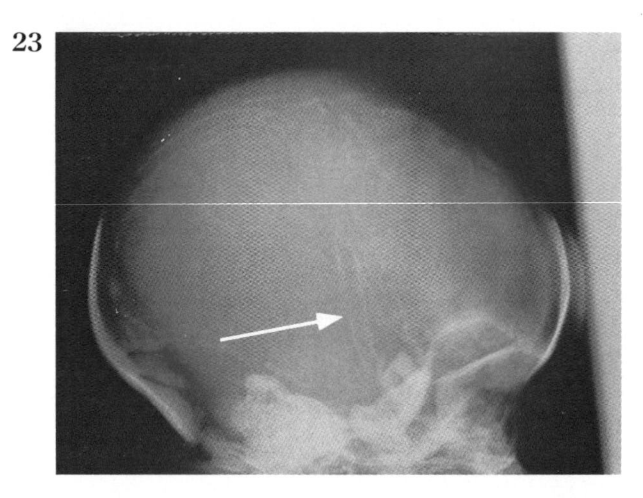

23 A lateral skull X-ray of a child with congenital toxoplasmosis. Intracerebral calcification is clearly visible.

A coccidian protozoan parasite, *T. gondii* is an obligate intracellular pathogen. It undergoes its full reproductive cycle only in the feline intestinal tract. Infection can arise either from ingestion of oocysts from cat faeces, or from ingestion of undercooked meat containing encysted bradyzoites. Infection in the mother is usually asymptomatic, but it may present as a glandular fever-like illness. Infection of the fetus can occur whether or not the mother is symptomatic. Fetal infection can result in intrauterine death (6%), but of live-born infected cases, the majority (75%) are asymptomatic. In 16% of cases, there is mild disease, and in 8% there is severe disease. Signs of severe disease include intracerebral calcification (**23**) with subsequent microcephaly (**24**) and mental retardation, and chorioretinitis (**25**).

Infection developing in pregnancy can be treated using spiramycin or pyrimethamine, which may limit fetal infection. Opinions vary as to the benefits of treating the congenitally infected neonate, since encysted bradyzoites, which can reactivate at a later date, will not be affected by antimicrobial chemotherapy.

24

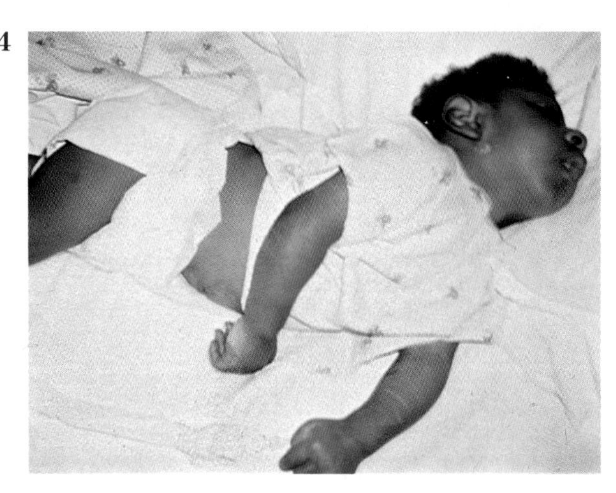

24 A child with microcephaly and opisthotonos following *in utero* infection with *T. gondii*.

25

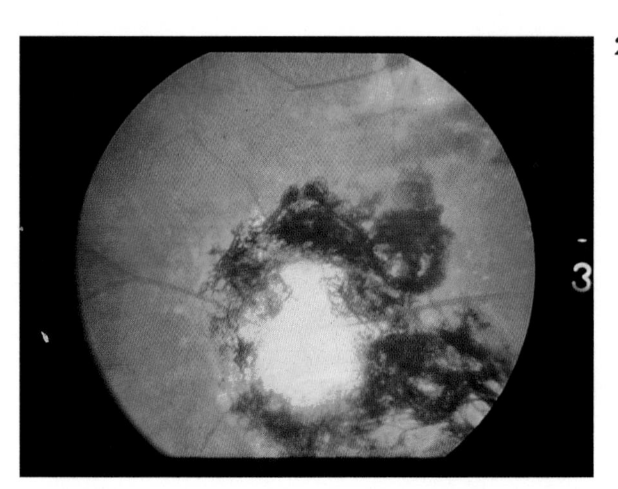

25 Chorioretinitis in a child with congenital toxoplasmosis.

Rare pathogens

There are sporadic reports of maternal poliomyelitis associated with fetal infection and growth retardation. However, it appears that, although contraindicated in pregnancy, oral poliovirus vaccine does not cause fetal malformation. The γ-herpesvirus Epstein–Barr virus (EBV) is not associated with congenital damage, but transplacental infection does occasionally occur.

The spirochaete *Borrelia burgdorferi* is transmitted by ticks (e.g. *Ixodes dammini* in the USA, and *I.ricinus* in Europe), and causes erythema chronicum migrans (**26**), which is one manifestation of Lyme Disease. Infection in pregnancy can cause fetal infection that is apparently associated with cardiac defects. Treatment is with high-dose penicillin.

As its name implies, the ewe abortion agent (*Chlamydia psittaci*) infects sheep placentae and fetuses, causing abortion. This agent can also infect pregnant women, leading to placentitis, chorioamnionitis (**27**), premature delivery and stillbirth. It can also lead to septic shock in the mother. Farmers' wives are at particular risk of such infection.

Transmission of tuberculosis from mother to infant via the placenta or amniotic fluid does occur, but very few cases have been reported (<200).

26

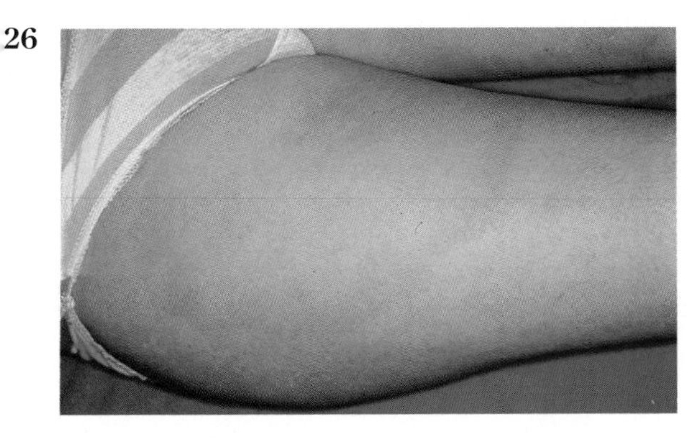

26 Erythema chronicum migrans, the rash typical of Lyme disease.

27

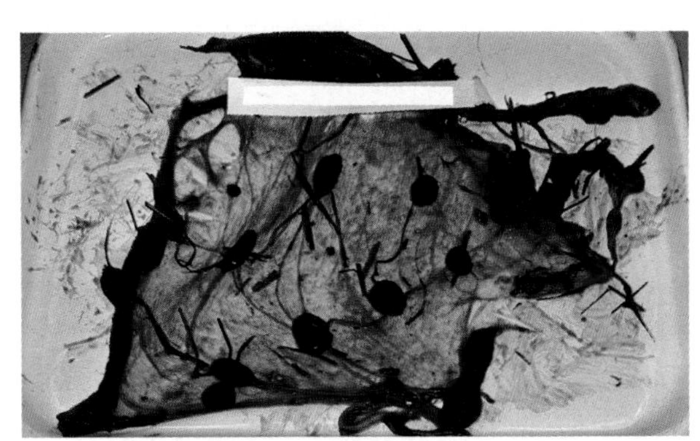

27 Placental membranes from a fetus aborted due to maternal infection with the ewe abortion agent (*C. psittaci*).

Infections acquired during delivery

Infections are acquired during delivery either by organisms that ascend through intact or ruptured membranes from the vagina, or as the neonate passes through the birth canal (**Table 4**). In general, infections that present within the first 48 hours of life are likely to have been acquired in this way. However, micro-organisms with long incubation periods, such as hepatitis B virus, are exceptions to this rule.

Table 4. Infections Acquired During Delivery.

Viruses	*Bacteria*	*Parasites*
Human herpesvirus 1 and 2	*Chlamydia trachomatis*	Plasmodium
Hepatitis B virus	*Neisseria gonorrhoeae*	Trypanosomes
Human immunodeficiency virus	*Mycobacterium tuberculosis*	Cryptosporidium
Cytomegalovirus	*Mycoplasma hominis*	
Enteroviruses	*Ureaplasma urealyticum*	
Rotavirus	Group B streptococcus	
Human papillomavirus	*Salmonella* spp.	
	Campylobacter spp.	
	Escherichia coli K1	

Herpes gestationis

The female genital tract can be infected either with herpes simplex virus type I (human herpesvirus (HHV) 1) or with type II (HHV 2), although infection with the latter is more common. After a primary infection, the virus tracks back along sensory neurons to the sacral dorsal root ganglia, where it remains latent. However, this latency is not permanent and the virus reactivates, passing back down the neuron either to be shed asymptomatically or, more often, to produce genital tract ulceration.

If the neonate is born through a sea of herpes simplex virus, it is at risk of developing severe infection. Unlike in later life, this infection is not usually limited to the skin and mucous membranes; rather, it disseminates throughout the body, causing hepatitis (**28**), pneumonitis and, most often, encephalitis (**29**). Encephalitis due to HHV 2 tends to be widespread and necrotizing, whereas that due to HHV 1 is more often focal. In approximately 80% of cases the neonate presents with skin vesicles; 60% of those affected will have central nervous system (CNS) signs including fits, a bulging fontanelle, decerebrate rigidity, or coma.

Early diagnosis requires a high index of suspicion, and specific diagnosis depends upon demonstrating herpes virus by electron microscopy and/or culture. Untreated neonatal herpes encephalitis has a very high mortality (up to 70%) and survivors often have high morbidity. Intravenous treatment with adenine arabinoside or acyclovir has greatly improved the prognosis.

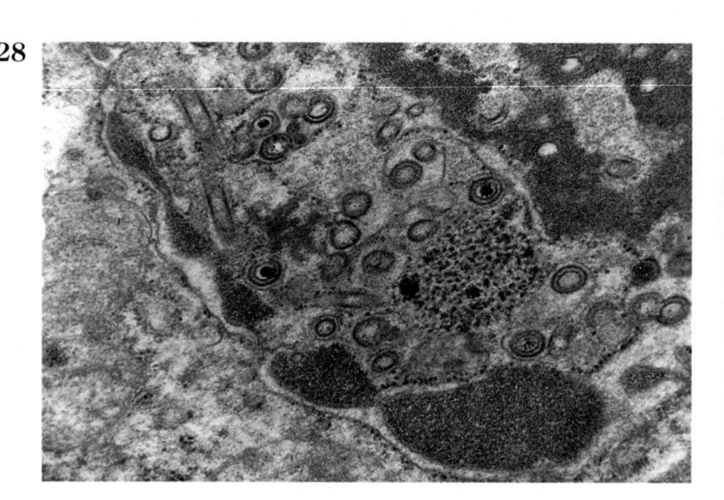

28 Thin-section electron micrograph of a hepatocyte from a fatal case of Herpes simplex hepatitis (× *20,000*).

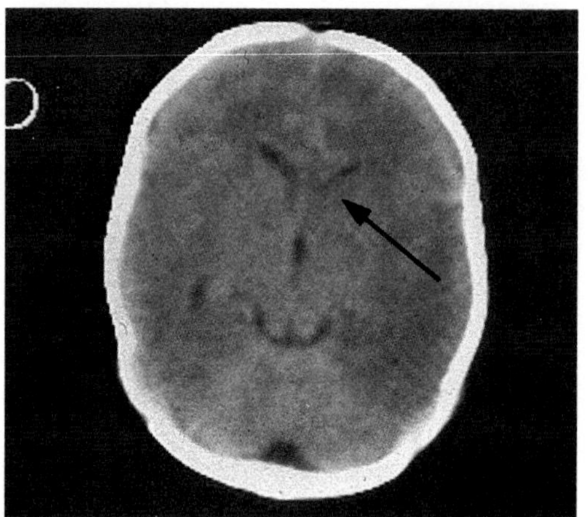

29 CT scan of the skull of a neonate with Herpes simplex encephalitis. Note the compressed ventricles.

Hepatitis B virus

A solely human pathogen, hepatitis B virus (**30**) is a hepadnavirus that is maintained by over 200 million carriers worldwide. Vertical transmission from carrier mother to neonate at birth is one of the most important routes of infection.

As transmission is by blood to blood contact, during delivery there is ample opportunity for maternal blood to gain access to the neonatal circulation. Hepatitis B surface antigen (HBSAg) is detectable in an affected infant's blood 2–5 months after delivery. Most often, the infant does not show clinical features of hepatitis, but becomes a chronic carrier who, in turn, can eventually pass on infection vertically. Currently, great efforts are being made to try to interrupt this vertical transmission. As a consequence, mothers are screened during pregnancy, and neonates born to mothers who are carriers are given hepatitis B vaccine, which is, in effect, a subunit vaccine consisting of

HBSAg particles (either derived from human carrier plasma, or genetically engineered in yeasts), and/or human hepatitis B immunoglobulin. These precautions prevent the neonate from becoming infected in the majority of cases, and may thus gradually diminish the numbers of carriers worldwide.

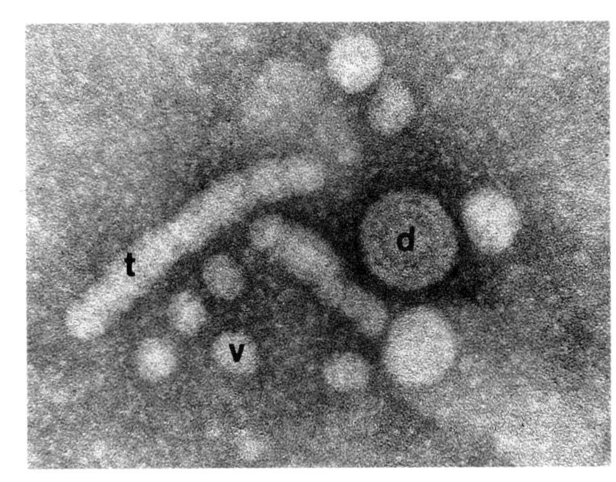

30 Negative-stain electron micrograph of serum from a child infected with hepatitis B virus. A Dane particle (d) and tubular (t) and vesicular (v) surface-antigen particles are present (× *110,000*).

Enteric viruses

Because viruses such as rotavirus and enteroviruses are excreted in large numbers in faeces, they may be acquired by the neonate following contamination of the maternal perineum. Enteroviruses such as ECHO 11 cause meningitis, encephalitis and the clinical features of sepsis neonatorum. Rotavirus infection is usually asymptomatic, with only 20% of neonates developing diarrhoea.

Ophthalmia neonatorum

Most cases (52%) of neonatal conjunctivitis are due to *Chlamydia trachomatis* or *Neisseria gonorrhoeae*, but pneumococci and *Staphylococcus aureus* are also potential pathogens.

C.trachomatis (serotypes D–K) is an obligate intracellular bacterial pathogen (**31**). Infection in the mother may be asymptomatic or it may present as urethritis, vaginitis or cervicitis. Neonatal conjunctivitis can produce a purulent exudate (**32**), intense inflammation (**33**) and periorbital oedema (**34**). The average incubation period is 7 days. Diagnosis is made by obtaining scrapes or swabs from the palpebral conjunctivae (**33**) and then detecting *C.trachomatis* by culture (**35**), which takes 3 days, or by antigen detection, which takes 3 hours. Treatment is with tetracycline ointment to both eyes and erythromycin orally for 1–2 weeks. Erythromycin is given to eradicate organisms from the nasopharynx. If untreated, infection may proceed to chlamydial pneumonia, which occurs, on average, 3–5 months later. It should also be remembered that if the neonate is infected, the mother must be too. She will also need treatment since *C.trachomatis* can spread to cause pelvic inflammatory disease.

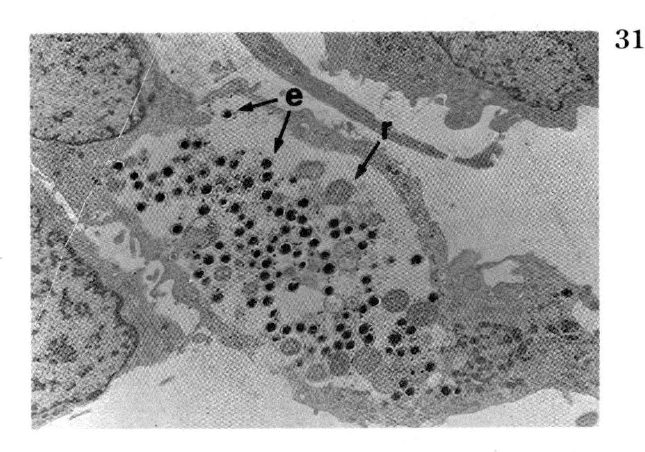

31 Thin-section electron micrograph of a McCoy cell with a large inclusion containing reticulate (r) and elementary (e) bodies of *C. trachomatis* (× *3,000*).

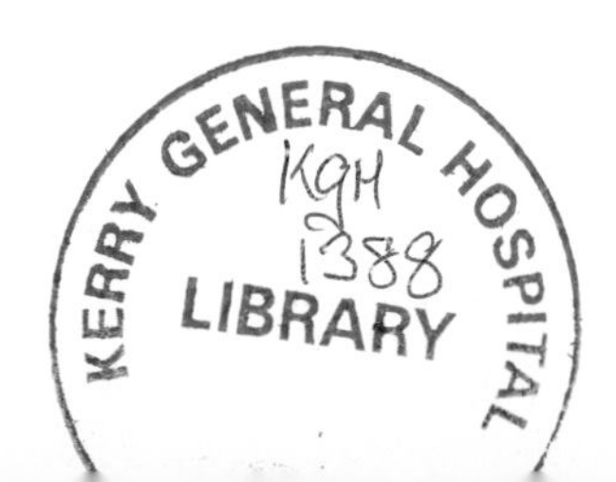

32

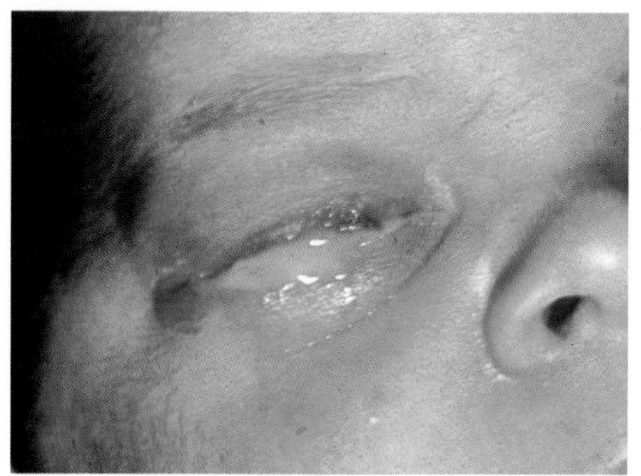

32 A neonate with a purulent ocular discharge due to *C. trachomatis*.

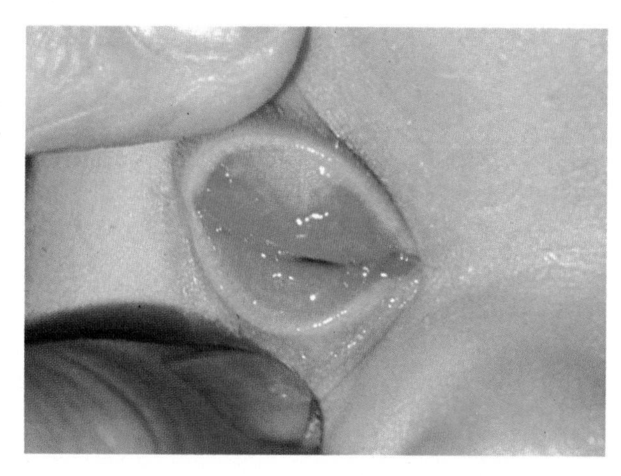

33 A neonate with the eyelid everted to show palpebral inflammation due to *C. trachomatis*.

34

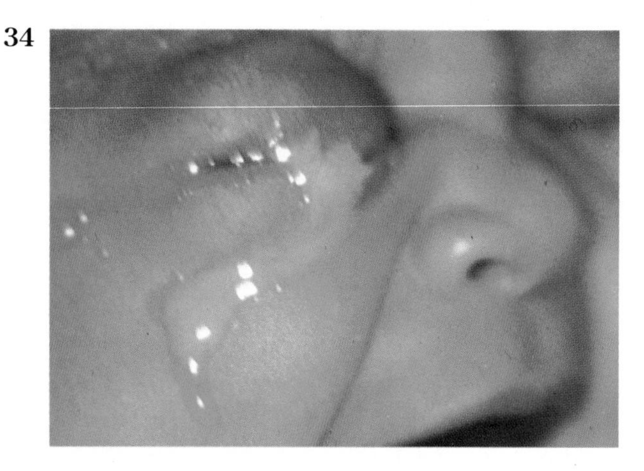

34 A neonate with periorbital oedema due to *C. trachomatis*.

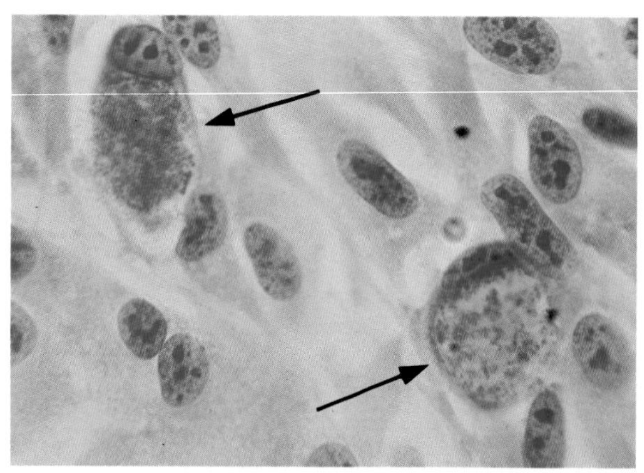

35 McCoy cells stained by Giemsa, demonstrating two large inclusions packed with *C. trachomatis* (× *1,000*).

36

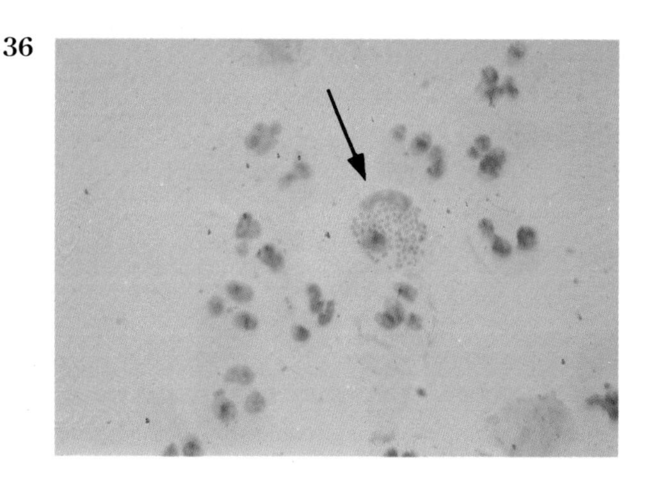

36 Gram-stained film of pus from a neonate with gonococcal ophthalmia. Numerous pus cells are present, one of which is filled with gram-negative cocci (gonococci) (× *1,000*).

Neisseria gonorrhoeae (**36**) is also acquired from the symptomatic or asymptomatic mother. However, gonococcal ophthalmia has a shorter incubation period than the chlamydial type, appearing within 2 days of birth. Untreated gonococcal ophthalmia leads to keratitis, anterior uveitis, perforation and blindness. Diagnosis is easily made by culture, gram-stained film of pus, and antigen detection, although results from an antigen-detection test must be interpreted with caution. Resistance to both penicillin and tetracycline encoded on plasmids has developed. A third-generation cephalosporin given parenterally or gentamicin given topically is usually curative.

Mycoplasma

Both *Mycoplasma hominis* (**37**) and *Ureaplasma urealyticum* can be part of the normal flora of the female genital tract, as well as being potential causes of pelvic inflammatory disease and non-gonococcal urethritis.

U.urealyticum has been associated with chorio-amniotic infection and premature delivery. Both agents have also been associated with respiratory tract and ventricular shunt infections, especially in premature neonates. Diagnosis is by culture both in broth and on solid media (**37**). *U.urealyticum* is sensitive to erythromycin, but the sensitivity of *M. hominis* to antimicrobials is much more variable and occasionally no agent other than tetracycline is effective.

37

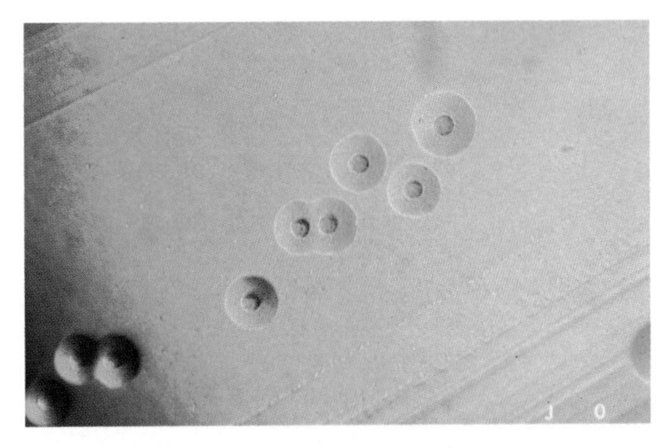

37 Colonies of *M. hominis* growing on solid media, demonstrating the typical 'fried-egg' colonial morphology.

Streptococcus agalactiae

The group B streptococcus (*S.agalactiae*) is a β-haemolytic gram-positive coccus (**38**) that is part of the normal vaginal flora of a proportion of women. Infection presents in the neonate in a very dramatic way, usually within the first 12 hours of life. The neonate becomes desperately ill with tachypnoea, respiratory distress and shock. Response to treatment can be equally dramatic, and either ampicillin or penicillin G is the drug of choice.

38

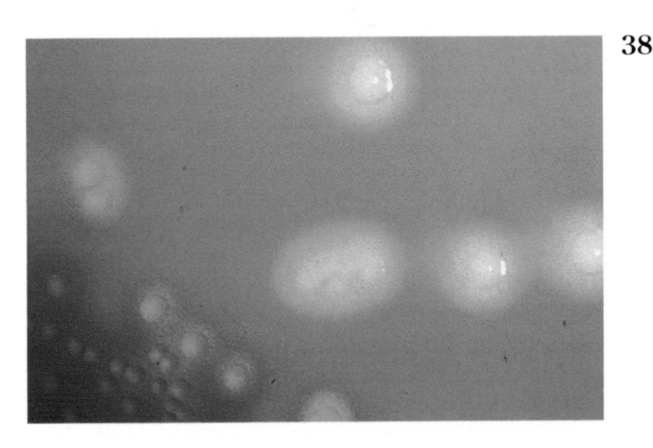

38 *S. agalactiae* (group B streptococcus) colonies on blood agar, demonstrating β-haemolysis.

Enteric bacteria

Neonates born to mothers excreting food-poisoning *Salmonella* spp. or *Campylobacter* spp. are at risk of acquiring infection via the contaminated maternal perineum or vagina. It is uncommon for these bacteria to cause diarrhoea but in the pre-term infant they can be associated with septicaemia and meningitis. *Escherichia coli* K1 is a capsulate bacterium (**39**), the capsule of which is a homopolymer of N-acetyl-neuraminic acid (exactly the same as for the group B meningococcus). As the capsular polysaccharide is also a self-antigen, this particular bacterium is a powerful pathogen, being able to avoid phagocytic killing and recognition by the humoral immune system. The only other defence mechanism is provided by the alternative complement cascade, in which the premature neonate is, of course, deficient.

39

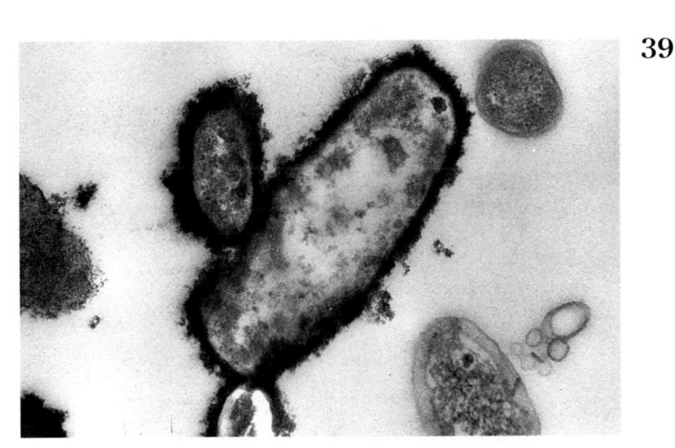

39 Thin-section electron micrograph of *E. coli* K1 stained with ruthenium red to demonstrate the capsule (× *7,000*).

Postnatally acquired infection

Acquired from the environment (animate or inanimate) in the neonatal intensive care unit (NICU), these infections are numerically the most important. It is estimated that between 10% and 22% of neonates in NICU will have septicaemia.

Infection can be due to viruses, bacteria or fungi, but bacterial infections tend to predominate. The types of pathogen and their antimicrobial susceptibility do vary, and close surveillance of them must be maintained. In the second quarter of the century, infections with *Staphylococcus aureus* and β-haemolytic streptococci were predominant in NICU. In the third quarter, possibly with the advent of penicillins, gram-negative bacteria, such as *Escherichia coli*, *Klebsiellae* and *Pseudomonas* spp., became predominant. Latterly, aminoglycoside-resistant coliforms, together with *Citrobacter* spp., *Enterobacter* spp. and *Serratia* spp. all resistant to third-generation cephalosporins, have increased in importance.

Finally, there has been a gradual increase in the incidence of infection with coagulase-negative staphylococci such as *S. epidermidis*. The mortality due to infections in NICU does appear to be decreasing, perhaps due to a combination of factors including better antimicrobial chemotherapy and the increased incidence of infection with low-level pathogens, such as *S. epidermidis*.

It is unusual for infections to be localized, and most present non-specifically. However, the results of infection can be catastrophic. Consequently, intravenous antimicrobial chemotherapy (with, for example, a combination of ampicillin and gentamicin) is begun pre-emptively. On average, only 10–15% of suspected infective episodes prove genuine, thus rigid criteria must be established for stopping antimicrobial chemotherapy.

Omphalitis

The umbilical stump is a fertile culture medium for aerobic and anaerobic bacteria, especially if it is moist. As bacteria can be grown from the stump in the absence of infection, a clinical assessment of the cord and its surrounding skin must be made before omphalitis is diagnosed. The bacteria most often associated with omphalitis are anaerobes such as *Bacteroides fragilis* or *Clostridium perfringens* (**40** and **41**) and aerobes such as *Staphylococcus aureus*. If *C. tetani* gains access to the stump, neonatal tetanus can result (**42**).

40

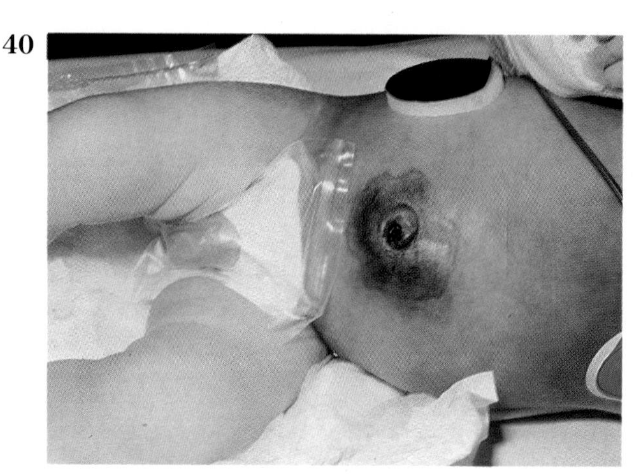

40 A neonate with fatal omphalitis due to *C. perfringens*.

4

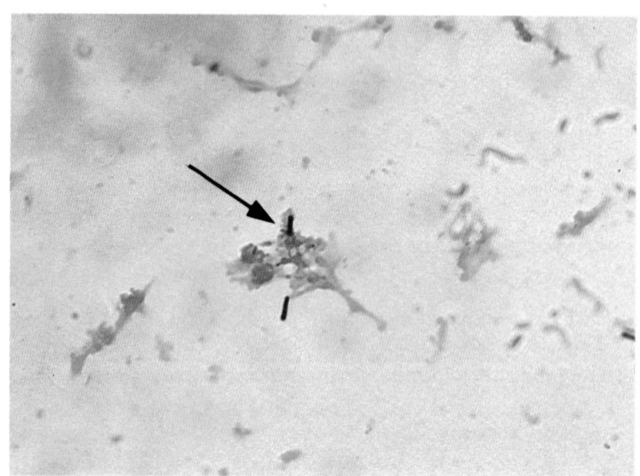

41 Gram-stained film of peritoneal fluid taken from the neonate shown in **40**. A gram-positive bacillus is visible next to a neutrophil that has been lysed, presumably by the bacterial phospholipase C (× *1,000*).

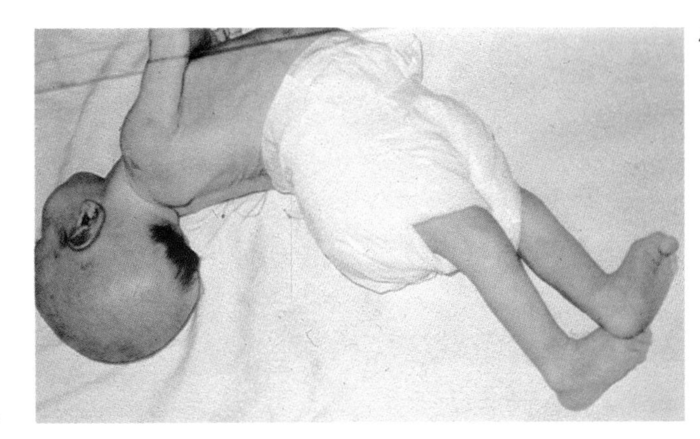

42 A neonate with tetanus.

Cutaneous infections

Skin abscesses, often due to *S. aureus,* can develop in the neonatal period. Such infections do, however, have a propensity to disseminate, causing septicaemia, arthritis and osteomyelitis. Infections with *S. aureus* strains of phage group II (3a, 3c, 55, 71) can be associated with toxic epidermal necrolysis or staphylococcal scalded skin syndrome (**43**). Such strains release an epidermolytic toxin (exfoliatin) that causes intraepidermal cleavage at the level of the granular cell layer, leading to extensive desquamation. In children outside the neonatal period the skin cleavage is limited to the formation of the localized bullous lesions of impetigo.

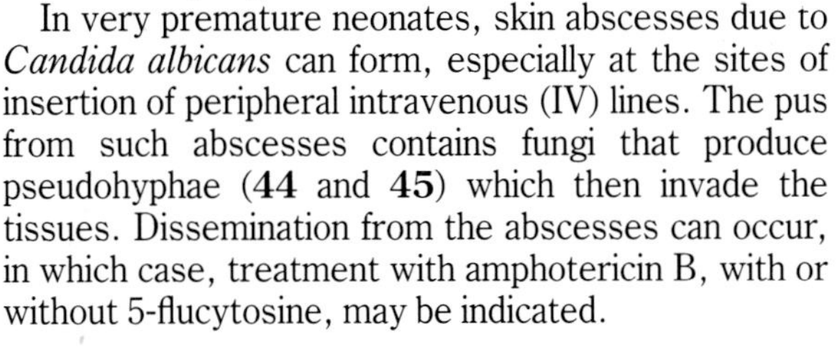

In very premature neonates, skin abscesses due to *Candida albicans* can form, especially at the sites of insertion of peripheral intravenous (IV) lines. The pus from such abscesses contains fungi that produce pseudohyphae (**44** and **45**) which then invade the tissues. Dissemination from the abscesses can occur, in which case, treatment with amphotericin B, with or without 5-flucytosine, may be indicated.

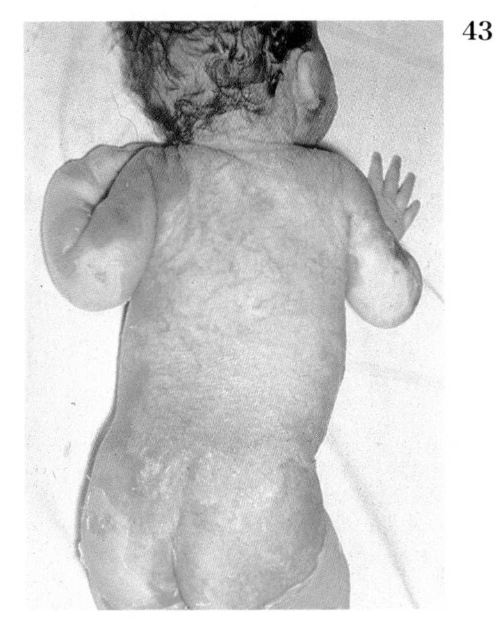

43 A neonate with staphylococcal scalded-skin syndrome. Note the extensive desquamation.

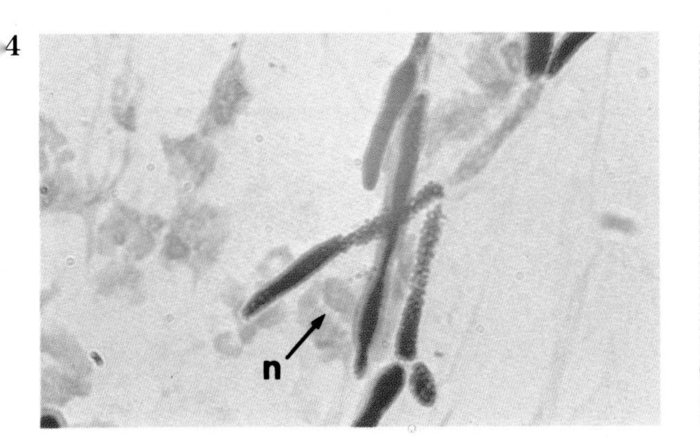

44 Gram-stained film of pus from a cutaneous abscess in a neonate. *C. albicans* with pseudohyphae and neutrophils (n) are present (× *1,000*).

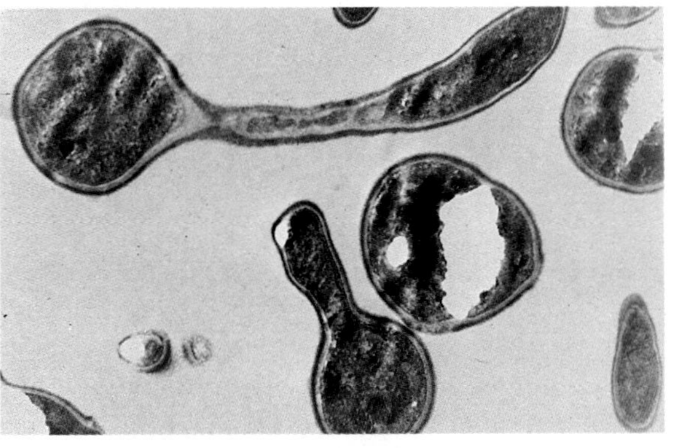

45 Thin-section electron micrograph of *C. albicans*, demonstrating pseudohyphae formation (× *2,000*).

Meningitis

Meningitis usually occurs as part of a septicaemic illness and the bacteria or fungi isolated from cerebrospinal fluid (CSF) reflect the general aetiological agents of neonatal septicaemia. However, group B streptococci, *Listeria monocytogenes* and *E. coli* K1 are especially important causes of meningitis. Management of such infections can be problematic and will depend upon the organism and its individual antimicrobial susceptibility. Treatment is further complicated by the difficulty of achieving therapeutic concentrations of aminoglycosides, such as gentamicin, in the CSF. Group B streptococci and *E.coli* are sensitive to third-generation cephalosporins, and *L.monocytogenes* is responsive to ampicillin. Since the neonate is an immune-compromised host, infection with seemingly innocuous bacteria such as *Bacillus licheniformis* can occur (**46**).

In very premature neonates, infection may result in ventricular haemorrhage and ventriculitis, with the bacteria trapped in the clot being unaffected by antibiotics.

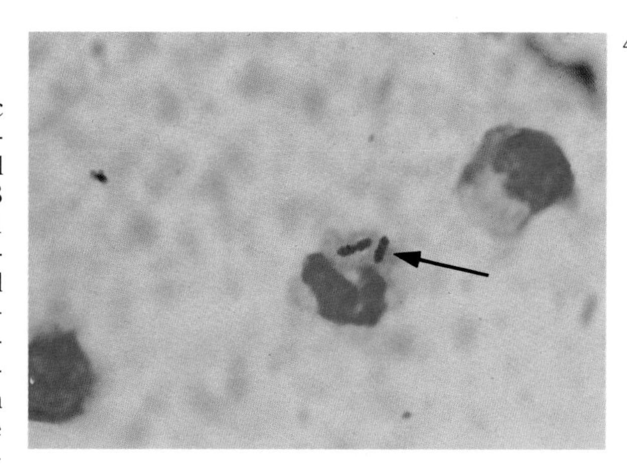

46 Gram-stained film of CSF from a neonate with meningitis due to *B. licheniformis*. Gram-positive bacilli are visible inside a pus cell (× *1,000*).

Shunt infections

Ventriculoperitoneal or ventriculoatrial shunts are inserted to drain CSF and relieve hydrocephalus (**47**). They consist of a ventricular catheter (which is inserted into the lateral ventricle) with a chamber (button) at its distal end for sampling and pumping the system (**48**). The chamber is connected to a valve that permits flow from the ventricles, opening at a set CSF pressure. The valve is then connected to another catheter, which is tunnelled under the skin to deliver CSF either into the peritoneum or into the atrium of the heart. Although shunt infections do not usually present in the neonatal period, the infecting micro-organisms gain access at the time of insertion of the system. It is estimated that approximately 10% of

47 A neonate with hydrocephalus.

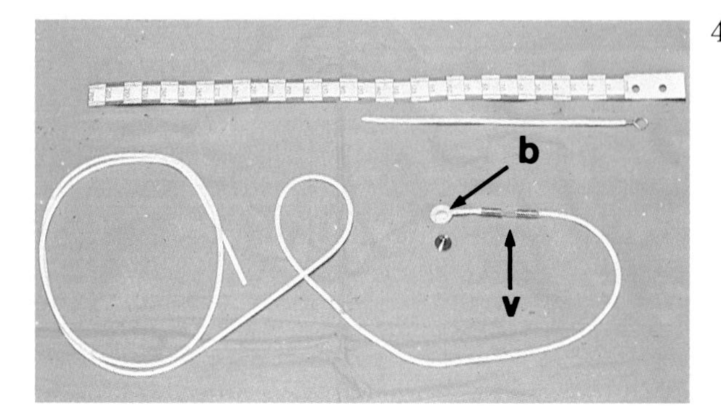

48 A ventricular shunt system, demonstrating the button (b), valve (v) and distal catheter.

such shunts will become infected. Most infections (90%) are due to coagulase-negative staphylococci, with other skin commensals (e.g. *S.aureus, Propionibacterium acnes, Corynebacterium jekeium*) accounting for most of the rest. Shunt infection is a misnomer since features of infection are the exception rather than the rule. Disease usually presents in the form of problems with shunt blockage and there is little inflammatory response in the CSF. Coagulase-negative staphylococci from the skin of the neonate or that of the theatre staff gain access at operation. The bacteria adhere firmly to the plastic catheter, growing to produce microcolonies that are enveloped in an extracellular slime released by the bacteria (**49**). The colony gradually enlarges, eventually blocking the shunt. Treatment involves exteriorization of the shunt system, drainage of CSF into sterile bags and intraventricular (or intrashunt) antibiotics. Because there is little inflammatory response, intravenously administered antibiotics do not achieve therapeutic levels. Vancomycin and gentamicin have been used with some success and little toxicity. It may be necessary to replace parts or all of the system, since bacteria in the microcolonies divide slowly and are protected by the slime layer.

49

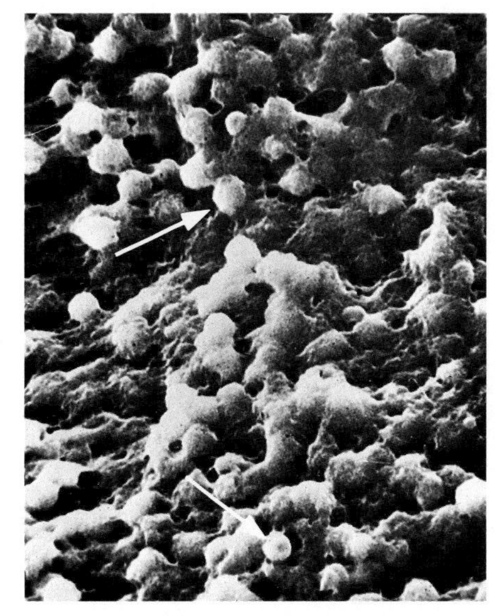

49 Scanning electron micrograph of the internal surface of a ventricular catheter colonized by *Staphylococcus epidermidis*. Cocci embedded in a sea of slime are clearly visible (× *2,000*).

Urinary tract infection

Urinary tract infection is more common in premature (3%) than in full-term neonates (0.5–1.0%) and there is a male preponderance. *E.coli* is the major pathogen, with those of capsular serotype K1, K2 and K12 being most frequently involved. Other virulence factors include the expression of P-fimbriae and haemolysins.

In the very premature neonate, urinary tract infection with *Candida* spp. can occur and may lead to the formation of fungus balls in the kidney (**50–52**), which can be very difficult to eradicate, often necessitating nephrostomy to drain the pus.

50

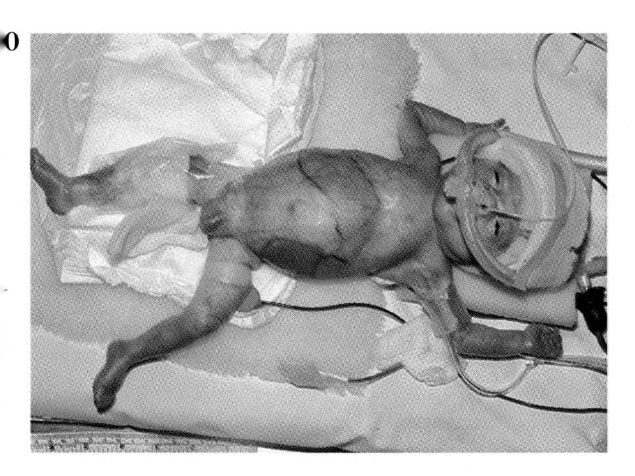

50 A young infant with renal, splenic and hepatic enlargement due to *C. albicans* infection of the renal pelvis and ureter.

51

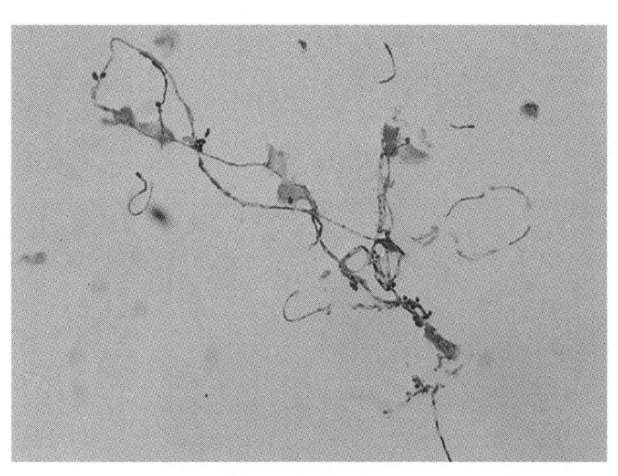

51 Gram-stained film of material drained from the renal pelvis, demonstrating *C. albicans* with pseudohyphae (× *400*).

52

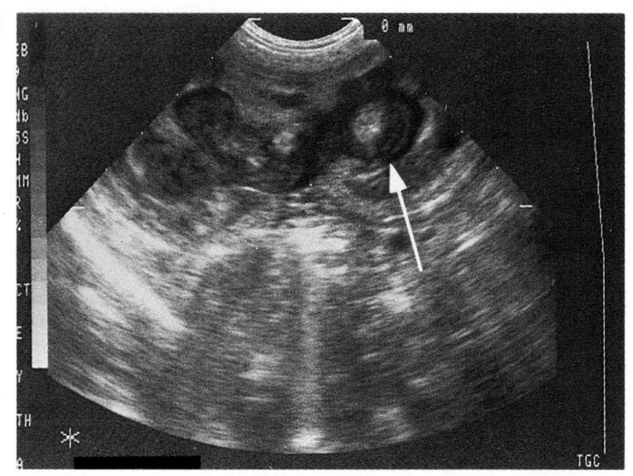

52 Ultrasound scan of the renal pelvis, demonstrating fungus (*C. albicans*) balls.

Necrotizing enterocolitis

In general, necrotizing enterocolitis presents in low birthweight infants, with lethargy, a distended abdomen, poor feeding and, in 25%, rectal bleeding. Its aetiology is unknown, but suggestions include ischaemic damage to the gut, followed by bacterial invasion. Radiologically it is characterized by the presence of intramural gas (**53**). It may also be seen as acute perforation with peritoneal gas and peritonitis.

At postmortem a gangrenous area of intestine (most often the terminal ileum and distal colon) is seen (**54**). The condition may lead to peritonitis and septicaemia, generally due to anaerobes such as *Bacteroides* spp. and aerobes such as *E.coli*. Thus, if perforation is suspected, appropriate antimicrobial chemotherapy (e.g. metronidazole and gentamicin) should be started.

53

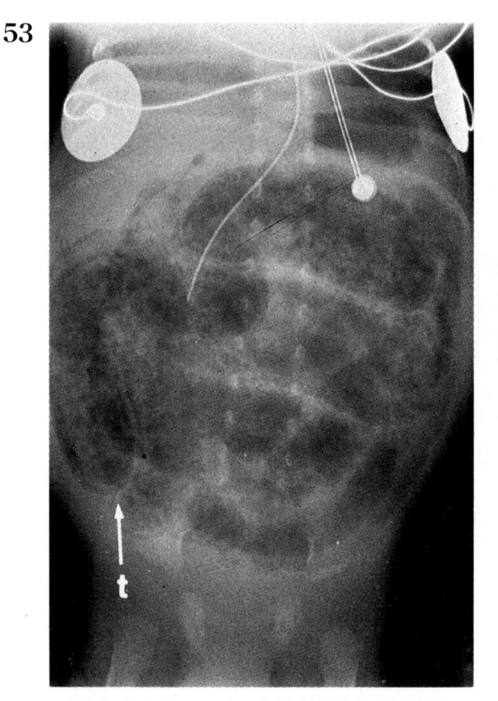

53 Abdominal X-ray of a neonate with severe necrotizing enterocolitis. Intramural gas is visible as 'tram lines' (t).

54

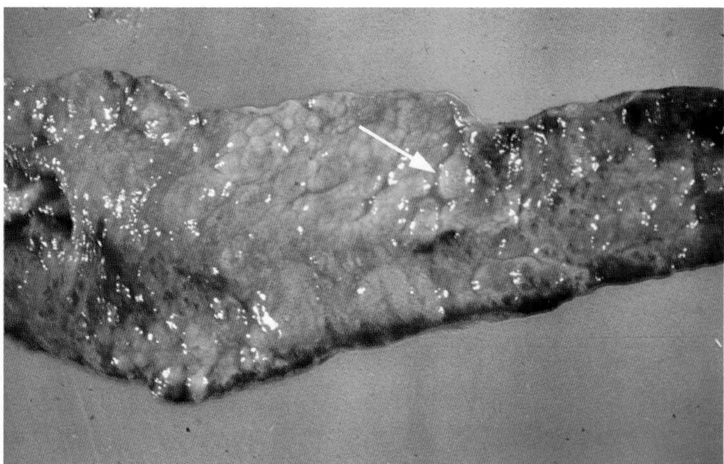

54 A length of colon from a neonate with necrotizing enterocolitis, showing gangrenous changes and intramural gas.

2 Gastrointestinal infections

In general the response of the gastrointestinal tract to infection is marked by abdominal pain, vomiting and diarrhoea. In addition, infection of the liver or biliary tract may lead to jaundice and perforation of the intestine to acute peritonitis.

Acute gastritis

In recent years it has been demonstrated that non-autoimmune (Type B) gastritis (**55**), both in children and in adults, is due to the spiral bacterium *Helicobacter pylori* (**56**). Originally named *Campylobacter pylori*, the organism was reclassified as *H.pylori* because it was genetically divergent and possessed sheathed flagellae with terminal bulbs (**57**). The main presentation is of upper abdominal pain, generally in children over 7 years of age. Approximately 15% of children attending an abdominal pain clinic can be shown to be infected with *H.pylori*. In developing countries, infection is much more frequent, occurs earlier, and may contribute to failure to thrive.

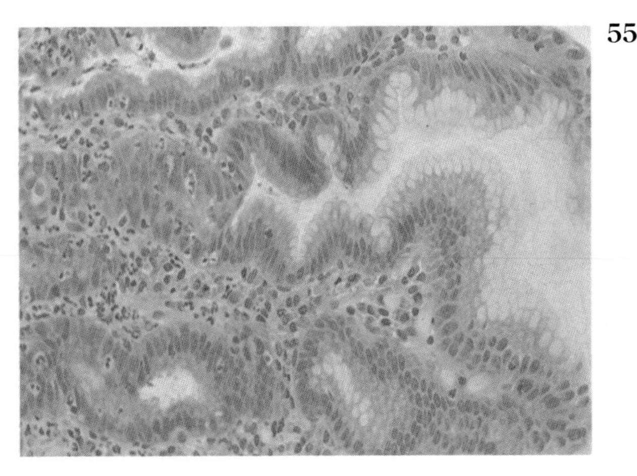

55 A section of gastric mucosa, demonstrating acute gastritis with infiltration by neutrophils (× *500*).

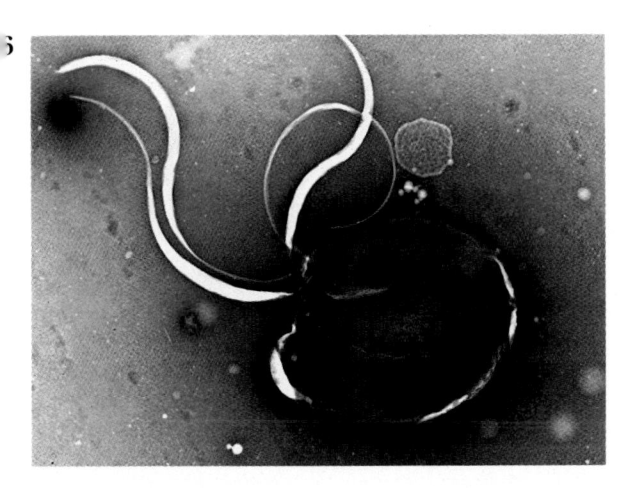

56 Negative-stain electron micrograph of *H. pylori* (× *3,500*).

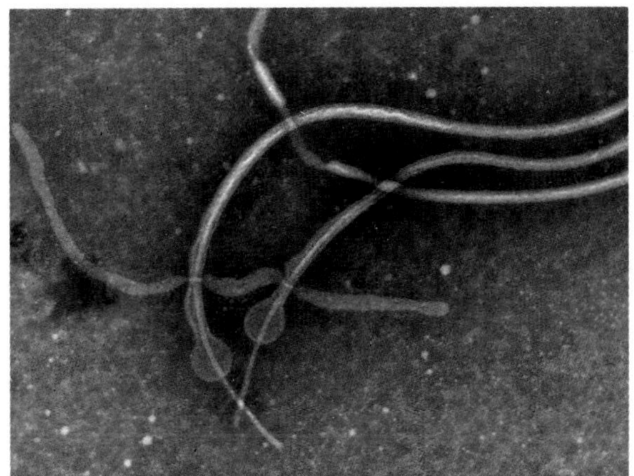

57 Negative-stain electron micrograph of *H. pylori* sheathed flagellae, showing the terminal bulb (× *10,000*).

Diagnosis is made by taking gastric and duodenal biopsies. These are cultured, examined histologically by acridine orange or Giemsa (**58**) stains, and subjected to a 'quick' urease test. *H.pylori* is slow growing and takes up to 5 days to produce colonies following microaerophilic incubation on enriched media. *H.pylori* adheres intimately to the gastric enterocytes beneath the mucous layer (**59**), producing a powerful urease which contributes to its pathogenesis. In adults, treatment with a combination of bismuth salts and an antibiotic (amoxycillin, erythromycin or metronidazole) has proved effective.

There is a strong association between *H.pylori* and peptic ulcer disease. However, peptic ulcer disease is uncommon in children.

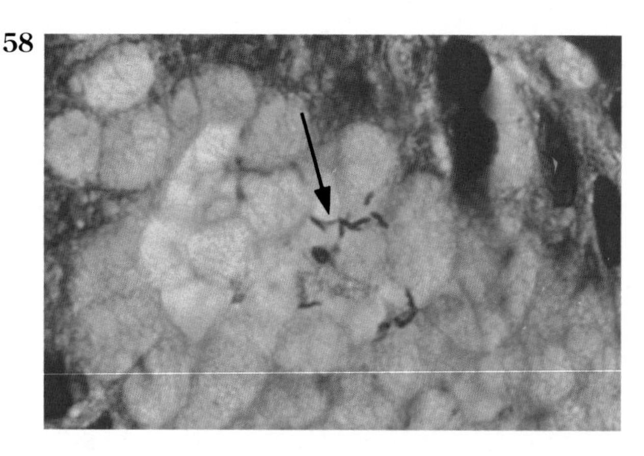

58 Giemsa-stained section of gastric mucosa, demonstrating *H. pylori* (× *1,000*).

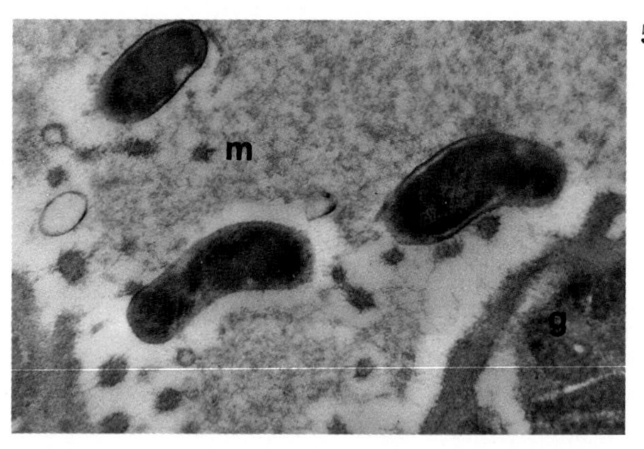

59 Thin-section electron micrograph of gastric mucosa, showing spiral *H. pylori* beneath the mucous layer (m), in close proximity to the gastric cell surface (g) (× *3,000*).

Gastroenteritis

Worldwide, diarrhoeal disease is one of the most common infective causes of death. Second only to acute respiratory tract infection, it is estimated to be responsible for 5–7 million deaths each year. The infection takes its heaviest toll among the very young and in developing countries. In such areas, gastroenteritis contributes greatly to malnutrition, further decreasing immunity to infection.

Two advances have contributed greatly to the prevention and management of diarrhoeal disease. Firstly, public health measures covering, for example, the separation of sewage from potable water supplies, have decreased the risk of transmission of disease. **60** shows a scene from Exeter around 1900. It can be seen that the toilets vented (through a hole in the floor) directly into the river, the water from which might be used for drinking, cooking and washing. By way of comparison **61** and **62** show scenes from present-day Bangladesh, with a similar toilet discharging directly into a pond, the water from which is also used for washing (people, clothes and buffalo) and cooking.

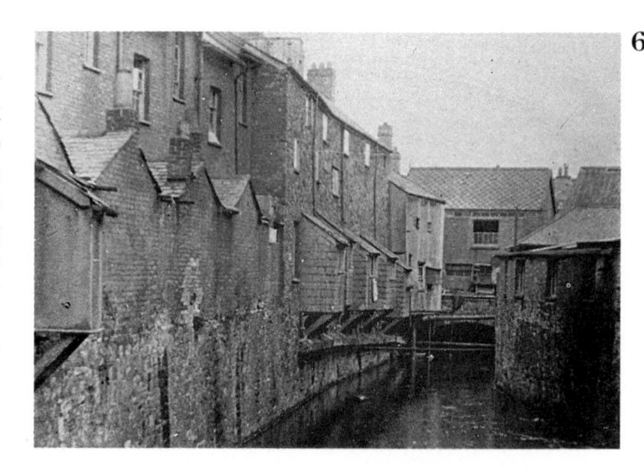

60 A scene from Exeter in 1900, showing toilets that discharge directly into the river.

61

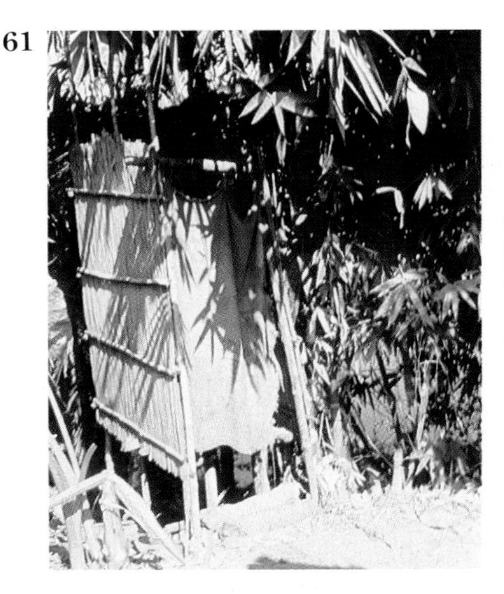

62

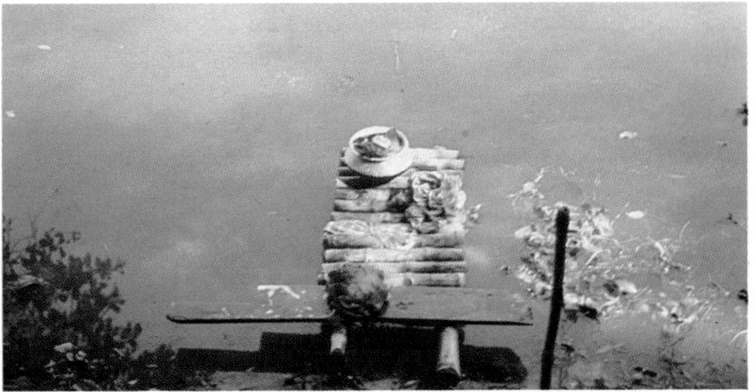

61 Present-day Bangladesh: a similar sort of toilet to those shown in **60**.

62 Another part of the pool into which the toilet shown in **61** discharges. It is also used for washing cooking utensils and buffalo.

The second advance has occurred in the management of diarrhoeal disease. Dehydration is the major life-threatening problem in gastroenteritis (**63**). If it is severe (>10%), it will present with extreme lethargy and later with alterations in conscious state, sunken eyes, loss of skin turgor, dry mucous membranes, oliguria, and a depressed fontanelle in very young infants (**Table 5**). Some infants may require urgent intravenous rehydration, but it is the development of oral rehydration therapy that has revolutionized the management of dehydration, especially in developing countries. Dehydration is particularly likely to occur if the infant experiences both diarrhoea and vomiting.

63

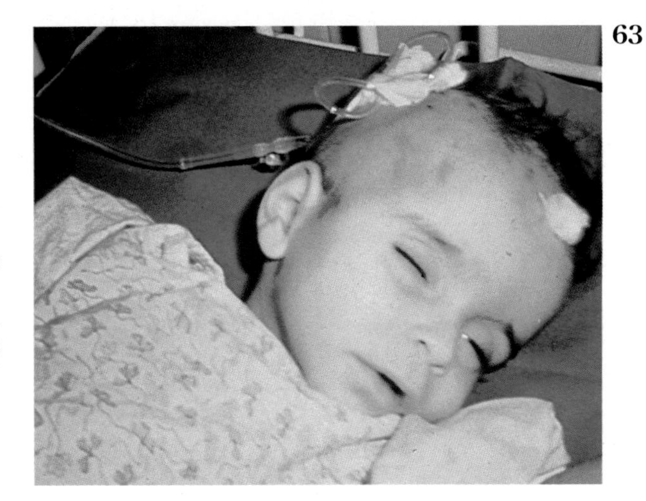

63 A child with severe dehydration and sunken eyes.

Table 5. Clinical Assessment of Dehydration.

Severity	*% Body Weight Lost*	*Clinical State*	*Signs*
Mild	<5	Not unwell	Dry mucous membranes Thirsty
Moderate	5–10	Apathetic	Sunken eyes and depressed fontanelle Tachypnoea, oliguria Loss of skin turgor
Severe	10–15	Shocked	Hypotensive Peripheral circulatory failure
Critical	>15	Moribund	Severely shocked, comatose

The definition of diarrhoea includes a change in both the frequency of defecation and in the character of the stool. In general the stool will asume the shape of the container into which it is placed (**64**). A large number of different viruses, bacteria and protozoa can cause gastroenteritis and it is not possible to differentiate between the different agents using clinical features alone. However, aetiological agents may be subdivided into three groups, those that produce vomiting alone, those that produce a non-inflammatory diarrhoea (with or without vomiting), and those that produce an inflammatory diarrhoea. The two types of diarrhoea can be distinguished by stool microscopy. An inflammatory diarrhoea will produce a stool containing pus cells (neutrophils) and erythrocytes (**65**). The characteristics of the two types of diarrhoea are shown in **Table 6**.

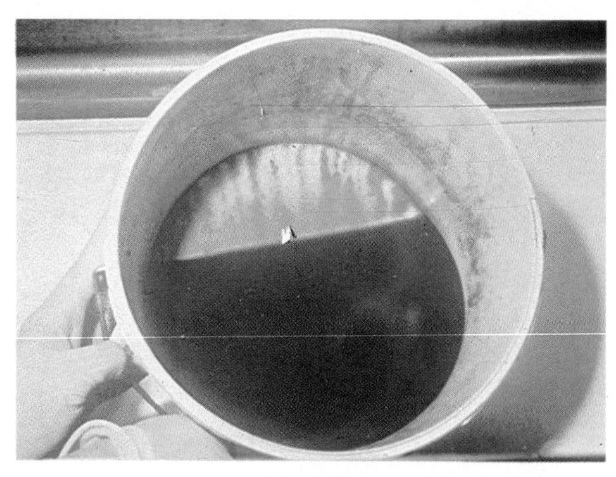

64 A diarrhoeic stool assumes the form of the container into which it is placed.

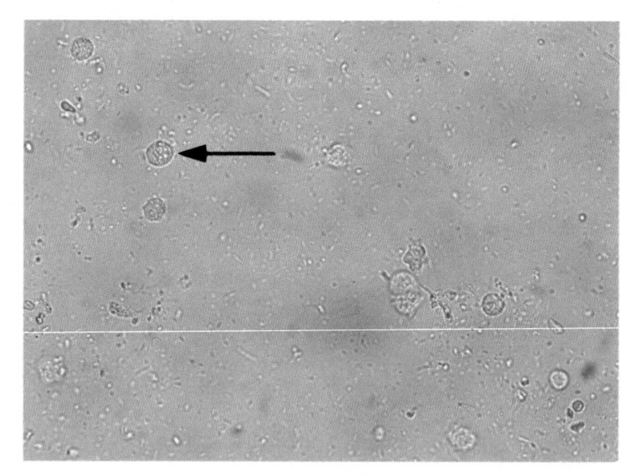

65 A wet preparation of a stool, showing pus cells (× *400*).

Table 6. Inflammatory and Non-Inflammatory Diarrhoea.

	Inflammatory	*Non-Inflammatory*
Symptoms	Abdominal pain Tenesmus, fever	Nausea, vomiting Abdominal pain and fever less prominent
Stool	Frequent, small volume Blood-stained Mucus	Voluminous Watery
Site	Distal small intestine Colon	Proximal small intestine
Mechanism	Invasion of enterocytes leading to cell death	Osmotic or secretory

Predominantly vomiting disease

In general, vomiting disease is due to ingestion of emetic toxins released by *S. aureus* or *Bacillus cereus*. With *S. aureus*, nausea, abdominal pain, vomiting and (later) diarrhoea develop 2–6 hours after ingestion of contaminated food. The usual pattern is that a food handler is a carrier of *S. aureus*, or has an infected lesion, and thus contaminates food (usually pre-cooked, or not cooked at all). Having gained access to the food, the organism then multiplies. Six enterotoxins (A–F) have been described, with optimal toxin production at temperatures above 35°C. Enterotoxins A and D are responsible for 70% of outbreaks; toxin F is also the toxin responsible for toxic shock syndrome. Infection will often present in mini-epidemics following a communal meal. Diagnosis is by detection of toxigenic *S. aureus* in food or vomitus, and of toxin (by enzyme-linked immunosorbent assay (ELISA) or latex particle agglutination (LPA)) in food or vomitus.

Bacillus cereus is a spore-forming gram-positive bacterium that grows readily on simple media. As its name implies, the spores of *B.cereus* can be found in cereal crops, such as rice. Outbreaks of infection are most often associated with fried or boiled rice from, for example, Chinese takeaway restaurants. The spores are able to survive frying and boiling. As the rice cools, vegetative organisms proliferate and release toxin. This process is enhanced by the presence of egg, beef or chicken in the meal. Specific diagnosis is by detection of toxigenic *B.cereus* in food or vomitus. The mode of action of the various emetic toxins is unclear, but they apparently work both locally on the gastric mucosa, and centrally on the emetic centre in the brain.

Treatment should not include the use of antibiotics.

Non-inflammatory diarrhoea

The pathogens that cause a non-inflammatory diarrhoea are shown in **Table 7**. For the majority, the principal site of action is the upper small intestine. A prime prerequisite for pathogens located here is the ability to adhere to the mucosal cells since transit through the small intestine is so rapid.

Table 7. Pathogens in Diarrhoea.

Non-inflammatory	*Inflammatory*
Viruses	
Rotavirus	Nil
Adenovirus 40/41	
Astrovirus	
Calicivirus	
Small, round, structureless virus	
Coronavirus	
Norwalk Agent	
Bacteria	
Enterotoxigenic *E.coli* (ETEC)	Enteroinvasive *E.coli* (EIEC)
Enteropathogenic *E.coli* (EPEC)	Enterohaemorrhagic *E.coli* (EHEC)
Bacillus cereus	Enteroaggregative *E.coli* (EAggEC)
Vibrio cholerae	*Aeromonas hydrophila*
Campylobacter spp.	*Campylobacter* spp.
Salmonella spp.	*Salmonella* spp.
Clostridium perfringens	*Yersinia enterocolitica*
	Clostridium difficile
	Shigella spp.
Protozoa	
Giardia intestinalis (lamblia)	*Entamoeba histolytica*
Cryptosporidium parvum	
Blastocystis hominis	

66

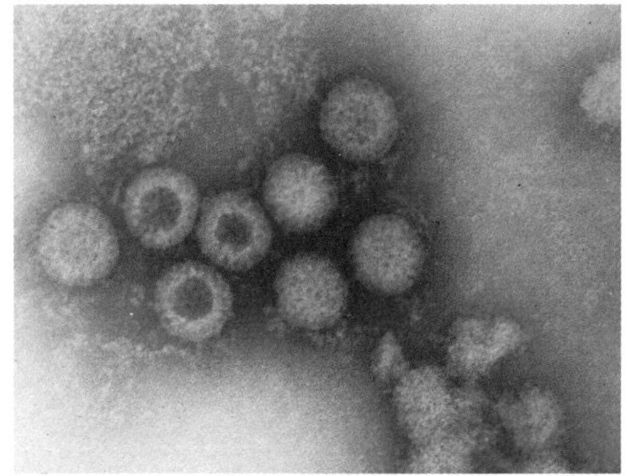

66 Negative-stain electron micrograph of a stool containing rotavirus (× *50,000*).

67

67 Rotavirus inclusions in duodenal enterocytes (× *5,000*).

In most surveys worldwide, rotavirus is the most common cause of gastroenteritis in infants, being responsible for 30–60% of cases. Rotavirus is a small (80 nm) unenveloped RNA virus with a genome consisting of 11 double-stranded segments. The virus has a double-shelled capsid, giving it a characteristic wheel-like (*rota* is Latin for a wheel) morphology (**66**). In temperate countries, infection peaks in the winter months (November to March). Patients present with vomiting and a watery diarrhoea with a characteristic milky odour. Rotavirus is a potent cause of dehydration, and management should be directed towards replacement of fluid and electrolytes. Infected patients excrete up to 10^{11} virus particles/ml faeces, and the infective dose is low (10^{1}–10^{2} particles). Consequently infection is spread very readily. The virus attaches to and penetrates the villus enterocytes of the small intestine but cannot infect the crypt cells. Initially the virus infects the enterocytes, and inclusions are formed within them (**67**). However, the brush border remains intact and the virus exits between the microvilli (**68**). Although the enterocytes are morphologically intact, brush border enzyme levels are markedly depressed. As infection proceeds, the enterocytes are killed and the villi become blunted, leading to malabsorption and an osmotic diarrhoea.

Diagnosis can be made using negative-stain electron microscopy (**66**) but this requires at least 10^{6} virus particles/ml faeces, and specialized equipment. Simpler methods include ELISA (**69**), LPA or polyacrylamide gel electrophoresis of rotavirus RNA that has been extracted directly from faeces (**70**). The last method has the advantage that it can also provide information on the similarities and differences between various rotaviruses. To date there is no uniformly effective human rotavirus vaccine available.

68

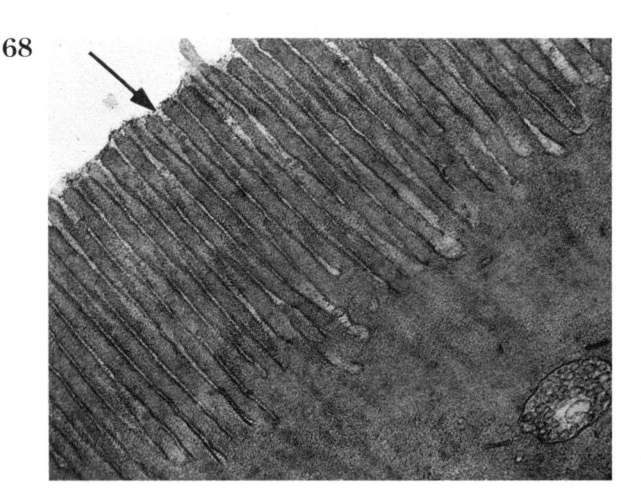

68 Rotavirus particles released from duodenal enterocytes. Note that the brush border is completely intact (× *7,500*).

69

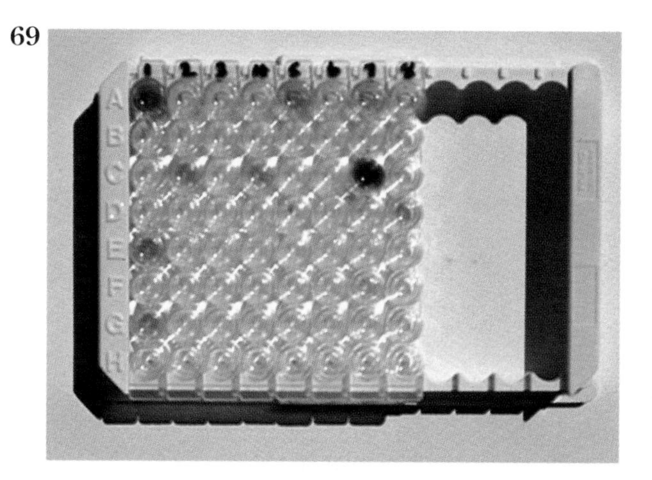

69 An ELISA for detection of rotavirus in stools.

70

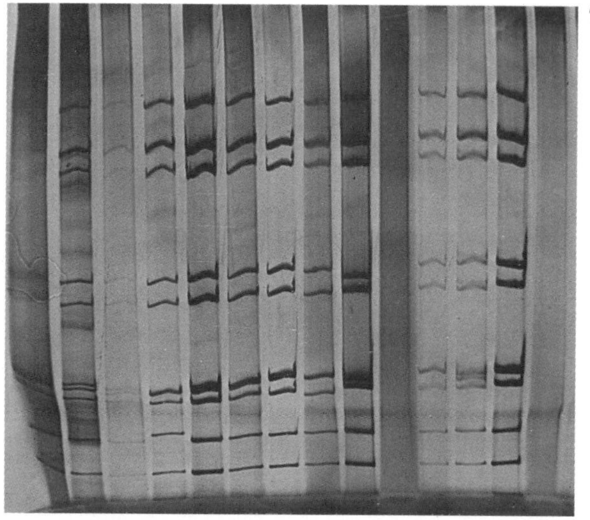

70 Polyacrylamide gel electrophoresis of rotavirus RNA extracted directly from faeces. Rotavirus genome has 11 double-stranded segments.

Astrovirus

Astrovirus is a very small (27 nm) round RNA virus that appears to have a star stamped on its surface (**71**). Infection is clinically indistinguishable from rotavirus gastroenteritis. It also has a winter peak that runs from October to February.

Adenovirus

There are 42 different serotypes of this small (80–90 nm) unenveloped DNA virus (**72**), but only types 40 and 41 cause gastroenteritis. Infection occurs throughout the year.

71

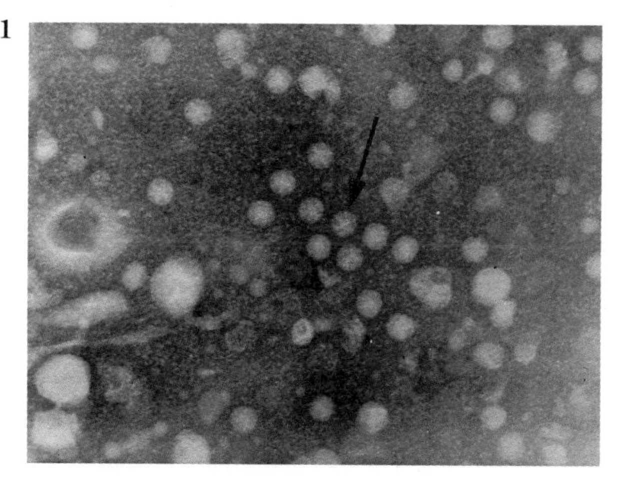

71 Negative-stain electron micrograph of a stool containing astrovirus (× *45,000*).

72

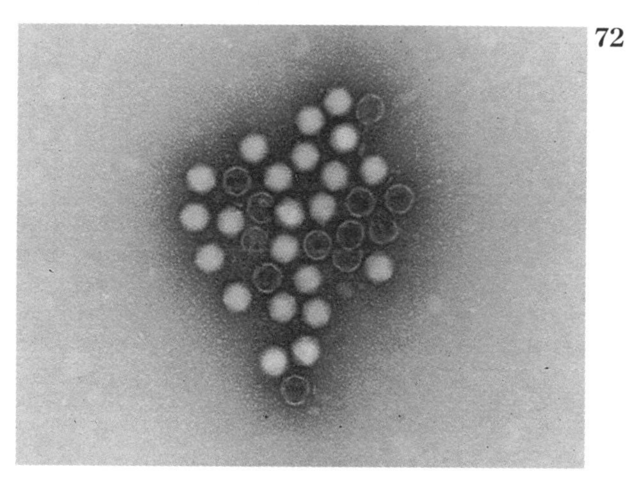

72 Negative-stain electron micrograph of a stool containing adenovirus (× *25,000*).

Calicivirus

A very small (29nm) unenveloped RNA virus, calicivirus has a characteristic morphology (**73**) with cup-shaped depressions in its surface (*calyx* is Greek for a cup). Infections occur throughout the year.

Coronavirus

Coronavirus is a rare cause of gastroenteritis. It is an enveloped RNA virus with club-shaped spikes on its surface (**74**).

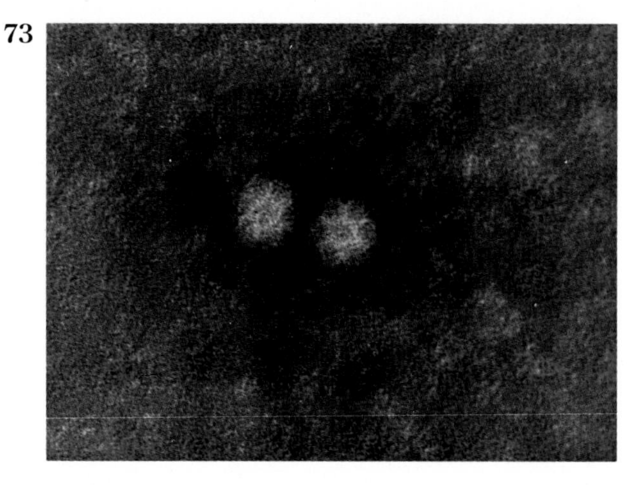

73 Negative-stain electron micrograph of a stool containing calicivirus (× *115,000*).

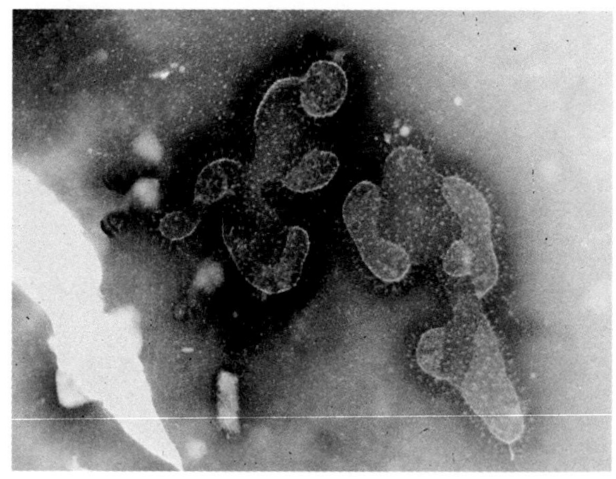

74 Negative-stain electron micrograph of a stool containing coronavirus (× *20,000*).

Norwalk agent

A small (26nm) round RNA virus which is named after a town in Ohio, USA, Norwalk agent is associated with Winter-vomiting disease but can also cause diarrhoea. It is excreted in large numbers in faeces but only for a short period after the onset of disease and diagnosis by electron microscopy can be difficult. An ELISA test for detection of virus in faeces is available.

Escherichia coli

An aerobic gram-negative bacterium, *E.coli* is part of the normal flora of the human intestine, and faeces contain approximately 10^7 colony-forming units (CFU)/ml. It is greatly to the credit of the UK paediatricians and microbiologists that *E.coli* was shown to be a cause of gastroenteritis. It was found that certain 0 serogroups of *E.coli* (e.g. 0111) were associated with epidemics of diarrhoea in children. Eventually it became clear that not all *E.coli* produced diarrhoea in the same way. Enterotoxigenic *E.coli* (ETEC) and enteropathogenic *E.coli* (EPEC) produce a non-inflammatory diarrhoea, whereas enteroinvasive *E.coli* (EIEC), enterohaemorrhagic *E.coli* (EHEC) and enteroaggregative *E.coli* (EAggEC) produce an inflammatory type.

E.coli sticks to the intestinal mucosa by means of two kinds of adhesins: fimbriae (or pili) or non-fimbrial adhesins. Fimbriae are protein spikes that stick out from the surface of the bacterium (**75**) and have an affinity for receptors on the enterocyte surface. ETEC may possess a variety of different fimbriae (e.g. CFA 1, CFA 2), which are used to adhere to the small intestinal mucosa (**76**). ETEC elaborates heat-labile (LT) and/or heat-stable (ST) toxins. LT activates adenyl cyclase in the enterocytes, raising levels of cyclic adenosine monophosphate (cAMP). In villous tip enterocytes, cAMP is antiabsorptive; in villous crypt enterocytes, it causes secretion of Na^+ and thus Cl^- and water. ST elevates levels of cyclic guanosine monophosphate (GMP) in enterocytes, which has an anti-absorptive effect. Thus, ETEC produces a secretory diarrhoea that is usually short-lived. ETEC is an uncommon cause of diarrhoea in children in developed countries, but it is a major cause both of travellers' diarrhoea and of diarrhoea in developing countries.

EPEC tends to produce a more chronic diarrhoea and, although common in the 1940s and 1950s, it is now an uncommon cause of diarrhoea in the UK. EPEC produces a characteristic ultrastructural lesion on the enterocyte brush border, called attaching effacement. The bacteria become firmly adherent to the mucosa, and can be demonstrated by gram film of duodenal biopsies (**77**). The EPEC then penetrates between the microvilli, attach firmly to the surface of the enterocyte, and cause the brush border to be shed by a process of vesiculation (**78**). A loss of absorptive area results, together with a loss of the brush border enzymes lactase, sucrase and maltase. Disaccharides in the diet must be cleaved to monosaccharides in order to be absorbed. Without the brush border enzymes, the disaccharides remain undigested, pass to the colon, and cause an osmotic diarrhoea.

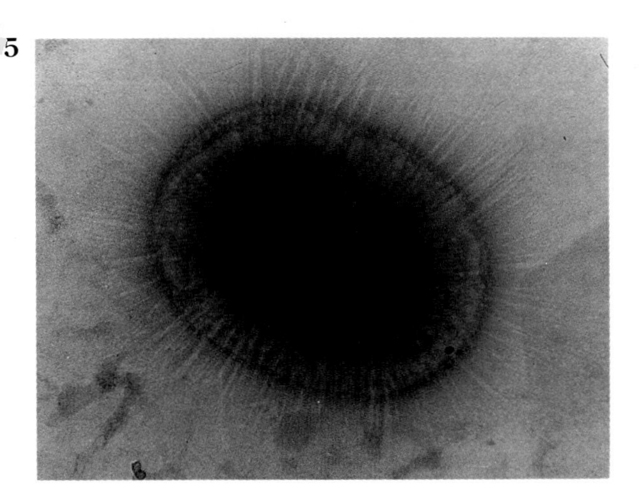

75 Negative-stain electron micrograph of an enterotoxigenic *E. coli* (ETEC), demonstrating the pili used to tether the bacterium to the small intestinal mucosa (× *14,000*).

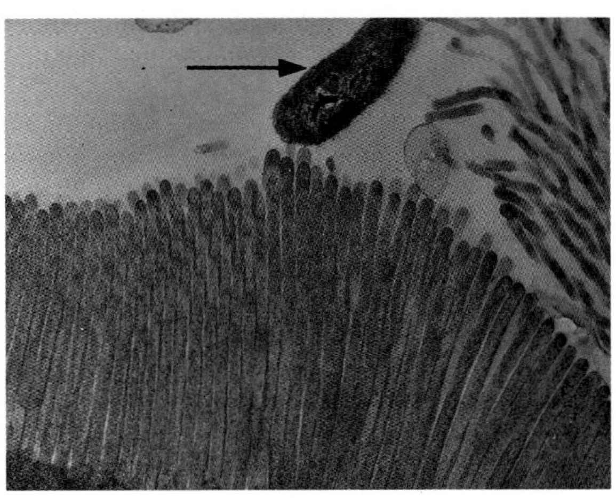

76 Thin-section electron micrograph of ETEC attached to jejunal mucosa (× *3,000*).

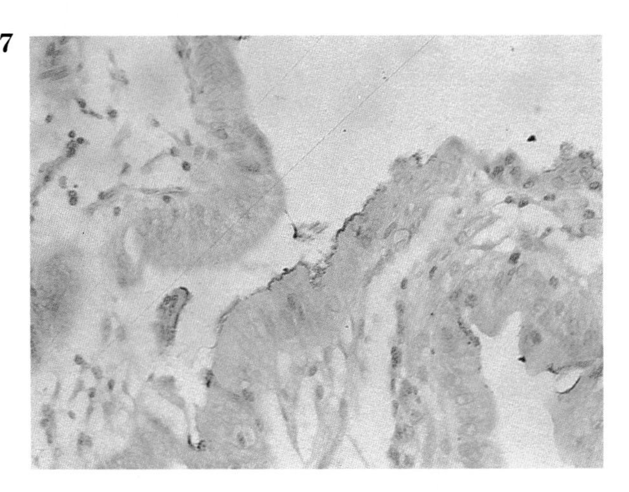

77 Gram-stained section of duodenal mucosa with numerous closely adherent enteropathogenic *E. coli* (EPEC) (× *1,000*).

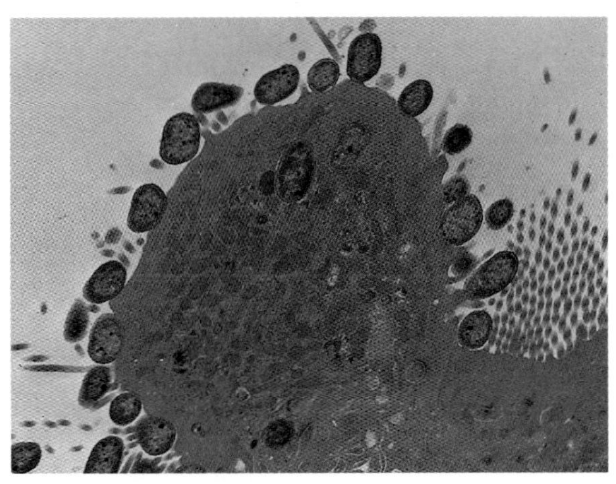

78 Thin-section electron micrograph of duodenum with numerous EPEC adherent to the mucosal surface, which has lost its brush border. This is termed attaching–effacement (× *1,800*).

Vibrio cholerae

Responsible for large outbreaks of diarrhoeal disease, particularly in developing countries, this curved motile gram-negative (**79**) bacterium produces a toxin with a structure and mode of action very similar to that of *E.coli* heat-labile toxin. A very fluid 'rice-water' (**80**) stool and profound dehydration result. As with most enteric infections, management does not include antimicrobial chemotherapy, but does involve urgent rehydration. The current cholera vaccine consists of whole killed bacteria, which is given subcutaneously. It is not highly effective.

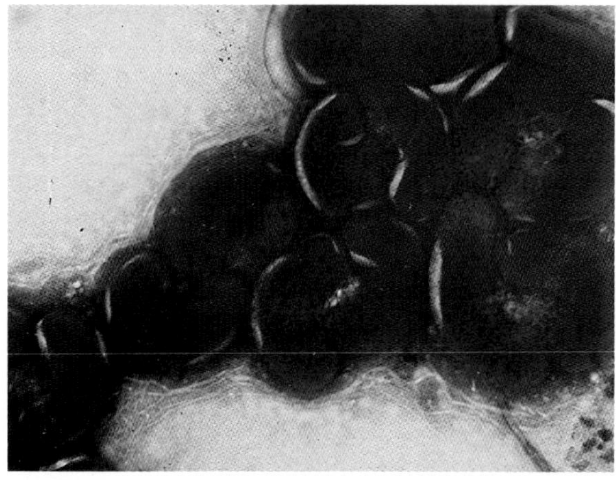

79 Negative-stain electron micrograph of comma-shaped *V. cholerae* (× *3,000*).

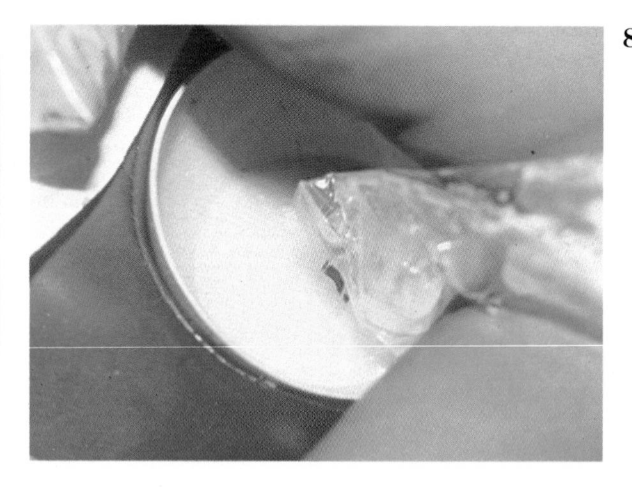

80 The typical 'rice-water' stool of cholera.

Clostridium perfringens

C.perfringens, an anaerobic gram-positive spore-forming bacterium (**81**), is a cause of food poisoning. Infection commonly follows ingestion of pre-cooked stews that have been incompletely reheated. The initial cooking kills vegetative bacteria, which then sporulate. The heated meat also provides good anaerobic conditions. As the stew cools, the spores germinate to produce large numbers of vegetative bacteria. If not reheated thoroughly, the bacteria survive and are ingested. In the gut, the bacteria sporulate and in doing so they release a structural spore protein that causes fluid accumulation in ileal loops. Abdominal pain and profuse watery diarrhoea occur, on average, 10–15 hours after ingestion of contaminated food.

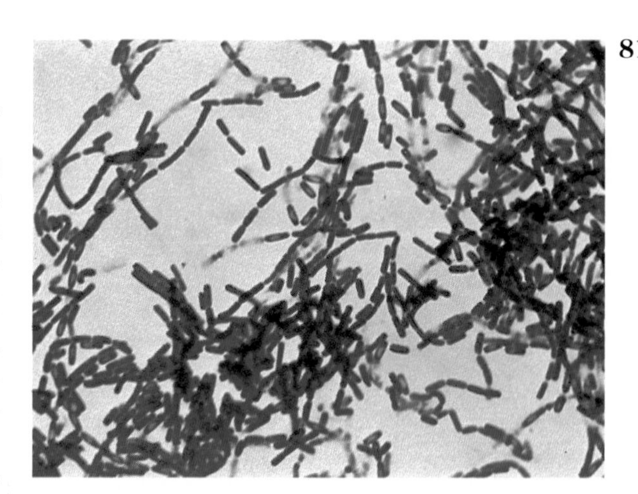

81 Gram-stained film of *C. perfringens* (× *1,000*).

Giardia intestinalis (*lamblia*)

This protozoan parasite, to which children seem to be more susceptible than adults, is an important cause of gastroenteritis. There is considerable variation in the response of patients to infection. Some children develop acute diarrhoea with abdominal pain, flatulence and an explosive watery foul-smelling stool. Others develop chronic diarrhoea with malabsorption and, occasionally, failure to thrive, and others are totally asymptomatic. Infected patients excrete cysts (**82**), which can remain viable for several months in their stools. Once ingested the cysts divide to produce two trophozoites (**83**), which attach to the brush border by means of an adhesive disc (**84**). How the parasites produce diarrhoea is unclear. Trophozoites can be seen following duodenal aspiration or in the stools of patients with acute diarrhoea. Treatment is supportive, involving the use of nitroimidazoles such as metronidazole. The whole family should be treated, since asymptomatic carriers in the family may reinfect the others.

82

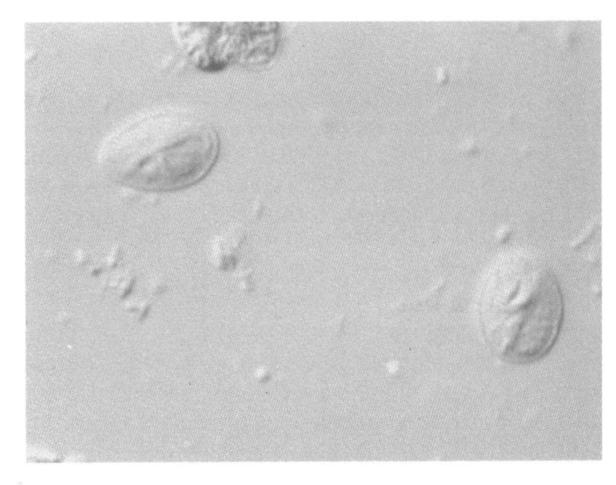

82 *G. intestinalis* (*lamblia*) cysts in faeces. Nomarski phase contrast (× *4,000*).

83

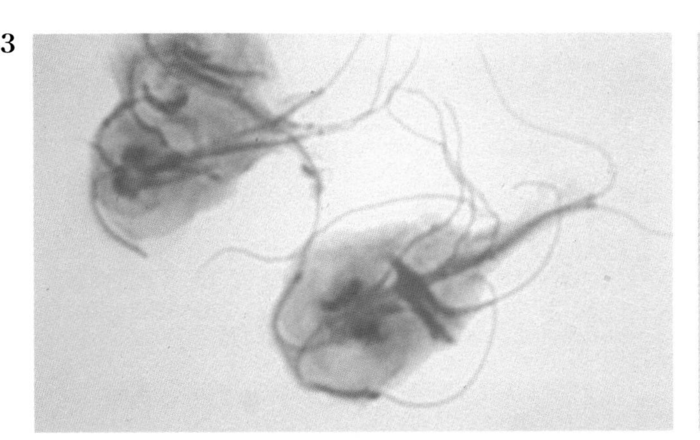

83 *G. intestinalis* (*lamblia*) trophozoites in duodenal aspirate (× *5,000*).

84

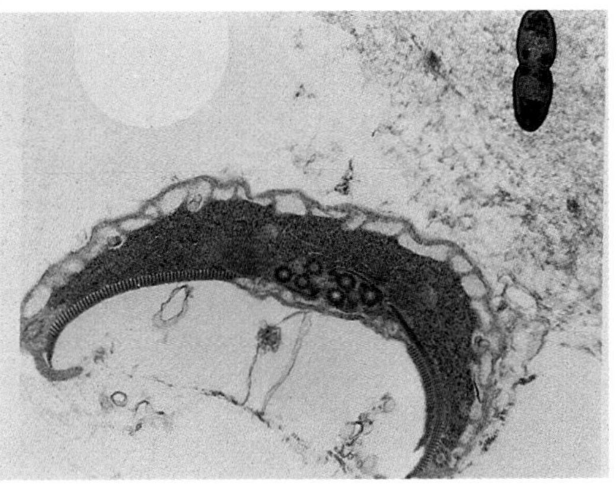

84 Thin-section electron micrograph of *G. intestinalis* (*lamblia*) demonstrating the striated adhesive disc (× *1,500*).

Blastocystis hominis

B.hominis, another protozoan parasite (**85**), has been associated with gastroenteritis, but it can also be found in asymptomatic individuals. Treatment (if necessary) is by metronidazole or trimethoprim.

85

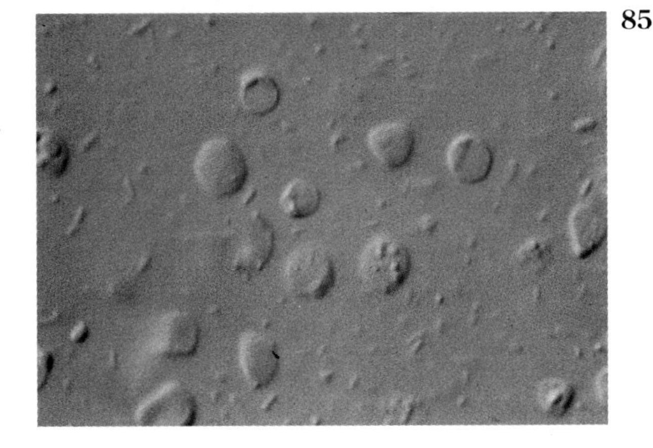

85 *B. hominis* with typical 'signet ring' forms. Nomarski phase contrast (× *4,000*).

Cryptosporidium parvum

C.parvum is a protozoan parasite that has been recognized as a human pathogen only in recent years. In most surveys it is recorded as being the second most common cause of gastroenteritis (after rotavirus) in children. In developing countries it is responsible for 6–17% of cases of gastroenteritis. In developed countries it accounts for 0.4–4.0% of cases. The infective form is the thick-walled oocyst (**86**), which is highly resistant to desiccation and to most disinfectants. In the stomach the four sporozoites escape through a suture in the oocyst's surface (**87**), maturing to become trophozoites which are found inside the enterocyte membrane but are separated from the rest of the cytoplasm by the so-called feeder organelle (**88**). How cryptosporidium produces diarrhoea is unclear, but it does not do so by causing inflammation. The infected patient excretes large numbers of oocysts, continuing to do so for 2–4 weeks after cessation of disease.

Specific diagnosis of cryptosporidiosis used to be made by demonstrating trophozoites on duodenal biopsy (**89**). A simpler and more convenient method is to demonstrate oocysts in stools, using basic staining techniques. Stains include safranin–methylene blue (**90**) and auramine phenol (**91**).

Cryptosporidium tends to produce a more prolonged diarrhoea than other enteric pathogens and consequently, is more often associated with failure to thrive. The stool is often green, watery and offensive. In immunocompetent children cryptosporidium is eventually eliminated but in the immunoincompetent it produces a profuse life-threatening disease that spreads to other organs to cause pneumonia, colitis and conjunctivitis. There is no effective anticryptosporidial drug, nor is a vaccine available.

86

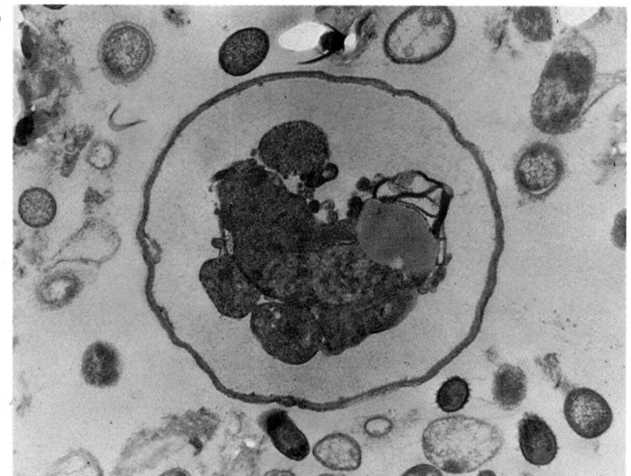

86 Thin-section electron micrograph of a *C. parvum* oocyst. The four sporozoites are sectioned in various planes (× *3,500*).

87

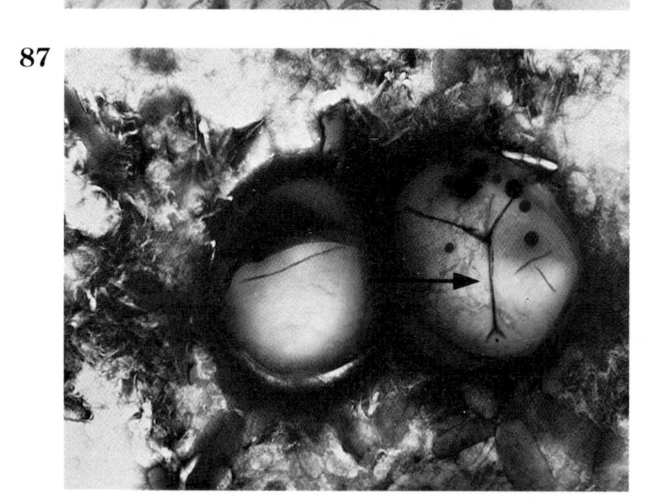

87 Negative-stain electron micrograph of *C. parvum* oocysts. The sutures through which the sporozoites escape are visible (× *2,000*).

88

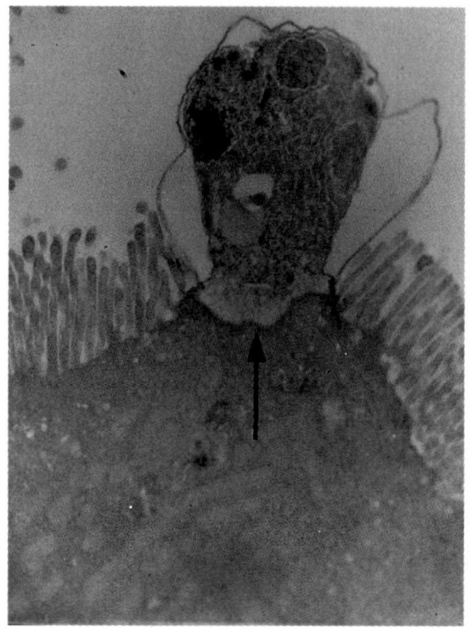

88 Thin-section electron micrograph of a jejunal enterocyte with *C. parvum* trophozoite. The organism is intracellular, but it is separated from the rest of the cytoplasm by a feeder organelle (× *11,000*).

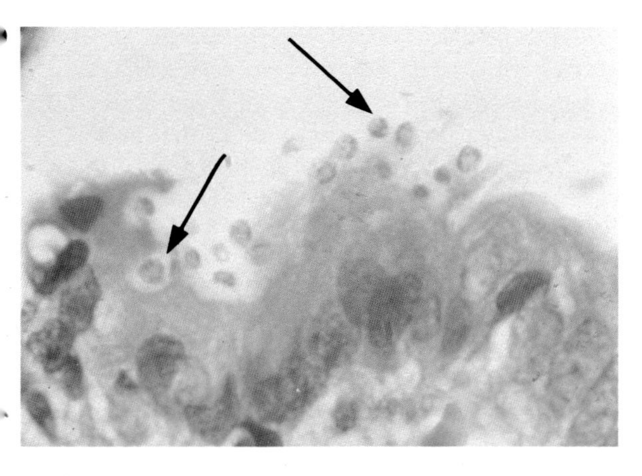

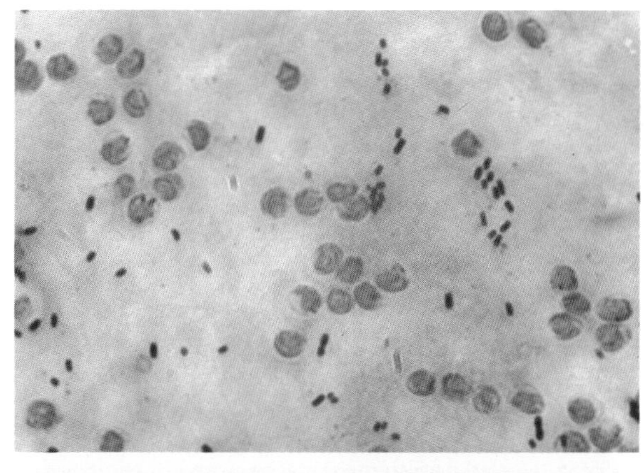

90

91

89 Section of jejunal biopsy showing *C. parvum* trophozoites (× *400*).

90 Faecal smear stained by safranin–methylene blue. Large numbers of pink *C. parvum* oocysts are present (× *400*).

91 Faecal smear stained by auramine phenol. The *C. parvum* oocysts fluoresce (× *800*).

Inflammatory diarrhoea

Although *Salmonella* and *Campylobacter* spp. elaborate toxins that cause non-inflammatory diarrhoea, both are most frequently associated with inflammatory diarrhoea (**Table 7**).

Enteroinvasive E.coli (*EIEC*)

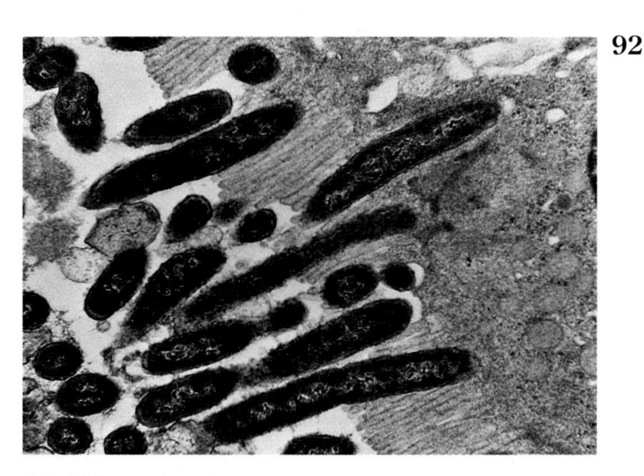

92

92 Thin-section electron micrograph showing enteroinvasive *E. coli* (EIEC) penetrating a colonic enterocyte (× *2,000*).

Enteroinvasive strains of *E.coli* are able to adhere to and penetrate the colonic enterocyte (**92**). Once inside the cell, the bacterium divides, eventually killing the enterocyte. This leads to areas of the colon being denuded of mucosa and there is an inflammatory response. The infection presents as a watery diarrhoea, with fever and abdominal pain. Although the stool does contain pus cells (and mucus may also be present), it is rarely frankly blood-stained. Infection is usually self-limiting.

The genes for pathogenicity are on a large plasmid carried by the *E.coli*, and they encode a surface protein. The genes have close homology to those of *Shigella* pathogenicity genes. DNA probes for specific diagnosis are available.

Enterohaemorrhagic E.coli (EHEC)

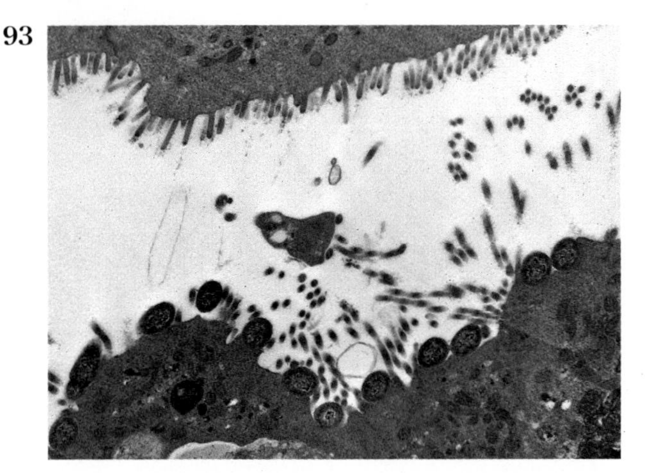

93 Thin-section electron micrograph showing attaching–effacement by enterohaemorrhagic *E. coli* (EHEC) on ileal mucosa (× *1,500*).

A recently discovered cause of gastroenteritis, these bacteria are also associated with the haemolytic uraemic syndrome. They are pathogens of cattle and pigs, and children may become infected following, for example, consumption of undercooked hamburgers. EHEC produce attaching effacement (**93**) of the brush border but this is limited to the terminal ileum and colon, in contrast to EPEC, which affect the whole of the intestinal tract. In addition, EHEC elaborate one or both of the toxins, verocytotoxins 1 and 2 (called Shiga-like toxins in the USA). These kill the colonic enterocytes, producing the haemorrhagic colitis. They also appear to promote the deposition of fibrin strands in capillaries, which leads to intravascular haemolysis and, eventually, to renal failure.

Although certain 0 serogroups (e.g. 0157) are associated with haemorrhagic colitis, specific diagnosis is made by detection of VT_1 or VT_2 and EHEC pathogenicity genes by DNA hybridization.

Enteroaggregative E.coli (EAggEC)

Enteroaggregative strains of *E.coli* produce large aggregates on the surface of cultured cells. Their pathogenesis and relative importance as an enteropathogen are unclear. However, they do appear to produce a chronic diarrhoea, particularly in children in developing countries. Microbiological diagnosis is made using a specific DNA probe.

Aeromonas hydrophila

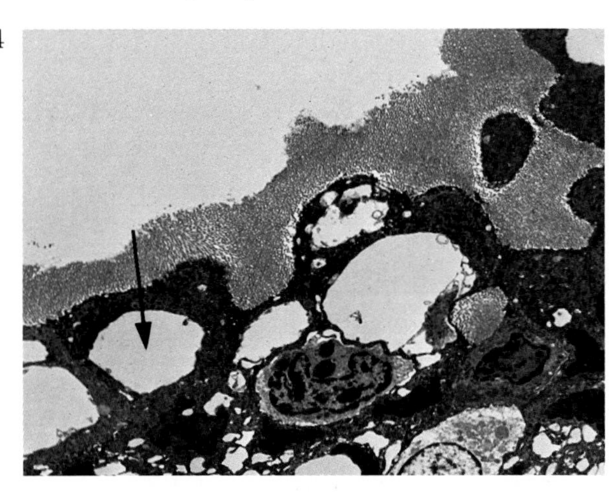

94 Thin-section electron micrograph showing the effects (vacuolation) of *Aeromonas hydrophila* on ileal enterocytes (× *1,000*).

A gram-negative bacterium, *A. hydrophila* is a recently recognized cause of gastroenteritis. The organism is ubiquitous in watery environments but not all isolates are able to produce disease. Infection is associated with production of enterotoxins and cytotoxins, which apparently produce vacuolation of colonic enterocytes (**94**). Peaks of infection occur during the summer months.

Campylobacter species

Three Campylobacter spp. have been associated with diarrhoeal disease: *C.jejuni* (types I and II), *C.coli* and *C.laridis*, which was first isolated from seagulls. They are short spiral bacteria that possess flagellae, which impart motility (**95**). Infection can be spread from person to person, as zoonoses or indirectly in food and water. The pathogenesis of infection is not entirely clear but both production of enterotoxins and mucosal invasion are involved. Treatment is usually supportive. However, occasionally bacteraemia may occur, in which case, treatment with erythromycin is indicated.

Bacteria can be isolated from faeces using selective media (e.g. Skirrow's) and microaerophilic conditions at 42°C.

95

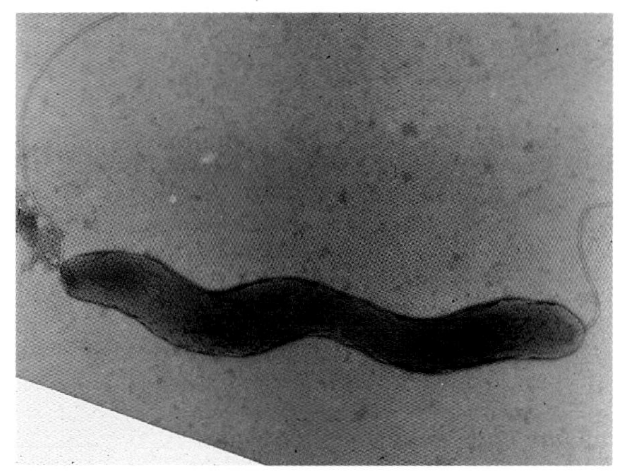

95 Negative-stain electron micrograph of *C. jejuni* (× *2,000*).

Salmonella species

The Salmonella spp. comprise a large family of gram-negative motile bacteria (**96**) that cause food poisoning. They can be part of the normal intestinal flora in chickens, pigs and cattle, and contamination of food products by intestinal contents may lead to the growth of these organisms, which, if ingested, cause profound diarrhoea. The Salmonellae are subdivided according to which O or somatic (lipopolysaccharide) and H or flagellar antigens they possess.

In the UK, *S.typhimurium* and *S.enteritidis* are the most frequently isolated of the 1,700 different serotypes. In general the infective dose is high (about 10^7 CFU), thus multiplication on food prior to ingestion is necessary. However, recent reports suggest that the infective dose for *S.enteritidis* (phage type 4), the organism found in eggs, is much lower (about 10^2–10^3 CFU). *S. typhi* produces enteric fever and rarely causes diarrhoea. Although infection is limited to the intestinal tract in most cases, *S.typhimurium*, *S.virchow* and *S.dublin* are able to produce bacteraemia. In such circumstances, antimicrobial chemotherapy with, for example, trimethoprim or ciprofloxacin is indicated. Bacteria can be isolated from food or stool samples using enrichment (selenite) and selective (XLD) media.

96

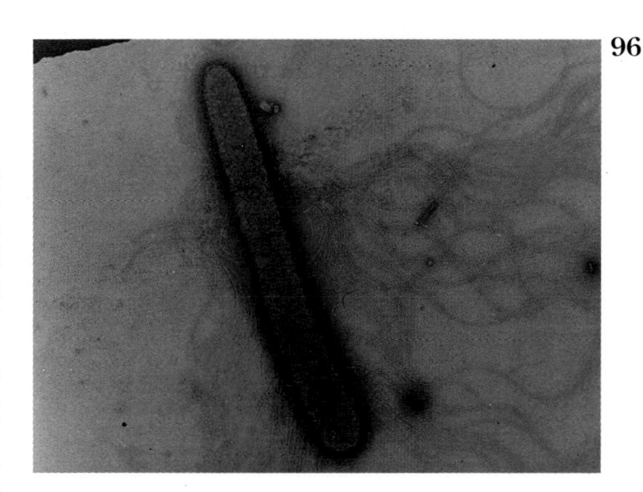

96 Negative-stain electron micrograph of *S. typhimurium*, with its numerous flagellae (× *2,000*).

Clostridium difficile

C.difficile is a cause of an antibiotic-associated diarrhoea that, in its severe form, presents as pseudomembranous colitis. It is an anaerobic gram-positive spore-bearing bacillus and colitis results from the release of its toxin(s). Its role in diarrhoeal disease in children is unclear. Infants, in particular, can excrete both the organism and its toxin in the absence of disease.

Yersinia enterocolitica

A gram-negative rod or coccobacillus, *Y.enterocolitica* is an infrequent cause of gastroenteritis in the UK. It may also cause acute mesenteric adenitis (as can *Y.pseudotuberculosis*). The diarrhoeal disease can last up to 3 weeks and is often accompanied by high fever and abdominal pain. The pathogenesis involves invasion of ileal and colonic enterocytes by the bacterium, and may also involve enterotoxins. In general the sources of the organism are food, water or animals.

Mesenteric adenitis usually presents without diarrhoea and is clinically indistinguishable from acute appendicitis. *Y.enterocolitica* is often recovered from the stools of affected patients, whereas *Y.pseudotuberculosis* is usually recoverable from lymph nodes or blood only. Antimicrobial treatment, if necessary, is with cotrimoxazole.

Shigella species

97

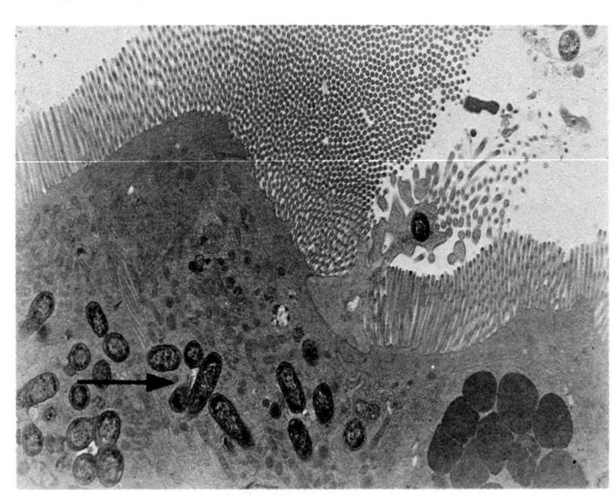

97 Thin-section electron micrograph of colonic enterocytes containing dividing *S. sonnei* (× *1,000*).

There are four serogroups of this non-motile gram-negative bacillus: *S.dysenteriae, S.flexneri, S.sonnei* and *S.boydii*. In the UK, *S.sonnei* is the most common cause of bacillary dysentery. It is solely a human pathogen, with infection spreading directly (usually from asymptomatic carriers) or indirectly (in food and water) from person to person. The infective dose is low (10–100 CFU). The pathogenesis involves invasion of colonic enterocytes (**97**). In addition, *S.dysenteriae*, in particular, produces shiga toxin, which inhibits protein synthesis.

Infections are usually associated with conditions of poor hygiene. They may occur in daycare centres, crèches, nursery schools and homes for the mentally retarded. Large spreading outbreaks occur following contamination of water and flooding, as has happened in Bangladesh. Management usually involves rehydration, but severe disease may require antimicrobial chemotherapy.

Entamoeba histolytica

98

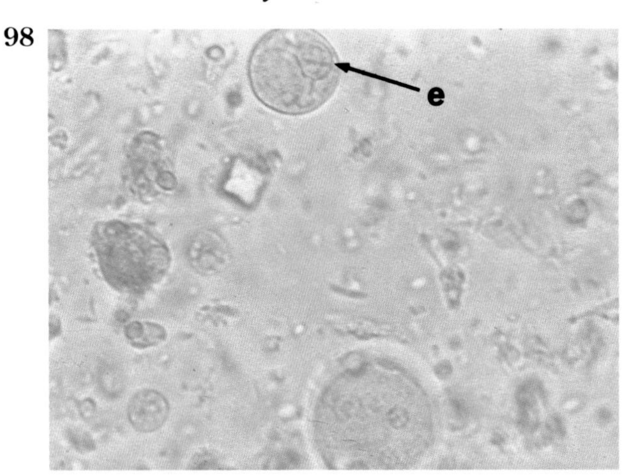

98 *Entamoeba* cysts in a stool. The upper cyst is of *E. histolytica*, and contains an erythrocyte (e); the lower cyst is of *E. coli* (× *200*).

E.histolytica is the cause of amoebic dysentery. This protozoan parasite has cyst (**98**) and trophozoite (**99**) stages in its life cycle. Infection is rare in the UK but is much more common in tropical countries. Diagnosis is reached by detection of cysts and by proctoscopic examination and biopsy. However, it must be remembered that not every patient who excretes *E.histolytica* has amoebiasis. Commensal forms do appear to exist. Infection produces friable haemorrhagic ulcers (**100**), and may spread to cause liver abscesses, which are responsible for almost half of the deaths in amoebiasis. The disease apparently does not have a worse prognosis in patients with AIDS. Treatment is with metronidazole or emetine.

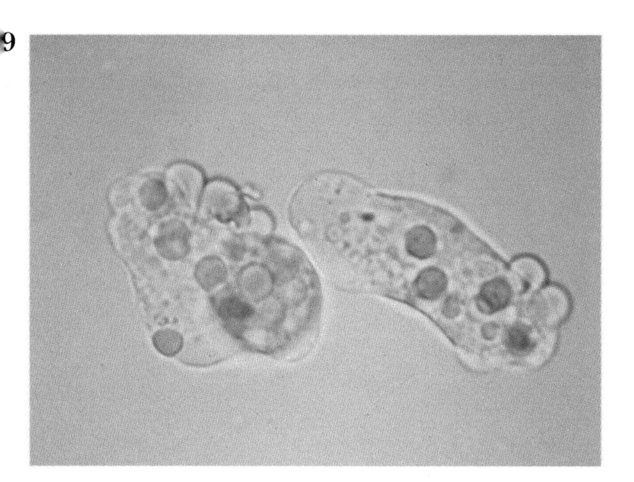

99 *E. histolytica* trophozoites containing erythrocytes (× *200*).

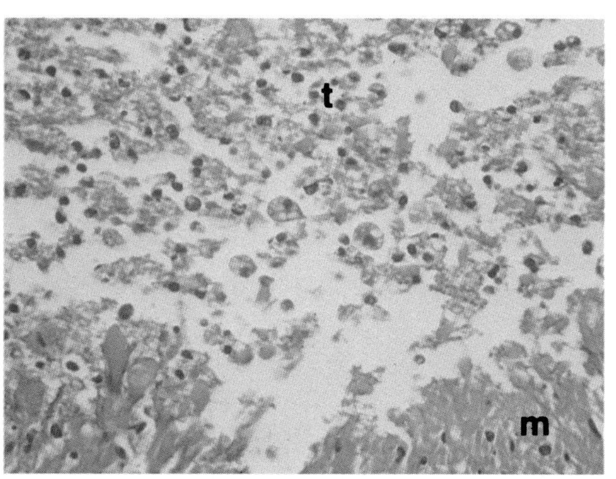

100 Section through an amoebic ulcer in the colon, showing ragged mucosa (m) and numerous trophozoites (t). (× *400*).

Acute appendicitis

Although appendicitis is not initiated by microbes, its complications may result in infection. Lymphoid hyperplasia, roundworms or even faecoliths (**101**) may block the appendix, leading to inflammation, gangrene and perforation of the appendix (**102**). Perforation may, in turn, lead to peritonitis or, more commonly, to the area being walled off, producing appendiceal, pelvic or subphrenic abscesses. The organisms associated with such abscesses are normally commensals in the intestinal tract. In particular, aerobes such as *E.coli*, anaerobes such as *Bacteroides fragilis*, and microaerophilic bacteria such as *Strepto-coccus milleri* (**103**) are often found either alone or in mixed culture. Treatment requires both surgical drainage and appropriate antimicrobial chemotherapy.

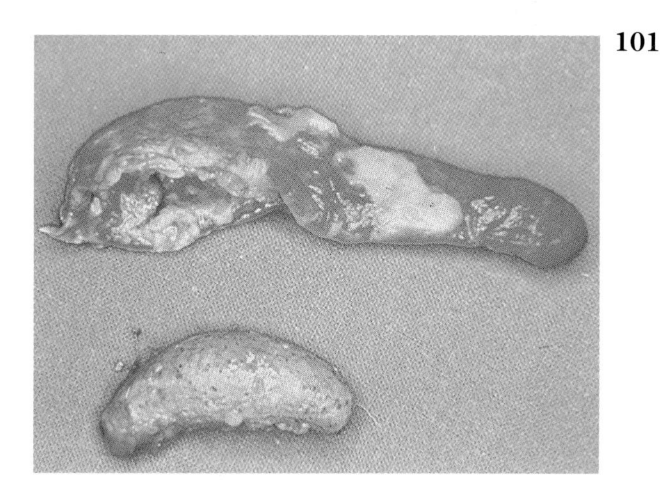

101 An appendix, together with the faecolith that it contained.

102

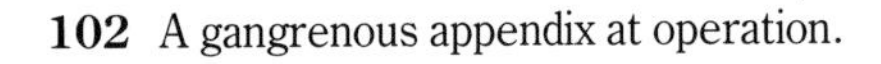

102 A gangrenous appendix at operation.

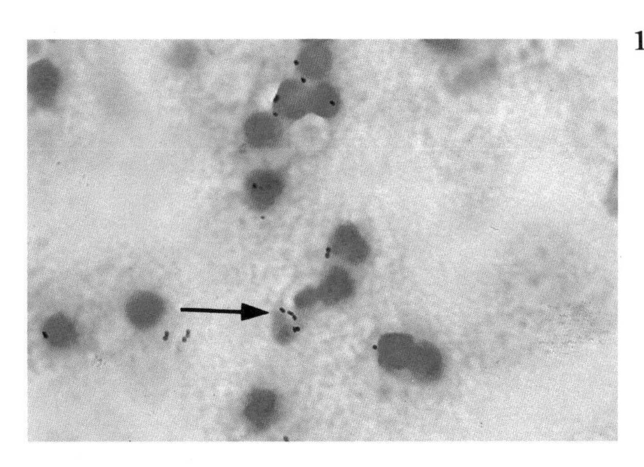

103 Gram-stained smear of pus from an appendiceal abscess, showing numerous pus cells and a few gram-positive cocci which, on culture, proved to be *S. milleri* (× *1,000*).

Enteric helminths

In this section, those helminths found in temperate zones are discussed. The tropical parasites are shown in Chapter 12. In most cases, infestation of the intestinal tract is asymptomatic and it is only, for example, when segments of tapeworms are excreted or worms migrate that it becomes apparent. In order to put this section into context, the range of helminths that infect man is shown in **Table 8**.

Table 8. Helminths Infecting Man.

Nematodes (roundworms)		
Intestinal	*Tissue*	
Ascaris lumbricoides	*Trichinella spiralis*	
Enterobius vermicularis (threadworm)	*Toxocara canis*	
Enterobius gregorii	*Wuchereria bancrofti*	
Ancylostoma duodenale (hookworm)	*Brugia malayi*	
Necator americanus (hookworm)	*Loa loa*	
Strongyloides stercoralis	*Onchocerca volvulus*	
Trichuris trichuria (whipworm)	*Mansonella* spp.	
Capillaria phillipinensis	*Gnathostoma spinigerum*	
Trichostrongulus spp.	*Dracunculus medinensis*	
Cestodes (segmented worms)		
Intestinal	*Tissue*	
Taenia solium	*Taenia solium*	
Taenia saginata	*Echinococcus granulosus* (hydatid disease)	
Diphyllobothrium spp.	*Multiceps multiceps*	
Hymenolepis spp.	*Diphyllobothrium* spp.	
Trematodes		
Intestinal	*Liver/Lung*	*Blood*
Fasciolopsis buskii	*Fasciola hepatica*	*Schistosoma mansoni*
Echinostoma spp.	*Opisthorchis* spp.	*Schistosoma haematobium*
Heterophyids	*Paragonimus westermani*	*Schistosoma japonica*

Nematodes

All nematodes are non-segmented (cf. segmented earthworms) cylindrical worms with tapered ends. All have a moderate to long lifespan (1–18 years), and some, e.g., *Strongyloides* and *Enterobius*, have auto-infective cycles. Diagnosis is usually made by demonstration of eggs in faeces, but occasionally an adult worm is noticed.

Ascaris lumbricoides

A creamy white roundworm (**104**), *A. lumbricoides* can be as long as 35 cm but males are shorter and slimmer. Worm loads can be extremely high (up to 1,000 per person), with mature females producing up to 200,000 eggs per day. Fertile eggs (**105**) are excreted and then mature in soil for 2–3 weeks. When ingested, the eggs hatch in the upper small intestine, liberating larvae. These penetrate through the intestinal wall to enter capillaries and lymphatics, travelling thence to the portal circulation. They then pass through the right chambers of the heart to the pulmonary artery and capillaries, breaking out of the blood vessels into the alveoli, bronchioles and bronchi. Having risen to the epiglottis, they descend the oesophagus to the intestine. Symptoms may arise during the migration, especially in children and in those patients with a heavy infestation. In such cases, adult worms may cause intestinal obstruction.

Treatment includes pyrantal palmoate, piperazine or mebendazole. Prevention will only be possible when human excreta are no longer allowed to contaminate food or water.

4

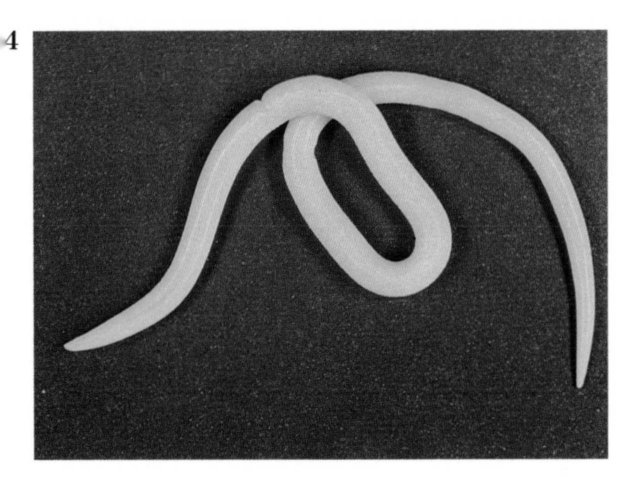

104 An adult *A. lumbricoides*.

105

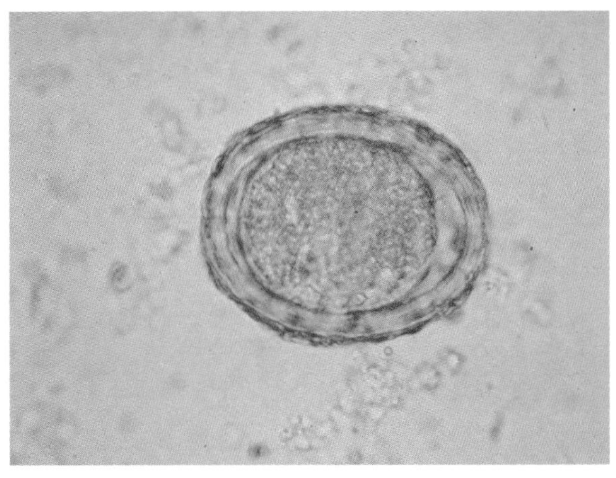

105 A fertile *A. lumbricoides* egg in faeces (× *160*).

Enterobius vermicularis

The threadworm or pinworm is one of the most common infestations of children and is frequently asymptomatic. The female worm is 8–13 mm long and about 0.5 mm in diameter. Adult worms live in the caecum and its environs. The gravid female worm (**106**) migrates to the anus and lays large numbers of eggs on the perineum. The eggs are fully embryonated and immediately infective when ingested. The worm can provoke pruritis ani and when the affected area is scratched, eggs are transferred to finger nails. Eggs may survive for weeks, and infection via contaminated dust, bedding or clothing can occur. When symptomatic, infestation produces irritability, perianal irritation, insomnia and anorexia. In female children, worms may migrate into the vagina and cause vaginal discharge.

Diagnosis is made by demonstration of eggs, although, occasionally, adult worms are seen in faeces. Application of transparent cellophane adhesive tape to the anus on waking will pick up eggs, visible by low-power light microscopy (**107** & **108**). Management involves administration of mebendazole or piperazine for the whole family, and thorough cleaning of bedding and clothes.

106

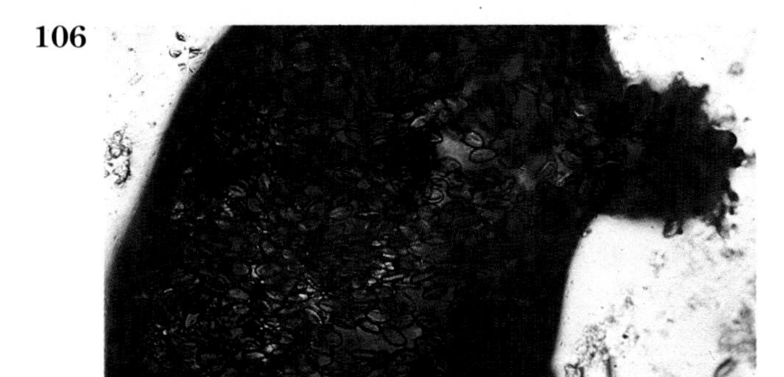

106 A gravid *E. vermicularis* worm packed with eggs (× *15*).

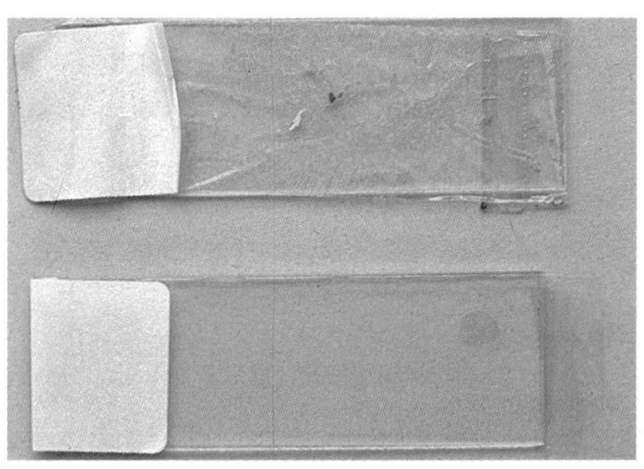

107 Cellophane tape slides for detection of threadworm eggs.

108

108 A threadworm egg with a larva visible inside (× *400*).

Hookworms

109

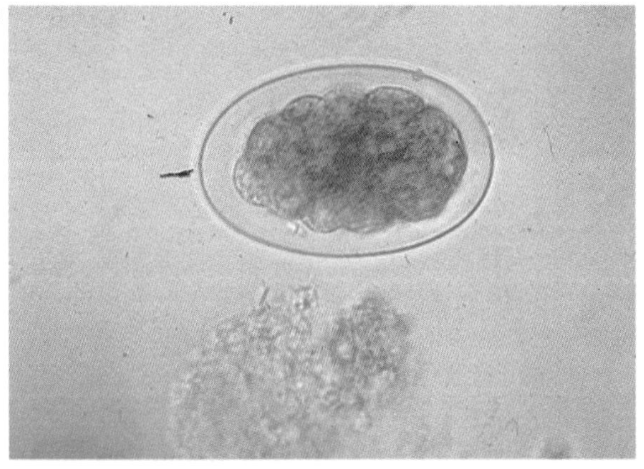

109 A hookworm egg (× *170*).

Ancylostoma duodenale is the only hookworm native to Europe, and is found principally around the Mediterranean. Eggs are excreted in faeces (**109**), where they hatch within 24–28 hours. The rhabditiform larvae grow and develop in the soil, using bacteria and organic material as nutrients. After about 7 days they change into filariform infective larvae, at which stage they have a further 2 weeks to find a host before they die. The worms infect humans by penetrating the skin (usually on the foot) and entering venules. They eventually reach the lungs, where they migrate up the trachea to be swallowed. They attach to the small intestinal mucosa, sucking blood and tissue fluids. *Necator americanus* is found in North and South America, as well as in Africa, south of the Sahara. It has a similar life cycle to that of *A. duodenale*.

When the hookworms penetrate the skin, an allergic reaction may cause 'ground itch' but infestation is usually asymptomatic. However, if large numbers of larvae reach the lung, pneumonitis may occur and, if a large number of worms parasitize the intestine, the blood and protein loss may be sufficient to cause anaemia and a failure to thrive. Treatment is with mebendazole and prevention is achieved by limiting skin contact with soil in endemic areas.

Strongyloides stercoralis

These parasites have a similar geographical distribution to that of hookworms. The females lay eggs that hatch in the intestine to release larvae which are then excreted in faeces. In soil the free-living nematodes are small (about 1 mm long). Eventually they develop into infective filariform larvae. Thereafter, the life cycle is similar to that of hookworms. The major difference is that the larvae produced in the intestine can mature to become infective while still in the intestine. As a consequence, amplification and persistent infection occur.

Gastrointestinal symptoms are rare, but malabsorption may occur with heavy infestation. Hyperinfection may lead to severe debilitation or even death. Diagnosis is made by demonstration of larvae in the stool (**110**).

110

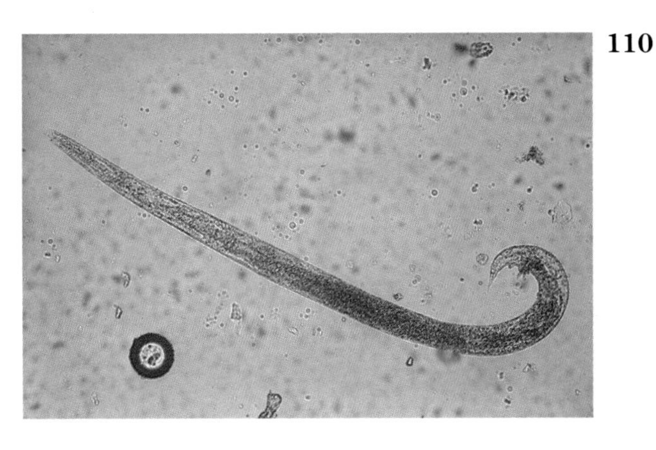

110 A filariform larva of *S. stercoralis* (× *100*).

Trichuris trichuria

Whipworm (**111**) infestation, which is rarely symptomatic, occurs in the large bowel. The parasite occurs worldwide, flourishing in conditions of poor hygiene. A heavy infestation may produce tenesmus, abdominal pain, bloody or mucoid diarrhoea and even rectal prolapse. Diagnosis is made by demonstration of the characteristic eggs (**112**). Treatment, if necessary, is with mebendazole.

111

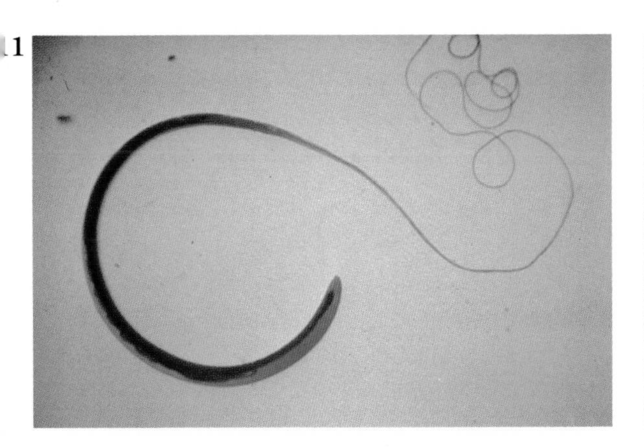

111 Adult whipworm (*T. trichuria*). (Copyright Liverpool School of Tropical Medicine (LSTM).)

112

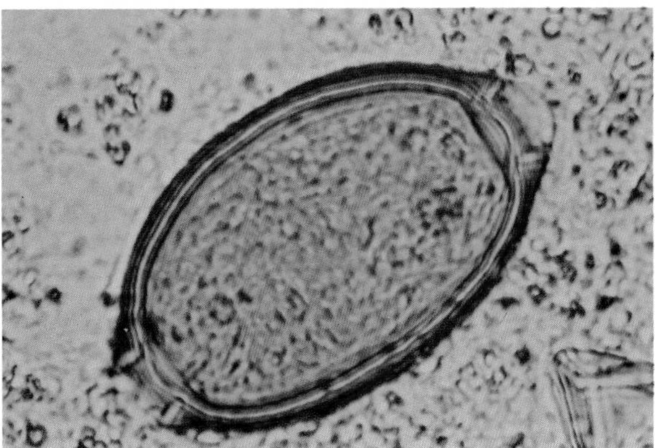

112 A *Trichuris* egg (× *480*).

Trematodes

The only non-tropical trematode is *Fasciola hepatica*. Infestation with this organism is rare and, since it is primarily a parasite of herbivores, it is generally confined to sheep rearing areas. It has an intermediate cycle involving aquatic vegetation, and infestation is linked to consumption of watercress. Metacercariae, ingested along with the plant, burrow through the intestinal wall, entering the bile ducts, where the adult worm is formed. Signs of infection include those of biliary obstruction. Treatment is with praziquantel.

Cestodes

An accidental parasite of children, cestodes are segmented worms. In general, infection with the adult worm is confined to the gastrointestinal tract and is asymptomatic. Infection with larvae tends to produce severe and life-threatening disease.

Taenia saginata

T.saginata is the beef tapeworm. Embryonated eggs are ingested by cattle and larvae penetrate into the flesh of the cow, developing into an infective cysticercus. It is the consumption of raw or improperly cooked meat that transfers infection to man.

The cysticercus develops into an adult worm in the intestine, and can reach a length of 25m. The head or scolex (**113**) attaches to the intestinal mucosa and derives nutrients from it. The worm grows by production of new segments (**114**); these segments mature and become sexually active (they are hermaphrodites). The terminal part of the worm contains gravid segments full of eggs. Diagnosis is made by demonstration of eggs or segments of worm in the faeces. Treatment is with niclosamide or praziquantel.

The fish tapeworm (*Diphyllobothrium latum*) and the pig tapeworm (*Taenia solium*) have similar life cycles, but differ in the morphology of their gravid segments (proglottids). In addition, *T.solium* can cause cysticercosis. The treatment is similar to that for *T.saginata*.

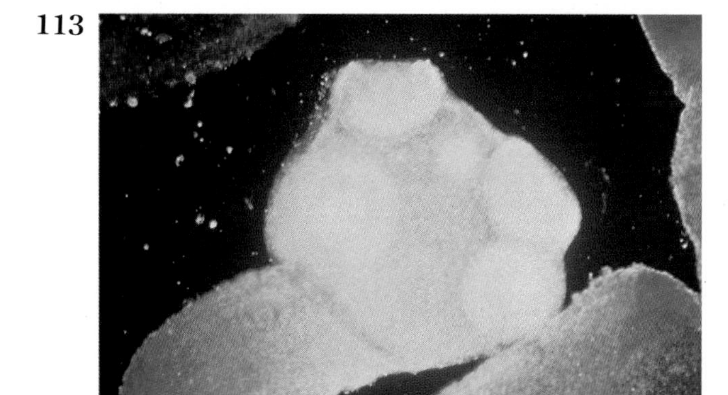

113 The scolex of *T. saginata*, the beef tapeworm. (Copyright LSTM.)

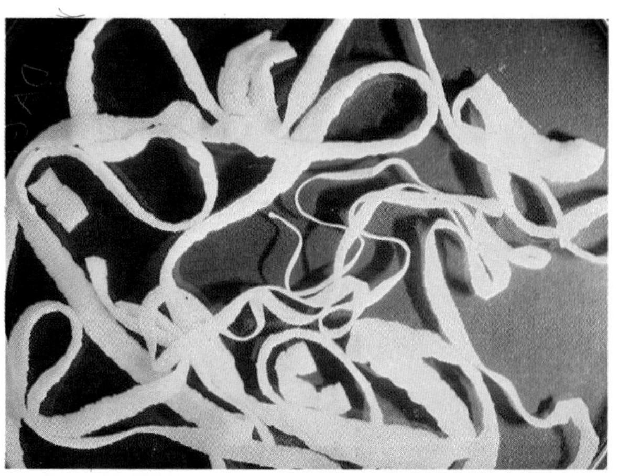

114 An adult tapeworm. (Copyright LSTM.)

Cysticercosis

Infection follows ingestion of *T.solium* eggs that have contaminated food (rather than of pork containing cysticerci). The egg disintegrates in the intestine and the larvae penetrate the intestinal wall to enter blood vessels. Cysticerci lodge in many sites in the body, particularly in skeletal muscle, and form small, fluid-filled bladders containing the parasite. Light infection is usually asymptomatic and the cysts may calcify in muscle (**115**). However, they may gain access to the brain, causing severe disease. Death of cysticerci may exacerbate the disease due to the intense inflammatory reaction it provokes. Diagnosis depends upon recognition of a clinical problem, radiological demonstration of calcified cysts and identification of the organism in surgically removed cysts. Treatment involves surgery and praziquantel with or without dexamethasone (to suppress the inflammatory response).

115

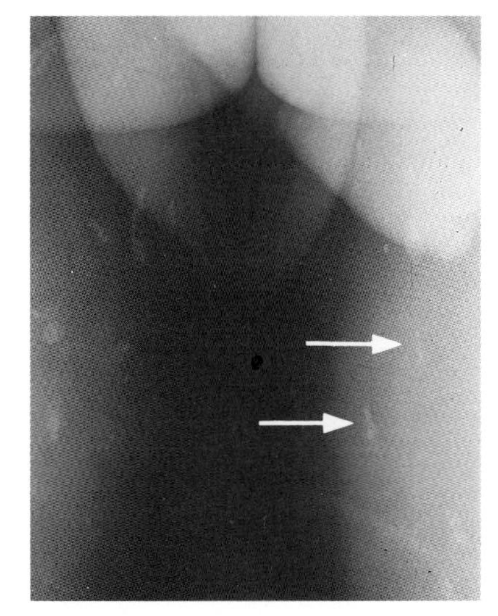

115 X-ray of the upper thigh, showing multiple calcified cysticerci.

Echinococcus granulosus

The canine tapeworm is an accidental pathogen for man and is the cause of hydatid disease. The disease occurs primarily in herbivores, especially in sheep, when dog faeces that contain eggs contaminate fodder. The sequence of events is similar to that encountered in cysticercosis but *E.granulosus* has a predilection for liver and occasionally, for bone. The cysts grow slowly but they are able to produce brood capsules and daughter cysts, thus, following ingestion of even a single egg, vast amplification can occur. Gradually, the daughter cysts and brood capsules break down, liberating a granular material called 'hydatid sand' (**116**). Clinical features of infection vary according to the site involved. Frequently infection is picked up on X-rays performed for unassociated reasons. Cysts are revealed as sharp calcified outlines, often with a fluid level (**117**). Serological tests are available and useful, but the Casoni skin test is less helpful. Examination of cyst contents demonstrates hydatid sand. Treatment is surgical, but recurrence is a possibility. Mebendazole provides a useful alternative treatment.

116

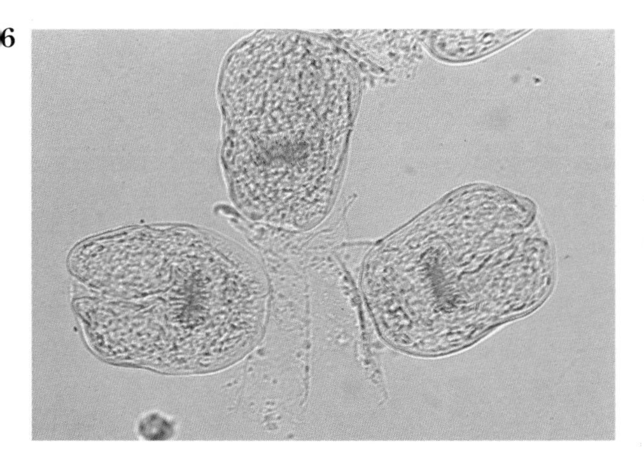

117

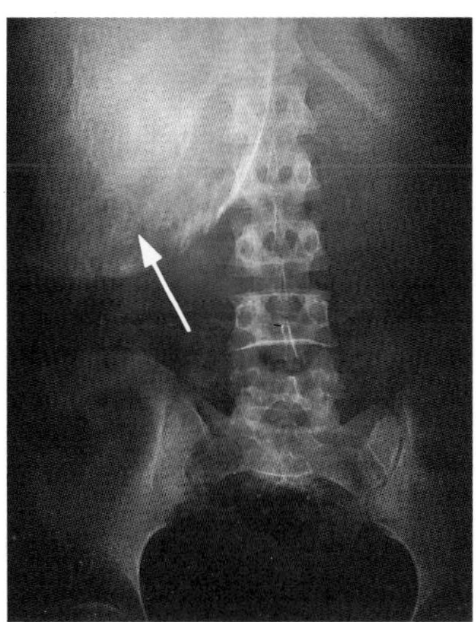

116 Hydatid sand showing three daughter cysts (× *100*).

117 Abdominal X-ray, demonstrating a large hydatid cyst in the liver.

Hepatitis

118

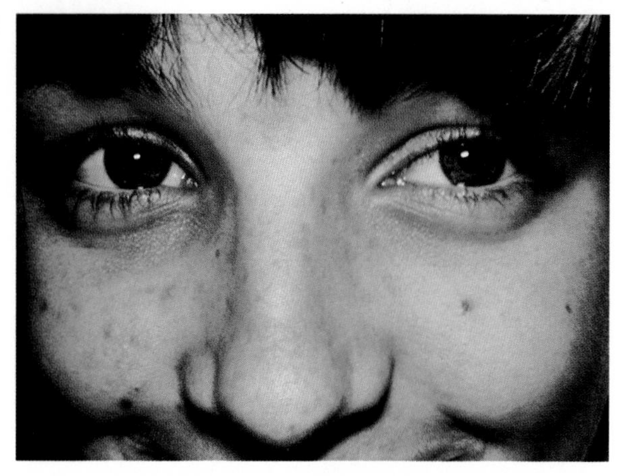

118 A jaundiced girl with yellow sclera.

The clinical presentation of hepatitis is a result of the destruction of hepatocytes. Infection in children is subclinical in up to 50% of cases, with jaundice being one of the major clinical features. The skin and the sclera in particular, assume a yellow tinge (**118**), and urine appears amber or brownish (**119**). Biochemical tests show a rise in both conjugated and unconjugated bilirubin in serum, together with a rise in serum levels of hepatocyte enzymes, such as alanine aminotransferase. In addition, anorexia, weakness, fever, headache, abdominal discomfort and nausea are reported by many patients.

Hepatitis can be caused by a large number of pathogens (**Table 9**). However, only the hepatitis viruses are dealt with here.

119

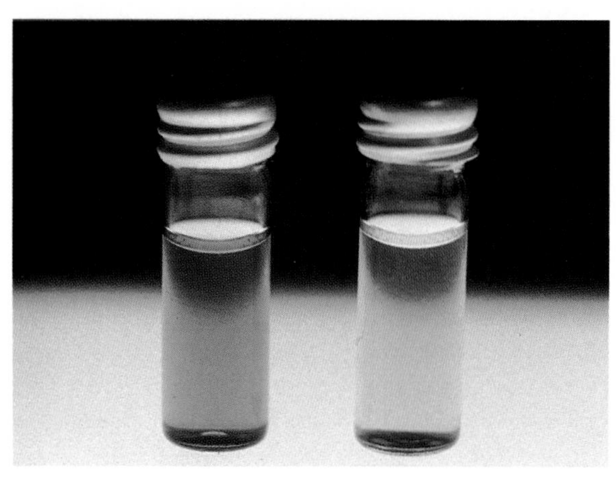

119 A comparison of normal urine with that (brown) from a child with jaundice.

Table 9. Pathogens in Hepatitis.

Hepatitis Viruses	*Other Pathogens*
Hepatitis A	Epstein–Barr Virus
Hepatitis B	Cytomegalovirus
Hepatitis C	Herpes simplex virus
Hepatitis D	Varicella–zoster virus
Hepatitis E	Adenovirus
Other	Coxsackie viruses
	Mumps virus
	Yellow fever virus
	Rubella virus
	Leptospira spp.
	Listeria monocytogenes
	Ascending cholangitis
	Treponema pallidum
	Toxoplasma gondii

Hepatitis A virus (HAV)

HAV causes infective hepatitis. The virus is spread faeco-orally and has an incubation period of about 30 days (range: 15–50 days). It is a small (27nm) RNA virus in the picornavirus family, and has been renamed Enterovirus 72 (**120**).

In developed countries, disease occurs in epidemics; in developing countries, it is endemic. Common source epidemics following, for example, consumption of improperly cooked shellfish (mussels, oysters) or of raspberries contaminated with human faeces have been described. The attack rate within households can be high. Infection is usually mild to subclinical, and fulminant hepatitis is rare (< 0.5% of cases). Just before jaundice occurs, virus is excreted in faeces and, to a lesser extent, in urine. Viral excretion is usually short-lived (up to 2 weeks).

Diagnosis is made by detection of IgM anti-HAV in serum. HAV does not cause chronic hepatitis, nor has a carrier state been detected. There is no specific therapy, and prophylaxis relies on passive immunization. However, a polypeptide vaccine should soon be available.

120

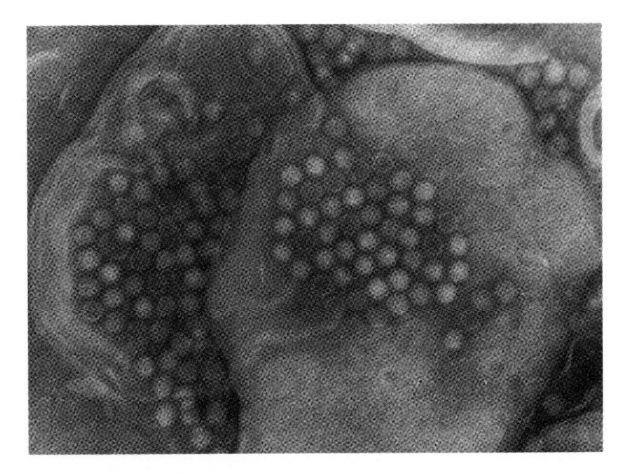

120 Negative-stain electron micrograph of faeces containing HAV (× *55,000*).

Hepatitis B virus (HBV)

HBV is the causative agent of serum hepatitis. An enveloped DNA virus, it has a diameter of 42 nm. Transmission occurs by blood-to-blood contact, with an average incubation period of 90 days (range: 60–180 days). The virus is solely a human pathogen, which is maintained by persistent carriers. In such carriers, virus produces a persistent infection in the hepatocytes. Whole enveloped virus (Dane particles) and lipid vesicles carrying hepatitis B surface antigen (HBSAg) are released into the blood stream (**30** & **121**). The Dane particle is infective but the HBSAg particles, which can be spherical (20–25 nm) or filamentous (up to 700 nm long), are not. Dane particles carry HBSAg, HBCAg (core antigen) and HBeAg (infectivity related antigen). Detection of HBSAg in asymptomatic patients indicates that they are likely to be carriers. If HBeAg is also detected, the patients are high-risk carriers, that is, infection can be transmitted by a small volume of blood. However, if they have HBe-antibody, they fall into an intermediate-risk group. If they have HBSAg alone, they are a low-risk carrier and it is probable that infection will be transmitted only if a large volume of blood is transferred, as in a transfusion. HBV infection is symptomatic more often than HAV infection. Approximately 1% of those infected with HBV will develop fulminant life-threatening infection, with around 10% becoming chronic carriers. Persistent infection is much more likely to occur if infection occurs in the first year of life or in the immunocompromised. Long-term sequelae in chronic carriers include the development of chronic hepatitis, cirrhosis and hepatocellular carcinoma. Although no antiviral agent is available, the HBSAg vaccine has proved highly effective in preventing infection.

121

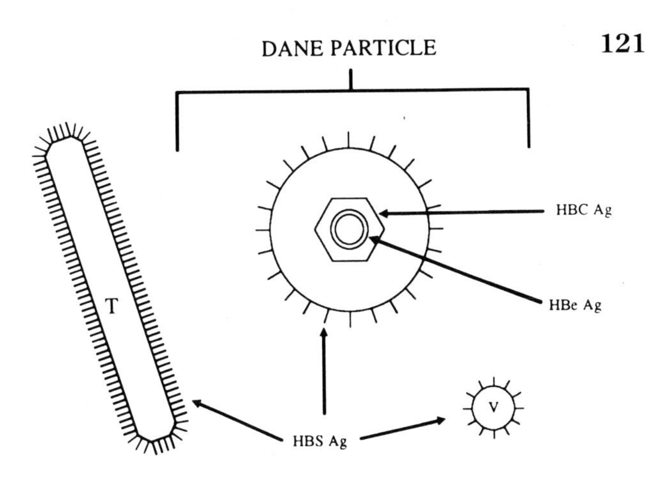

121 Diagramatic representation of HBV (B) and the vesicular (V) and tubular (T) forms of surface antigen particles.

Hepatitis C virus (HCV)

After the original identification of HAV and HBV, it became apparent that cases of viral hepatitis were occurring that were due to neither virus nor to any of the other pathogens listed in **Table 9**. However, these infections, which were termed non A non B (NANB) hepatitis, consisted of cases of hepatitis with different epidemiological characteristics (some were spread faeco-orally and some parenterally, with varying incubation periods). One form of NANB was transmitted parenterally to a chimpanzee, and plasma from the animal was used to produce a high-infectivity pool and a cloned cDNA library. The cDNA was used to express putative viral antigens which were screened using sera from patients with NANB hepatitis. Eventually, one cDNA sequence was found which produced an antigen that was reactive with the sera. This cDNA was shown to have been derived from a single-stranded RNA sequence, present only in NANB sera, and to be related to togavirus RNA sequences.

The virus has never been grown and diagnosis is made by detection of antibody against this genetically engineered protein, or of RNA sequences complementary to the cDNA. Approximately 80% of those with NANB hepatitis have developed antibody to HCV. The prevalence of antibody in the blood donor population ranges from 1% to 5%, increasing with age. There is evidence to suggest that vertical transmission might occur.

Hepatitis D virus (HDV)

Originally known as the Delta agent, HDV is an incomplete virus that can only replicate fully in the presence of HBV. It is a small enveloped RNA virus (35–37nm) and coinfection with HBV or subsequent infection of an HBV carrier can produce fulminant hepatitis. Transmission of infection is as for HBV.

Hepatitis E virus (HEV)

HEV is an unenveloped RNA virus (32–34nm) that is similar to calicivirus. It is another cause of NANB hepatitis and is spread faeco-orally. Epidemics of infection occur and the virus apparently has a high mortality in pregnant women.

3 Infections of the oropharynx and upper respiratory tract

Infections of the upper respiratory tract and oropharynx are responsible for more visits to the doctor than any other single condition. Although they cause a great deal of morbidity and misery, upper respiratory tract infections are seldom fatal; indeed, they are often mistreated or overtreated.

Infections of the oropharynx

Aphthous ulcers (canker sores)

Aphthous ulcers are shallow painful lesions, usually not more than 1 cm in diameter, which usually occur on the ventral surface of the tongue, gingival margin and mucobuccal fold. They have a white base of fibrinous exudate (**122**).

The ulcers may be single or occur in crops. The aetiology is unknown, but a topical application of tetracycline speeds the healing process.

122

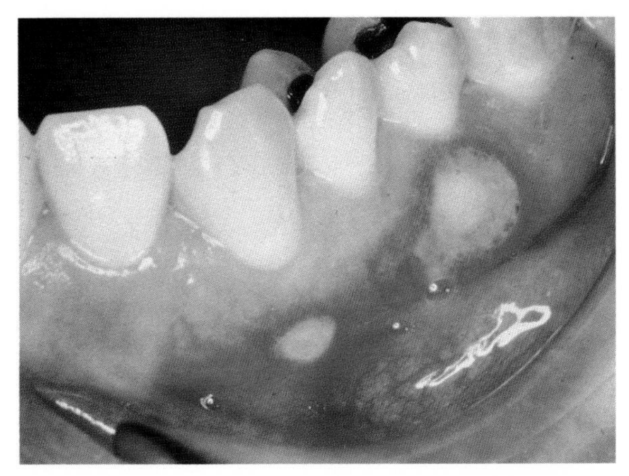

122 Aphthous ulcers on the gingiva. They may occur singly or in clusters.

Gingivitis

Gingivitis is an infection of the gums and the soft tissue of the alveolar margin. It results from poor dental hygiene and is frequently associated with dental caries. The gums become reddened and bleed easily when the teeth are brushed (**123** & **124**). Gingivitis may be a presenting symptom of acute leukaemia, diabetes mellitus, and nutritional and vitamin deficiencies, as well as being due to certain drugs, such as phenytoin (**125**).

Good oral hygiene and regular tooth and gum brushing are the best methods of treatment and prevention.

123

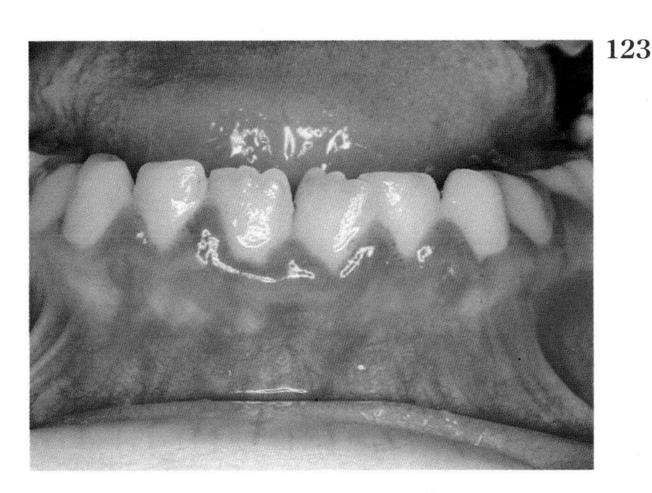

123 Gingivitis. Inflammation and puffiness of the gingiva are clearly visible.

124

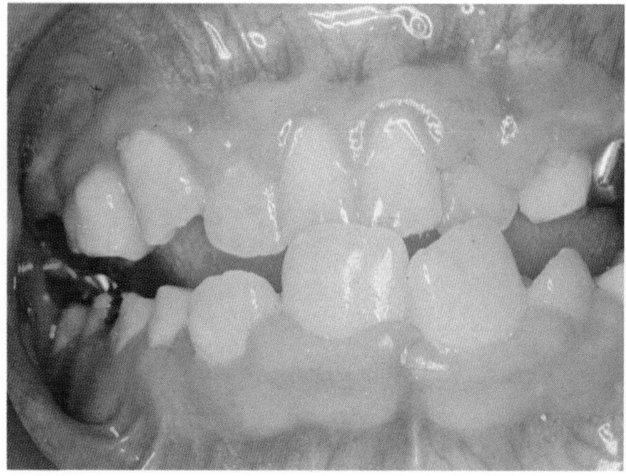

124 Gingivitis. Puffiness of the gum margins from chronic inflammation due to poor oral hygiene can be seen.

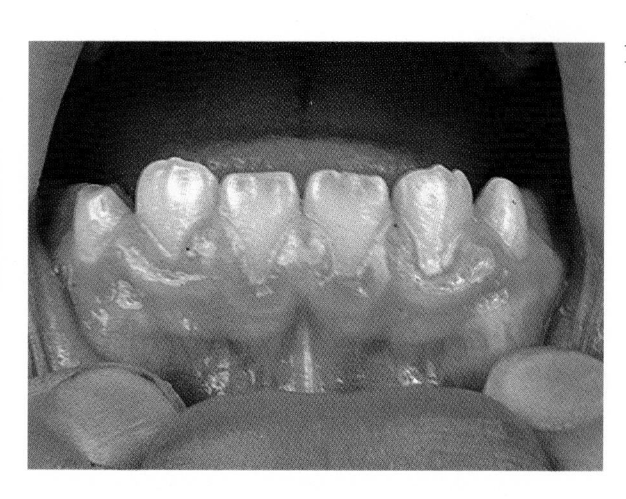

125 Gum hypertrophy and inflammation due to phenytoin.

Vincent's infection (acute ulcerative gingivitis, Trench mouth, cancrum oris)

Vincent's infection is an acute infection which usually affects the gingiva but may spread to other areas of the oropharynx. It is caused by the synergistic interaction of two organisms, *Fusiformis fusiformis* and *Borrelia vincentii*. Infection in the debilitated and malnourished child may progress to tissue ulceration and destruction, a condition known as cancrum oris (**126** & **127**).

Cancrum oris often follows measles infection in a severely malnourished child. Urgent treatment with penicillin is necessary, together with management of the underlying cause of debility in the child.

126

126 Vincent's infection has caused cancrum oris in this malnourished refugee child.

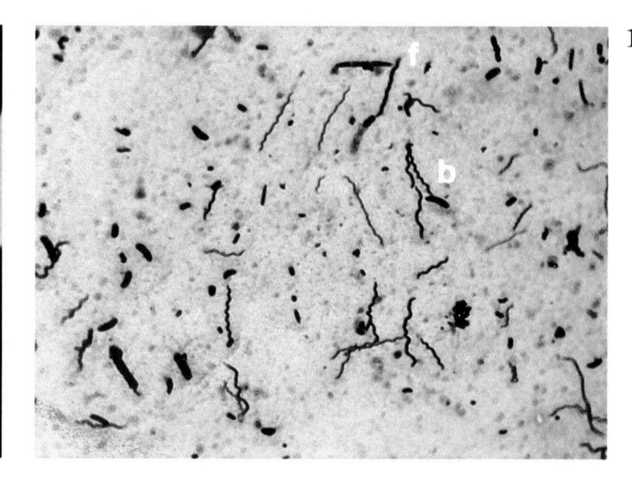

127 *F. fusiformis* (f) and *B. vincentii* (b) shown by silver impregnation stain. They cause cancrum oris (× *1,000*).

Herpetic gingivostomatitis

Herpetic gingivostomatitis is caused by a primary infection with herpes simplex virus type I. It presents with acute inflamed bullous lesions of the mouth and gums, which progress to painful ulcers (**128 & 129**). Pain may prevent a child from taking food or fluids, necessitating hospital admission for rehydration. The infection is self-limiting over 7–10 days, but the time may be shortened by the topical or oral use of acyclovir.

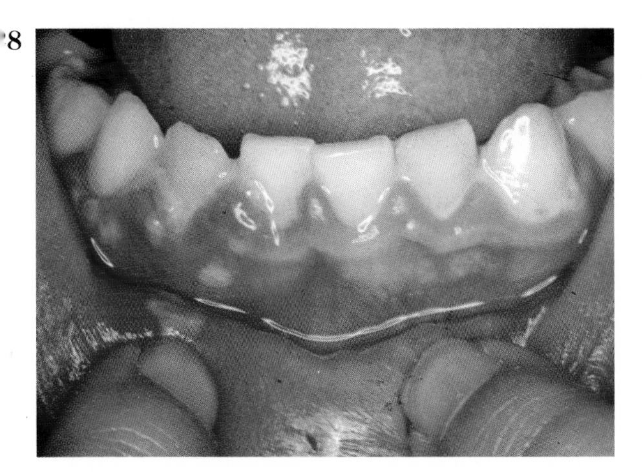

128 Herpetic ulcers on the gingiva and lower lip.

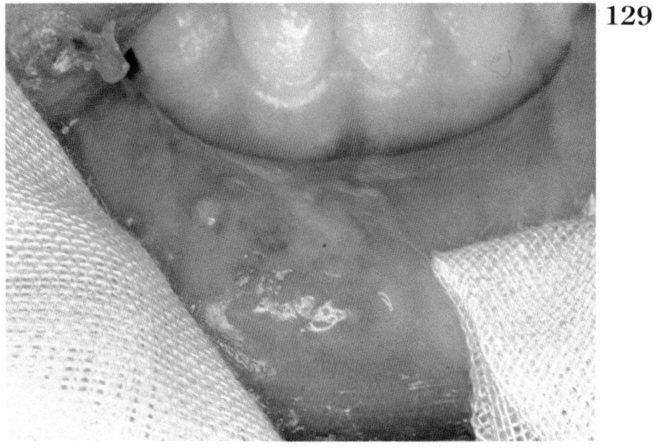

129 Herpetic ulcers, with crusting of lesions on the lower lip.

Papilloma virus

Occasionally, the papilloma virus (a DNA virus) may be spread to the mouth by a child sucking a finger or thumb on which a wart is present (**130 & 131**). These lesions usually resolve spontaneously without treatment.

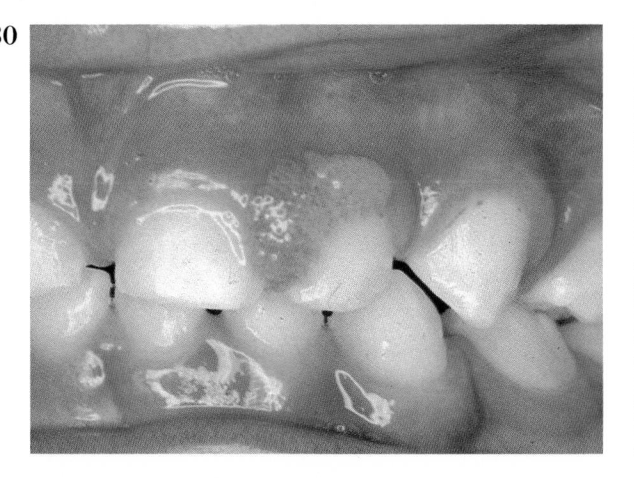

130 Papilloma virus has been transmitted to the upper gingival margin by thumb-sucking.

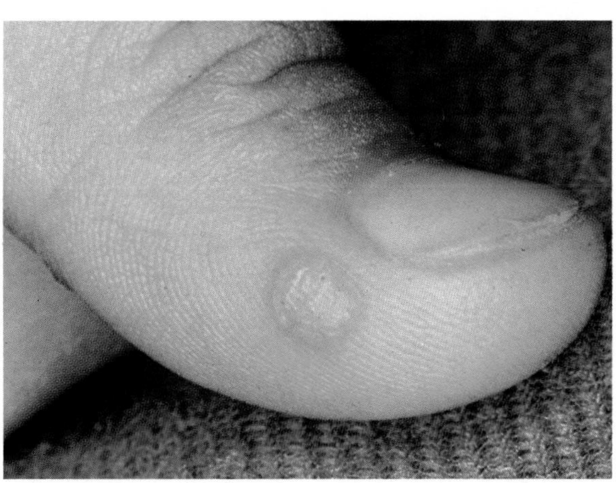

131 A wart on the thumb, caused by papilloma virus.

Ludwig's angina

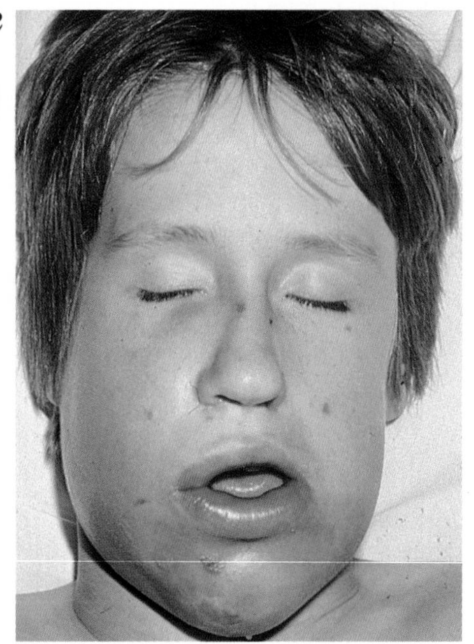

Ludwig's angina is a severe acute cellulitis of the sublingual region. It is usually caused by anaerobic organisms, such as *Bacteroides fragilis* or *Clostridium* spp. If not treated promptly, the infection may spread to the submandibular region and posteriorly, thereby causing respiratory obstruction (**132**).

Most cases will respond to a combination of penicillin and chloramphenicol. In severe infection systemic cefotaxime and metronidazole may be indicated.

132 Ludwig's angina secondary to a dental abscess.

Dental caries

Dental caries is a severe and chronic problem in some children. It is caused by a group of streptococci designated *Streptococcus mutans*. These organisms ferment dietary carbohydrates, causing the release of organic acids that erode tooth enamel. Feeding bottles that contain sweet drinks encourage caries, especially when they are left in a child's mouth during sleep (**133**).

Once the enamel has been eroded, cavities form; other bacteria, especially lactobacillis, then invade the pulp of the teeth, causing pulp infection (**134** & **135**). If untreated, the bacteria may destroy the tooth and invade the soft tissue, causing cellulitis and dental abscesses (**136**). Chronic infection in primary teeth may also interfere with secondary dentition.

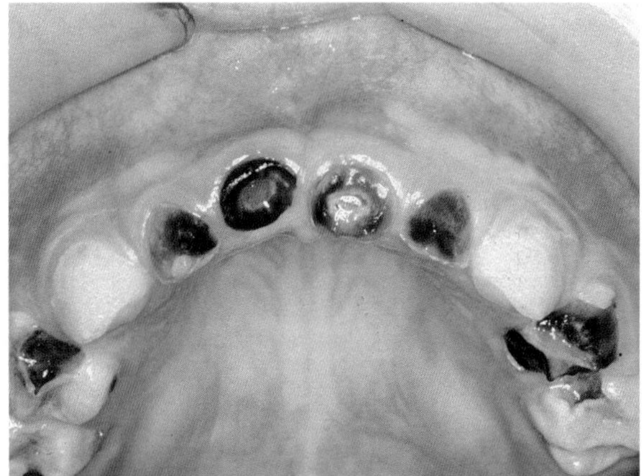

133 Advanced dental caries in the upper incisors, where the teat of the baby's bottle has been left during sleep.

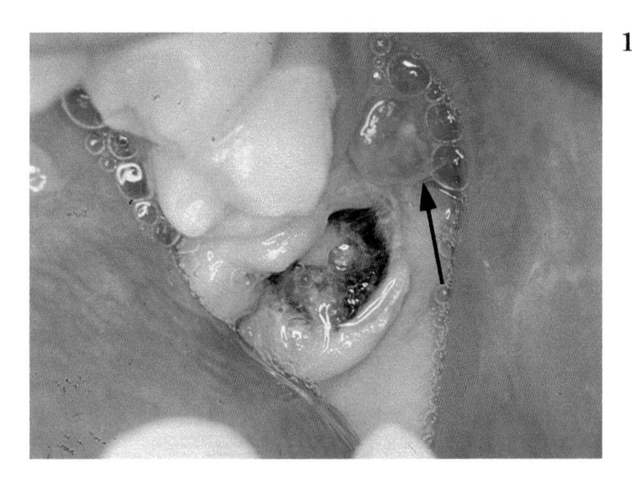

134 Caries of the lower first molar, with abscess and sinus formation.

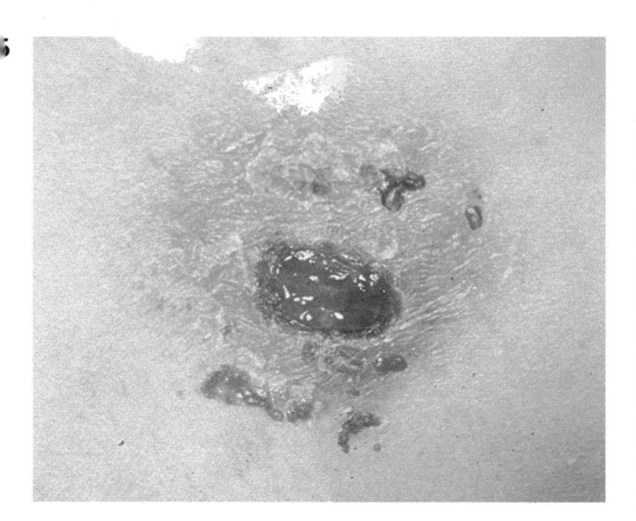

135 A sinus from a dental abscess discharging onto the cheek of the child seen in **134**.

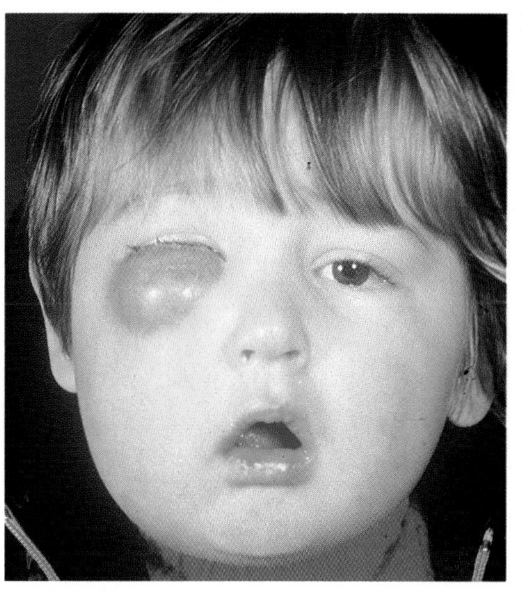

136 Cellulitis secondary to dental abscess of deciduous teeth.

fluoride, which is now routinely added to most water supplies at 1 p.p.m., and is given to children as a topical application in toothpastes. Good oral hygiene, a balanced regular diet and regular attendance at the dentist to detect early disease are also important preventative measures.

It should be noted that tetracycline may cause bands of yellow-brown discoloration across the tooth enamel if given to young children before secondary dentition has occurred. Such discoloration may be seen particularly in older children who were given the antibiotic for chronic respiratory disease, before it was realized that tetracycline caused staining by binding as a chelate with enamel and developing bone (**137**).

137

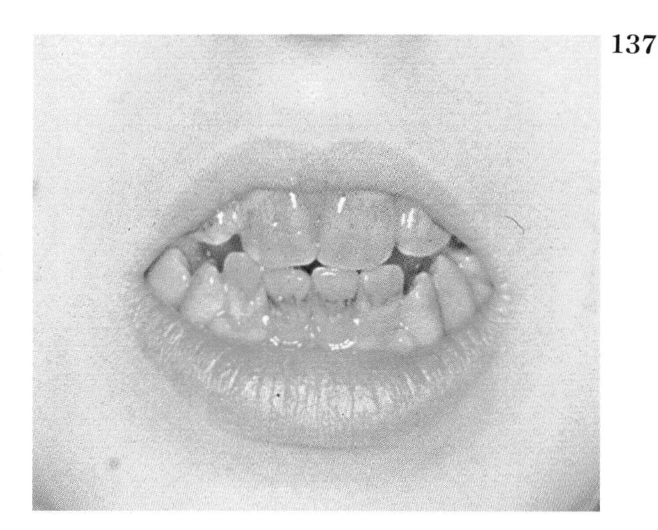

137 Tetracycline-staining of upper and lower incisors.

Oral candidiasis (thrush, moniliasis)

138

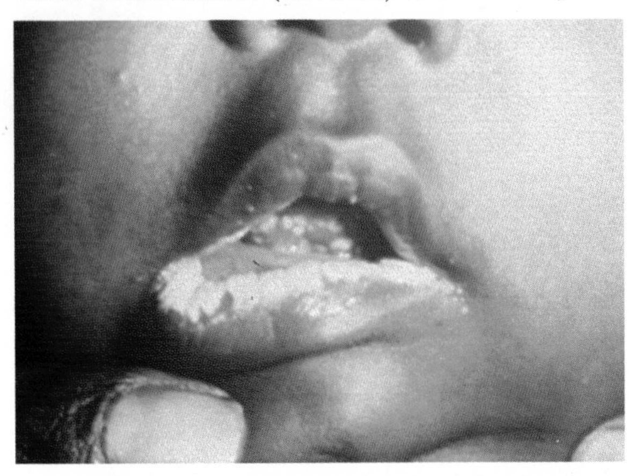

138 *C. albicans* infection of the buccal cavity.

Candida albicans infection is common in neonates, especially if they have had a course of broad-spectrum antibiotics. It may also occur in the immune-compromised child. Transmission initially occurs via the maternal birth canal, but the fungus may be transmitted from infant to infant through unwashed feeding teats and dummies.

The characteristic lesions are irregular white plaques that adhere to the buccal mucosa, tongue and other areas of the buccal cavity (**138**). The plaques can be removed from the mucosa, leaving an inflamed and often bleeding surface. In neonates, feeding becomes painful and the infant may stop altogether. Nystatin applied topically on a cotton swab four times daily will cure most babies in 2–3 days. Severe infection may be treated with oral fluconazole.

Acute viral rhinitis (the common cold)

Children are particularly susceptible to the common cold because their immunity, which derives from secretory IgA, is relatively immature and they have not encountered the viruses before. They are also exposed to a great many viruses through contact with the family and their peers at school. Upper respiratory tract infections occur most frequently between 6 months and 6 years of age. Up to the age of 6 months, babies have some passive immunity derived from their mothers. During the pre-school period, children have an average of around 8 or 9 viral upper respiratory infections per year, but this may rise to an average of 12 per year on admission to nursery school.

Many different viruses may cause the same symptoms of mucoid nasal discharge, low-grade fever and coryza (**Table 10**). Rhinoviruses are probably the most frequent cause of the common cold. There are over 100 different serotypes, and infection with one type does not appear to confer protection against another (**139**). Coronaviruses also play an important role (**140**). The most obvious clinical sign is a persistent mucoid nasal discharge which, over a few days, may become mucopurulent (**141**). The fever is usually of a low grade, but occasionally a febrile convulsion in the predisposed child may be precipitated. This usually occurs when the infection spreads to involve the middle ear, mastoids, sinuses or lower respiratory tract.

139

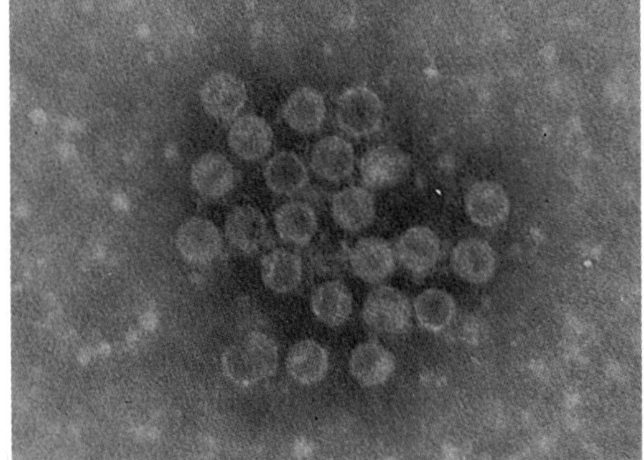

139 A negative-stain electron micrograph of rhinoviruses (× *50,000*).

Table 10. Agents Responsible for Upper Respiratory Tract Infection.

Viruses	*Bacteria*
Rhinoviruses (> 100 serotypes)	Group B Streptococcus
Coronaviruses	*Haemophilus influenzae*
Influenza viruses (A,B,C)	*Streptococcus pneumoniae*
Parainfluenza 1–4	*Corynebacterium diphtheriae*
Adenoviruses	*Mycoplasma pneumoniae*
Enterovirus (Coxsackie A and B, ECHO)	*Staphylococcus aureus*
Epstein–Barr virus	*Branhamella cartarrhalis*
Respiratory syncytial virus	*Chlamydia pneumoniae*

Usually the diagnosis is in little doubt, and investigations to define the particular virus responsible do not contribute to treatment. Immunofluorescence for respiratory syncytial virus and parainfluenza viruses may sometimes be helpful (**142**).

Treatment is essentially symptomatic. Antibiotics, antihistamines and decongestants are of little use and have many undesirable side effects.

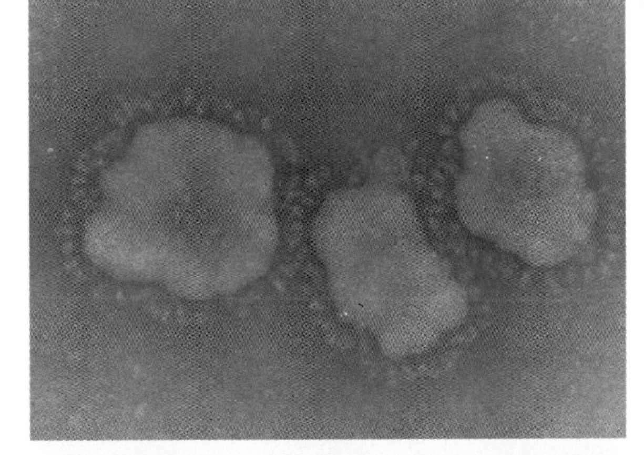

140 A negative-stain electron micrograph of coronaviruses (× *56,000*).

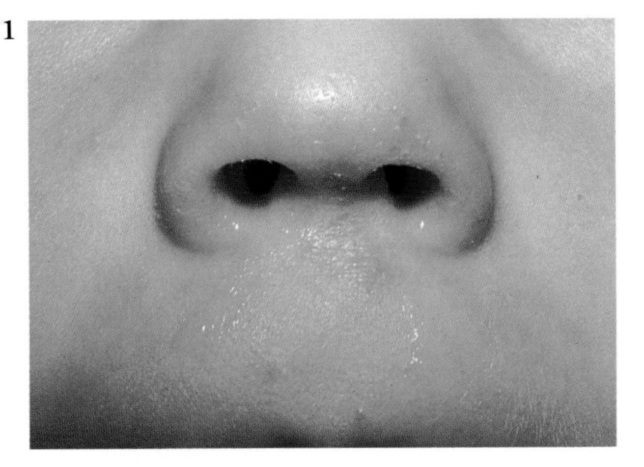

141 A mucoid nasal discharge, the main characteristic of the common cold.

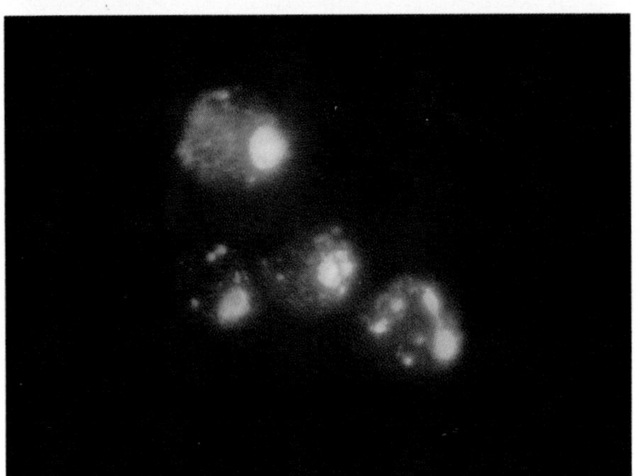

142 Immunofluorescence is used as a technique to diagnose respiratory syncytial virus (× *400*).

Acute purulent rhinitis

Occasionally, the mucoid nasal discharge of what was initially diagnosed as a viral upper respiratory tract infection may develop into a purulent discharge. If this persists, it indicates a bacterial superinfection. The most likely causative organisms are *Haemophilus influenzae, Streptococcus pneumoniae* and *Staphylococcus aureus*. Nasal diphtheria may present with a serosanguineous discharge (**143**).

If a unilateral discharge is present, a foreign body (**144**) in the infected nostril should be suspected. Provided that the discharge allows positive identification of the organism, a 7-day course of oral amoxycillin should successfully treat most cases.

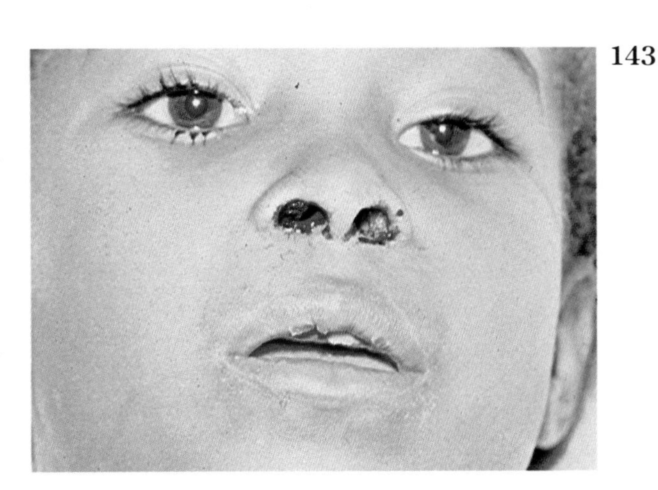

143 Nasal diphtheria demonstrating serosanguinous discharge.

144

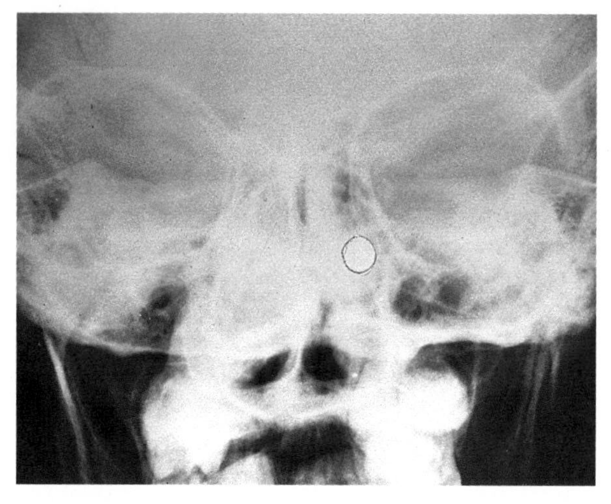

144 Skull X-ray demonstrating an air-gun pellet lodged far up the left nostril. This caused a unilateral nasal discharge.

Otitis media

Otitis media is one of the most common complications of upper respiratory tract infections. Because the Eustachian tube is shorter, more horizontal and more patent than in the adult, infants are more prone to the condition than older children. With the development of sinuses and the maturation of the skull, a functional valve is created, allowing better drainage from the middle ear and limiting ascending infection. The symptoms of acute purulent otitis media are severe earache, fever and irritability. When visualized, the tympanic membrane will have lost the light reflex and will appear dull or red in colour (**145**). If the drum perforates at this stage, the child will often experience relief from pain, and pus will be noted in the external auditory canal.

Although viruses may cause otitis media as part of an upper respiratory tract infection, bacteria are usually responsible for the acute purulent type. The most commonly detected organisms are *Streptococcus pneumoniae, Haemophilus influenzae* and *Staphylococcus aureus*. Other organisms may include *Branhamella catarrhalis* and *Mycoplasma pneumoniae*. Nasopharyngeal and throat swabs are not usually helpful since the organisms are part of the normal nasopharyngeal flora. A blood culture, however, may reveal the organism responsible, as intermittent bacteraemia (especially pneumococcal bacteraemia in infection with *S.pneumoniae*) may occur. Prompt treatment with a 7-day course of an appropriate oral antibiotic should successfully treat most cases.

145

145 Acute otitis media is characterized by an inflamed tympanic membrane, with loss of the light reflex.

Table 11. Complications of Otitis Media.

Complications
Hearing loss
Perforation
Chronic suppurative otitis media
Mastoiditis
Cholesteatoma
Labyrynthitis
Intracranial abscess

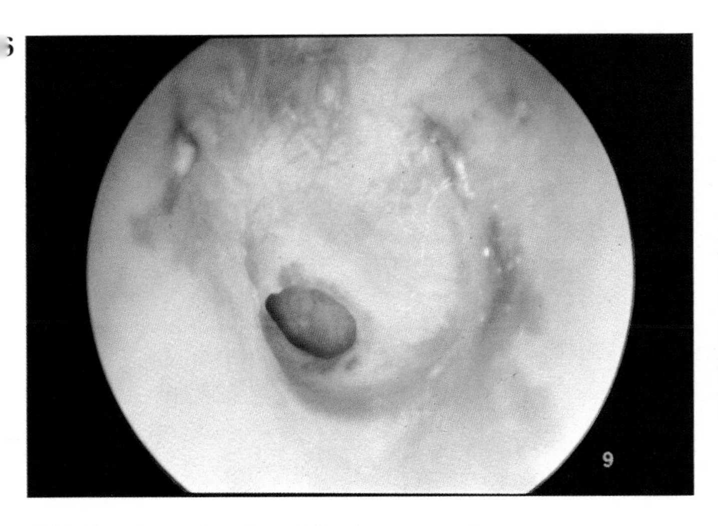

146 A perforated eardrum following rupture due to pressure necrosis from pus in the middle ear.

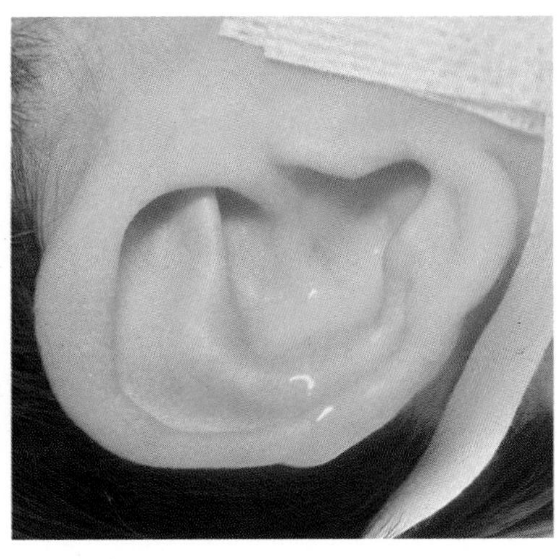

147 Pus discharging from the pinna following perforation.

Complications of otitis media are listed in **Table 11**. The most common complication is probably an acute perforation of the drum (**146**). Once the pus has discharged through the perforation, rapid resolution of pain usually occurs. The pus may be seen dripping from the pinna (**147**).

One consequence of repeated middle ear infection may be the development of chronic secretory otitis media or 'glue ear', so called because of the viscous fluid that fills the middle ear. A meniscus may be observed behind the drum. Chronic secretory otitis media results in conductive hearing loss, and is managed by inserting grommets to allow the fluid to drain and the middle ear to dry out (**148**).

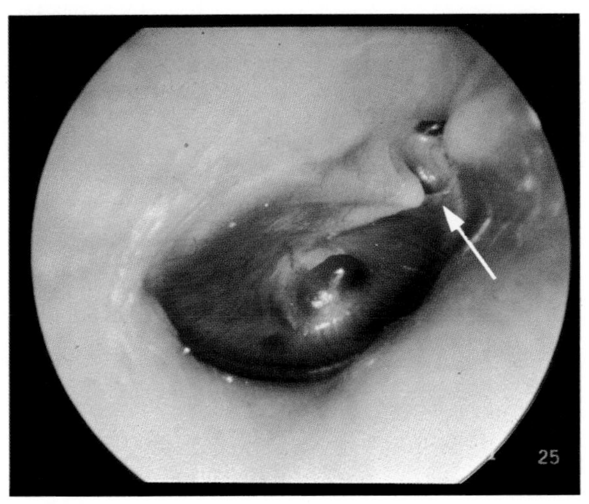

148 Chronic secretory otitis media. A meniscus of fluid can be seen in the middle ear.

Mastoiditis

Mastoiditis is usually a complication of otitis media, and represents an osteitis. It occurs after the age of 2 years, by which time the mastoid air cells have developed. The organisms most frequently responsible for infection are *Streptococcus pyogenes*, *S.pneumoniae* and *Staphylococcus aureus*. In long-standing disease, gram-negative organisms, such as *Pseudomonas aeruginosa*, and anaerobic bacteria may cause chronic mastoiditis. The clinical presentation is often one of a child complaining of severe post-auricular pain with fever. There is usually exquisite tenderness over the mastoid, and the pinna of the ear may be pushed forward (**149 & 150**). An X-ray of the mastoids will show increased opacity of the mastoid air cells (**151 & 152**).

Acute mastoiditis is a serious and painful condition which requires urgent treatment. Since the bone is inevitably involved, systemic broad-spectrum antibiotics are needed; they should be followed by at least 4 weeks of oral antibiotics. If complications such as meningitis, lateral sinus thrombosis or suppurative labyrinthitis threaten, surgery may be indicated.

149

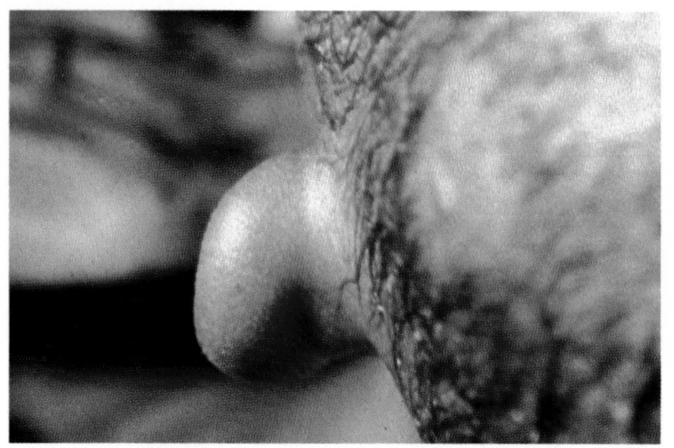

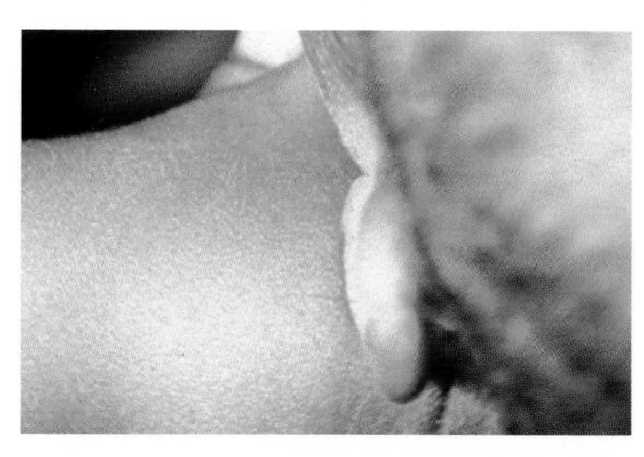

149 Acute mastoiditis with the left ear pushed forward.

150 The same child as shown in **149** after treatment.

151

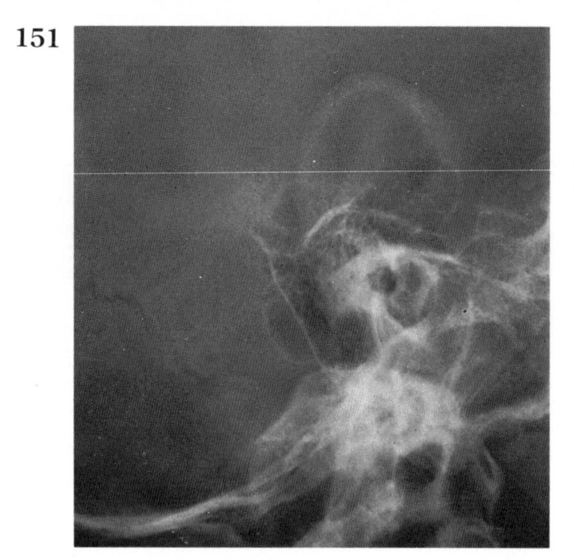

152

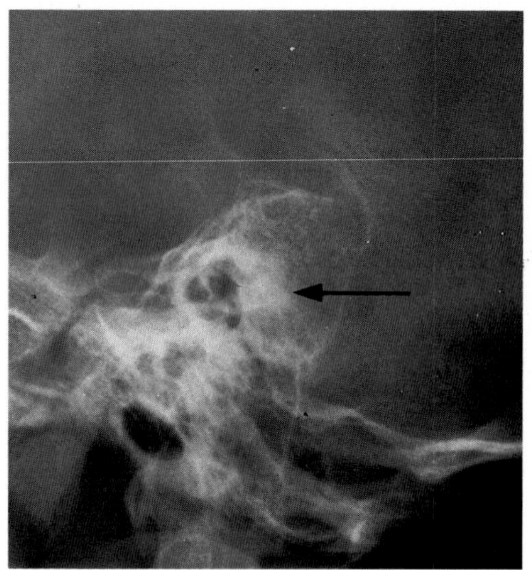

151 X-ray of normal right mastoids.

152 X-ray of the child shown in **151**, demonstrating radio-opaque left mastoids due to inflammation.

Sinusitis

The sinuses are poorly developed at birth. The ethmoid sinus is present, but the maxillary sinus only becomes evident on X-ray at the age of 6 months. Between the ages of 4 and 9 years the frontal sinus becomes visible on X-ray (**153**). Infection of the ethmoid sinuses tends to occur in children of 1–5 years of age. It can present with periorbital cellulitis (**154**).

Frontal sinusitis is unusual before the age of 10 years. Upper respiratory tract infections are the most common antecedent events precipitating sinusitis. The resulting inflammation causes oedema of the mucosa, which obstructs the ostea causing stasis. Superinfection with bacteria then occurs. The organisms most likely to cause infection are *S.pneumoniae*, *H.influenzae* and *S.pyogenes*. *B.catarrhalis* and anaerobes may also rarely cause acute sinusitis.

If a purulent nasal discharge is present, a fresh specimen should be obtained and cultured. X-ray of the affected sinus may demonstrate opacity and even fluid levels (**155**).

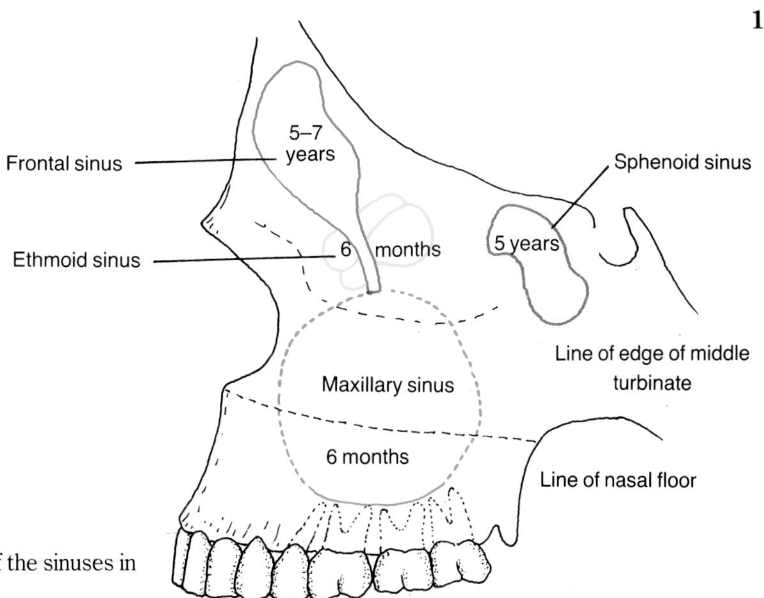

153 The approximate appearance of the sinuses in childhood.

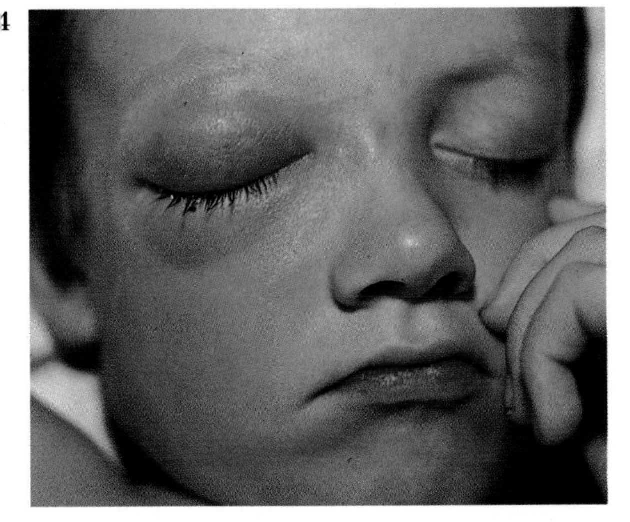

154 Ethmoid sinusitis, presenting with cellulitis over the saddle of the nose, with spread to the periorbital region.

155

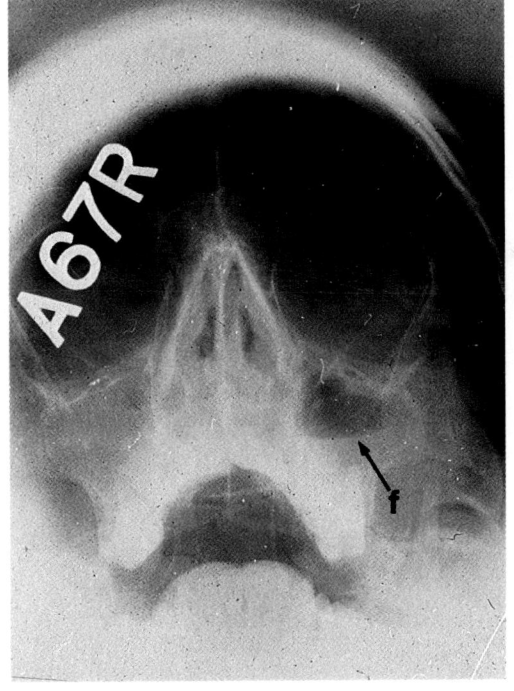

155 A plain X-ray demonstrating complete opacity of the left maxillary sinus, with a fluid level (f) in the right maxillary sinus.

The important principle in the management of sinusitis is to establish good drainage from the sinus. Nasal decongestants may help, as may prompt administration of an antibiotic such as amoxycillin or trimethoprim. Pain relief is important and analgesics should be given where indicated. Rarely, symptoms may persist, in which case surgical treatment may be necessary. This is uncommon in children under 12 years of age. Surgical treatment may include lavage of the sinuses and, occasionally, surgical drainage.

Viral pharyngitis and tonsillitis

156

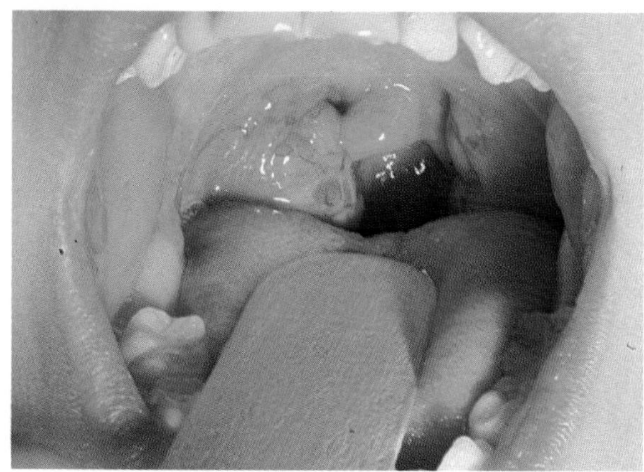

Viruses are responsible for the majority of attacks of pharyngitis and tonsillitis (**156**). They often form part of the syndrome of the common cold. The presence or absence of an exudate on the tonsils and pharynx does not necessarily distinguish a bacterial from a viral cause of pharyngitis.

156 A viral pharyngitis with mild inflammation of tonsils.

Acute streptococcal pharyngitis

157

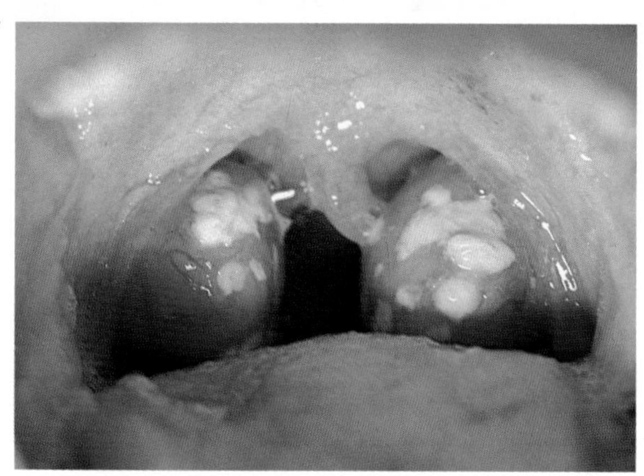

Streptococcus pyrogenes is responsible for approximately 10% of acute purulent sore throats (**157**). A white exudate may be detected in the crypts of the tonsils and on the pharynx. A throat swab should be taken and prompt treatment with penicillin should be started.

157 Acute *S. pyogenes* pharyngitis with pus in the tonsillar crypts and palatal petechiae.

Infectious mononucleosis (glandular fever)

Infectious mononucleosis is caused by the Epstein–Barr virus (EBV), which is a herpes virus (HHV5). Although glandular fever may occur in children under 3 years of age, it is more common in older children and in adolescents. The most common presenting symptom is that of a sore throat with cervical lymphadenopathy (**158**). Fever is also present and the child may have severe dysphagia. Examination of the pharynx may reveal a white exudate (**159**), and small submucosal haemorrhages are sometimes visible on the hard and soft palate (**160**).

Investigations should include a peripheral blood count. At least 20% of the lymphocytes may prove to be atypical (**161**). A heterophil antibody test may be used as a screening investigation. A raised titre of specific IgM anti-viral capsid antigen will indicate acute infection.

Management is mainly symptomatic. If dysphagia is severe, a short course of steroids for 3–5 days may give symptomatic relief. Antibiotics, particularly ampicillin, should not be given since they can precipitate a generalized hypersensitivity rash. It should be noted that cytomegalovirus and *Toxoplasma gondi* infection can cause a syndrome almost indistinguishable clinically from EBV infection. Such infections will be heterophil antibody-negative. Adenovirus 8 can cause a severe pharyngitis, occasionally seen in association with conjunctivitis.

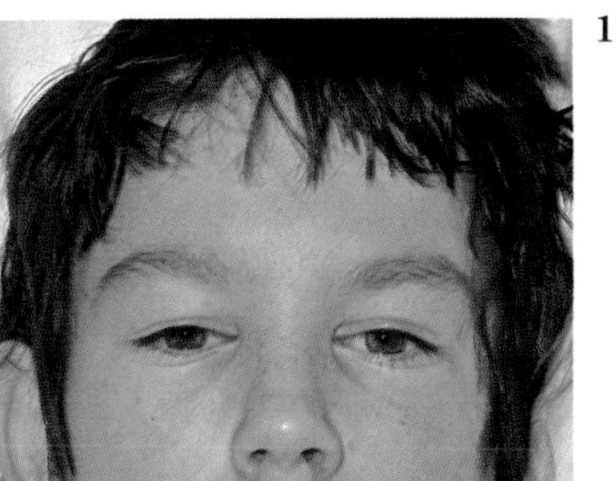

158 Glandular fever demonstrating right-sided cervical lymph node enlargement, with oedema of the surrounding tissue.

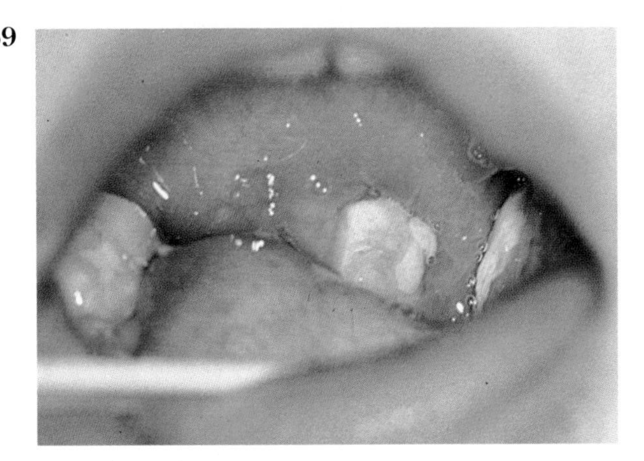

159 Glandular fever showing a white exudate in the pharynx.

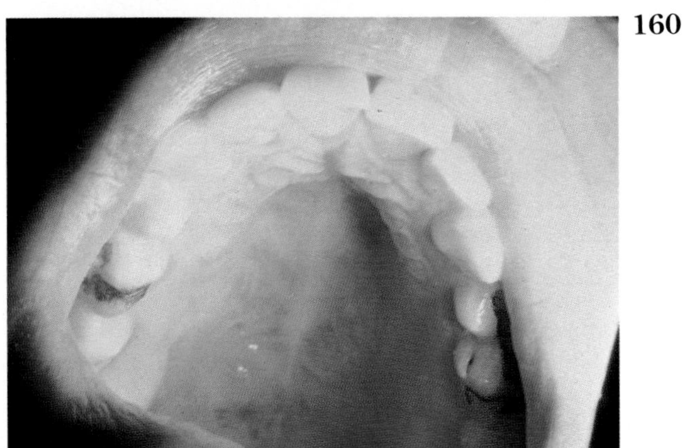

160 Glandular fever with submucosal haemorrhages on the palate.

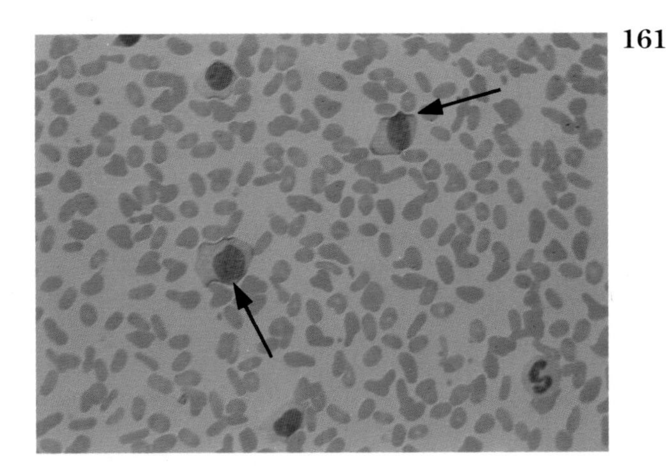

161 A blood film in glandular fever, demonstrating many atypical lymphocytes with large nuclei (× *300*).

Herpangina

Herpangina is caused by several group A coxsackie viruses (types 2–6, 8 and 10). It presents acutely with a painful sore throat. Initially, clusters of ulcers may be found in the pharynx. The clusters then coalesce to form a large ulcer, which can involve the soft palate and uvula, as well as the pharynx itself (**162**).

162

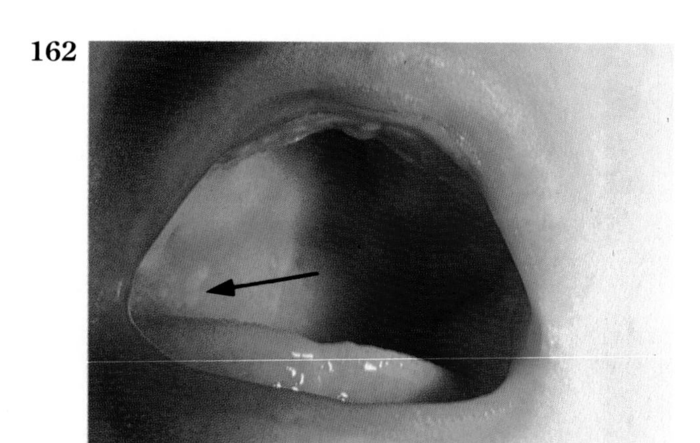

162 Herpangina demonstrating painful coalescent ulcers surrounded by inflammation.

Hand, foot and mouth disease

Hand, foot and mouth disease is a viral infection caused by coxsackie viruses A5, A10 and A16. Small, discrete ulcers may appear on the tongue, oral mucosa and pharynx (**163**) as well as vesicles on the palms of the hands and soles of the feet.

163

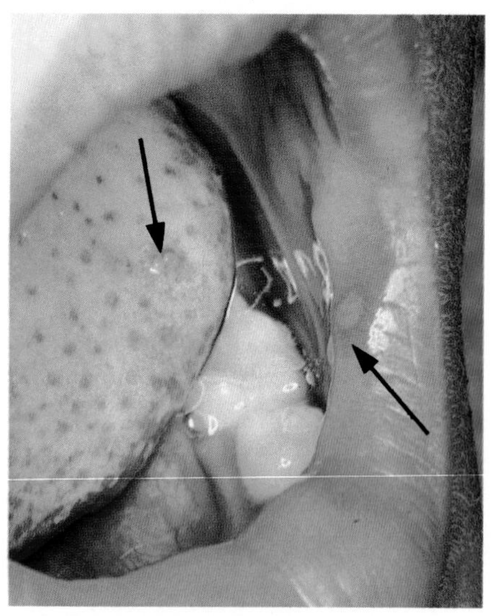

163 Coxsackie infection. Discrete ulcers on the tongue and lower lip, which is characteristic of hand, foot and mouth disease, is visible.

Peritonsillar abscess (quinsy)

164

164 Peritonsillar abscess demonstrating displacement of the uvula across the midline to the left.

Peritonsillar abscesses, which are nearly always unilateral, are usually caused by β-haemolytic streptococci. Normally, the soft palate and the uvula are displaced across the midline from the affected side. The abscesses tend to occur in children over 2 years of age. There may also be dysphagia and fever (**164**).

The majority of cases respond to prompt administration of antibiotics, although surgical aspiration may be necessary. Because recurrence of quinsy is so common, the occurrence of an abscess is an indication for tonsilectomy.

Retropharyngeal abscess

Retropharyngeal abscesses may present in a similar fashion to peritonsillar abscesses, but there are some important differentiating features (**Table 12**). The retropharyngeal type occurs in children under 2 years of age. Children often present with dysphagia, fever, and hyperextension of the neck to relieve impending obstruction. On examination of the throat, the swelling in the retropharyngeal space does not cross the midline and the uvula is not usually deflected.

Immediate systemic antibiotics are necessary for treatment, and surgical intervention may be necessary to prevent airway obstruction or carotid artery erosion (**165**).

165

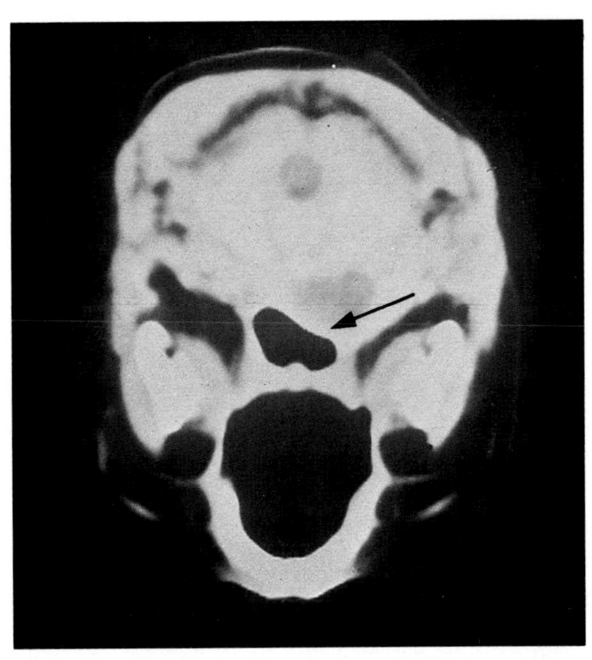

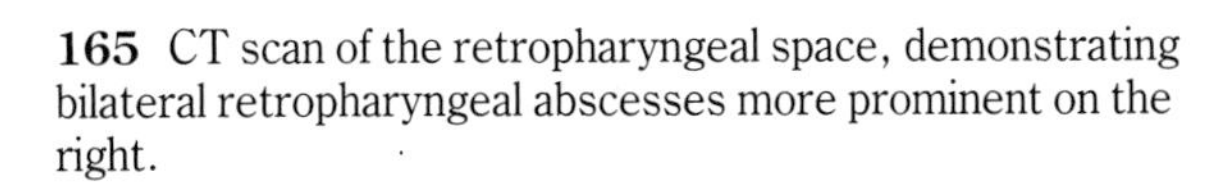

165 CT scan of the retropharyngeal space, demonstrating bilateral retropharyngeal abscesses more prominent on the right.

Table 12. Distinguishing Features of Retropharyngeal Abscess and Peritonsillar Abscess.

	Retropharyngeal abscess	*Peritonsillar abscess*
Age	Under 2 years	Over 2 years
Crosses midline displacing uvula	No	Yes
Hyperextension of neck	Yes	Occasionally
Obstruction of airway	Yes	Yes
Danger of infiltration into mediastinum	Yes	No
Blockage of Eustachian tube	No	Yes

Upper respiratory tract infections

The croup syndrome

Croup is caused by partial obstruction of the larynx. It manifests as inspiratory stridor and a cough, usually with a sudden onset. The most common cause of croup is viruses, but pre-existing causes, such as cord paralysis and aspiration of a foreign body, may also give the same symptoms (**Table 13**).

Table 13. Causes of Croup.

Viruses	*Bacteria*	*Other*
Parainfluenza viruses	*Corynebacterium diphtheriae*	Cord paralysis
Influenza virus	*Haemophilus influenzae*	Foreign body
Respiratory syncytial virus	*Staphylococcus aureus*	Acute smoke inhalation
Measles virus		Acute ingestion of caustic acid
Epstein–Barr virus		

Viral croup (laryngotracheobronchitis)

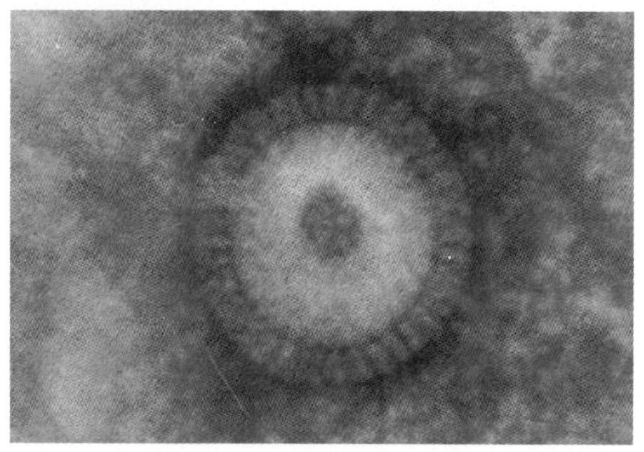

166 A negative-stain electron micrograph of parainfluenza virus, the agent most commonly responsible for laryngotracheobronchitis (× *100,000*).

The viruses that are most commonly responsible for croup are parainfluenza (**166**) and influenza viruses, respiratory syncytial virus, measles and adenoviruses. From a clinical point of view, it is important to distinguish viral croup from acute epiglottitis (**Table 14**).

Viral croup tends to occur in children under 3 years of age and is often preceded by an upper respiratory tract infection. Constitutional symptoms are less marked than those exhibited in acute epiglottitis, although the distinction is not always clear cut. Treatment includes nursing in a humidified environment. Temporary relief may be gained by giving nebulized adrenaline, and the early use of steroids may shorten the attack.

Table 14. Clinical Differences Between Viral Croup and Epiglottitis.

	Viral Croup Laryngotracheobronchitis	*Epiglottitis*
Usual cause	Parainfluenza virus	*Haemophilus influenzae* (b)
Age	Under 3 years	Over 3 years
Season	Autumn, winter	None
Fever	Variable, usually $< 39°C$	$> 39°C$
Onset	Often preceded by upper respiratory infection	Rapid, toxic
Dysphagia	None	Severe, with drooling
Neutrophil count	Usually normal	High

Acute epiglottitis

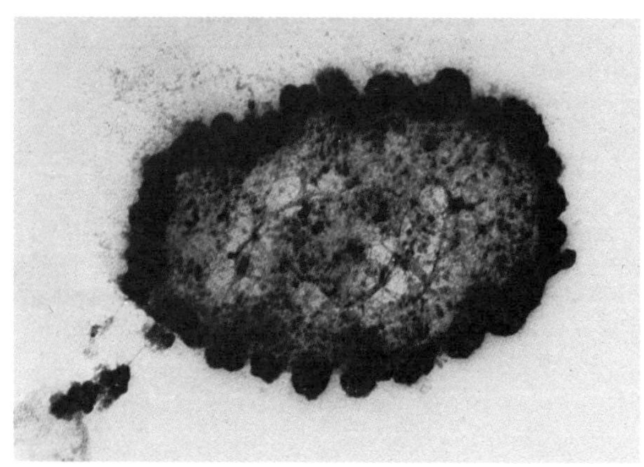

Acute epiglottitis is a most serious form of croup because it presents with great suddenness and there is a risk of obstruction (**167**). Caused by *H. influenzae* type b, it tends to occur in children over 3 years of age and is not related to season. In rare cases streptococci or pneumococci have been isolated and can cause epiglottitis.

167 A negative-stain electron micrograph of *H. influenzae*, demonstrating its capsule (× *13,000*).

If acute epiglottitis is suspected, examination of the larynx should not be attempted as it might precipitate obstruction. A lateral soft-tissue X-ray of the neck may reveal a swollen epiglottis, the so-called 'thumb' sign (**168**). However, if acute epiglottitis is suspected on clinical grounds, time should not be wasted on taking an X-ray. A blood culture should be performed. If elective intubation is anticipated, a naso-pharyngeal swab may be taken. Treatment with intravenous antibiotics should be started. When the symptoms resolve and swallowing becomes easier, oral antibiotics can be continued.

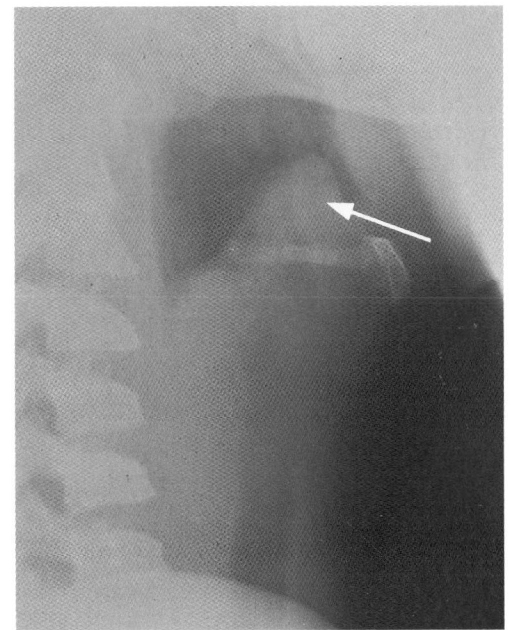

168 Lateral X-ray of an extended neck, demonstrating the 'thumb' sign of the swollen epiglottis.

Diphtheria

Diphtheria is a serious infection caused by a gram-positive rod *Corynebacterium diphtheriae*. Infection is spread by airborne droplets, usually from a child with nasal or laryngeal infection (**169**). *C.diphtheriae* usually attacks the upper airway, especially the pharynx and larynx, but colonization and infection of cutaneous sores may occur. *C.diphtheriae* produces a potent toxin which causes local tissue necrosis, as well as damage to the heart, peripheral nerves, adrenals and kidneys.

The toxin produces necrosis of cells and local inflammation by disrupting protein synthesis. Tissue necrosis is severe surrounding the area of colonization, and a fibrinous exudate, which contains erythrocytes, bacteria and inflammatory cells, is formed as a pseudo-membrane (**170 & 171**). Often, there is soft tissue oedema in the vicinity of infection which if it occurs in the cervical region is termed 'bull neck' (**172**). The pseudo-membrane can become detached, causing acute obstruction of the airways (**172**).

C.diphtheriae may be cultured on tellurite medium.

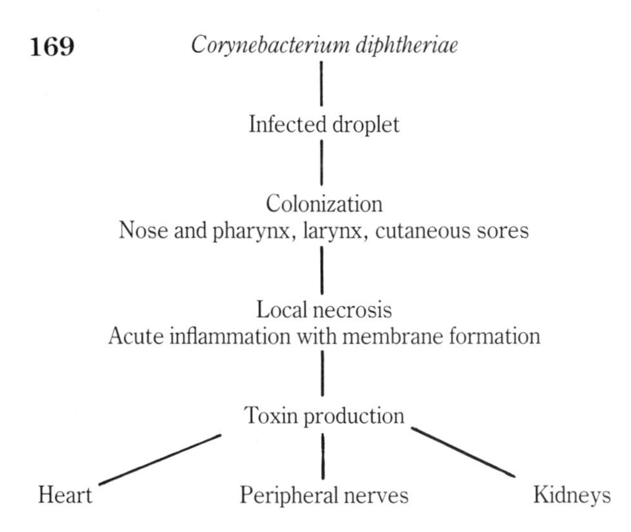

169 Pathogenesis of diphtheria.

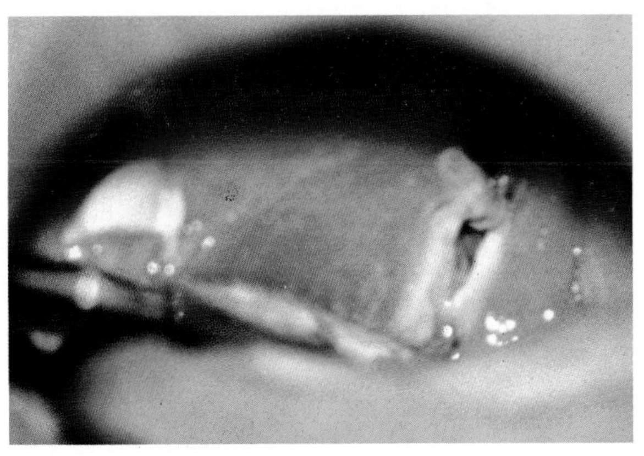

170 Pharyngeal diphtheria showing white membrane and very inflamed fauces.

The size and shape of the colonies may indicate whether the strain is responsible for high level toxin production. Nevertheless toxin production should be demonstrated using immunodiffusion (Elek test). The colonial characteristics do not always correlate with the severity of infection (**173**).

Treatment should aim to kill the organism with penicillin and to neutralize the toxin with antiserum. The Schick test may be used to detect contacts who are not immune and who therefore need active immunization. A positive reaction indicates that a person is non-immune (**174**).

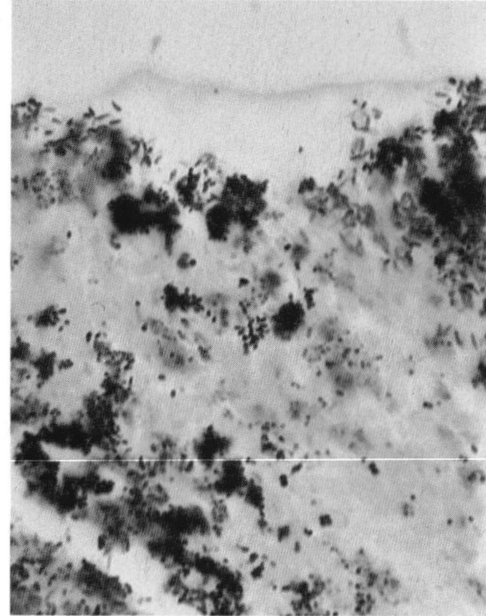

171 A gram stain of membrane demonstrating *C. diphtheriae* with a fibrinous exudate. The red and white blood cells are enmeshed (× *1,000*).

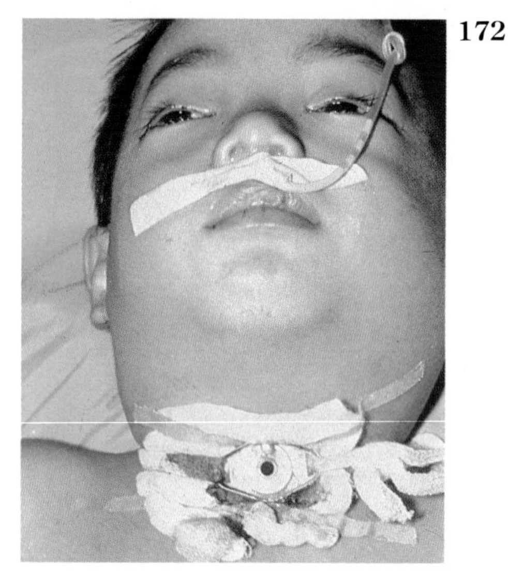

172 This diphtheritic child needed a tracheostomy to avoid obstruction. Note characteristic cervical oedema, often described as a 'bull neck'.

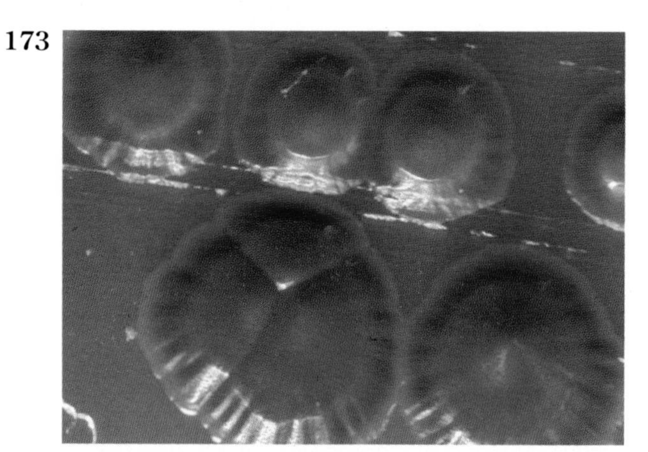

173 *C. diphtheriae* (*gravis*) growing on tellurite medium.

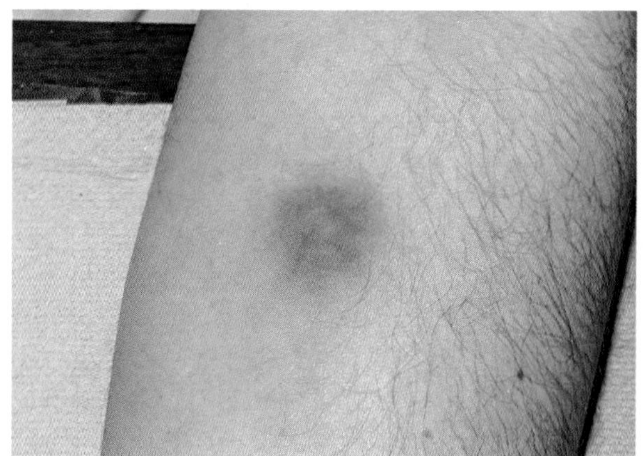

174 A positive Schick test indicating non-immunity to *C. diphtheriae*.

Acute bacterial tracheitis

Bacterial tracheitis is usually caused by *Staphylococcus aureus* or *H.influenzae* and is secondary to a viral infection. It presents with stridor and with symptoms similar to those of acute epiglottitis.

4 Infections of the lower respiratory tract

Throughout the world, lower respiratory tract infections are probably responsible for more deaths in children under 5 years of age than any other single clinical condition. The World Health Organization has embarked on a programme to control acute respiratory infections and to assess their severity by the use of simple clinical signs to score and identify pneumonia.

Viral pneumonias

In developed countries the organisms that most commonly cause pneumonia in children are viruses. Pneumonia may be associated with measles, chickenpox and influenza, or be due primarily to specific viruses, such as adenovirus and the respiratory syncytial virus (RSV). Viral pneumonias may clinically differ little from bacterial pneumonias. The onset of symptoms may be more gradual, as the child becomes increasingly breathless. Physical signs are usually present in both lung fields (**175**), and the resolution is also more gradual. Antibiotics have little influence on the outcome unless there is complicating bacterial infection. Pneumonias are often classified by their anatomical distribution or by the organism that causes them. Many remain difficult to classify; these are usually due to viruses.

175

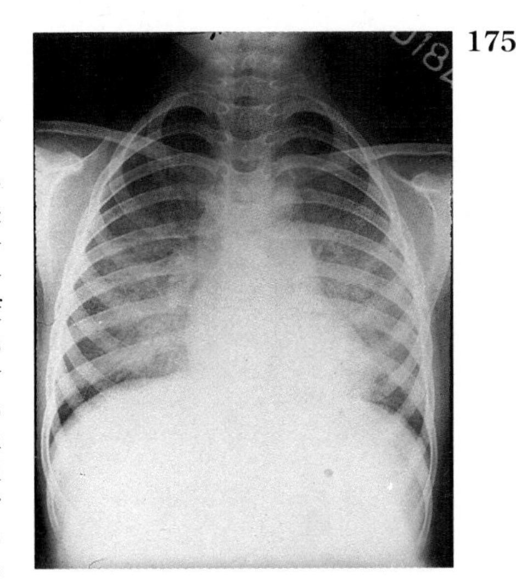

175 X-ray of a one-year-old child with viral pneumonia, showing diffuse infiltration in both lungs.

Bronchiolitis

Bronchiolitis is usually caused by RSV, an RNA paramyxovirus (**176**). Less commonly, adenoviruses (Types 1 and 6) (**177**) and parainfluenza virus can cause an illness indistinguishable from RSV infection.

RSV is spread by droplet, and infection is more common in winter and in spring. Acute bronchiolitis is mainly limited to children under one year of age, with a peak incidence at about 6 months, although the RSV can affect persons of any age.

The incubation period for RSV is 4–6 days. The virus causes oedema, epithelial necrosis, desquamation and increased mucous secretion in the bronchioles. This produces areas of atelectasis and air trapping in the lungs. Chest X-ray demonstrates increased translucency. Areas of consolidation (**178**) or lung collapse may be observed.

176

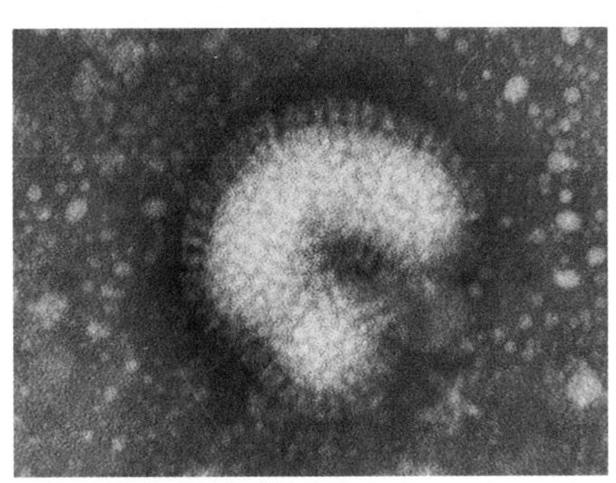

176 A negative-stain electron micrograph of respiratory syncytial virus (× *50,000*).

The clinical development of bronchiolitis usually extends over 6–8 days and presents with upper respiratory tract signs and symptoms including coryza, a dry cough and a low-grade fever that is usually below 38°C. The infant becomes progressively more breathless. An audible wheeze may be present, together with prolonged expiration, subcostal and intercostal recession, and predominantly abdominal breathing. In the most severe cases, cyanosis may occur and assisted ventilation may be necessary. Most cases resolve without complication.

With the use of an immunofluorescent test, the RSV can be rapidly identified from nasopharyngeal aspirates. Bacterial superinfection is uncommon but should be suspected if there is a secondary rise in temperature. In severe cases congestive cardiac failure may occur. Treatment is usually symptomatic, aiming at the maintenance of hydration and adequate nutrition. Oxygen may be necessary. The antiviral agent ribavirin may be used for severe infection in children who have an underlying abnormality such as congenital heart disease, bronchopulmonary dysplasia or immunological abnormalities.

177

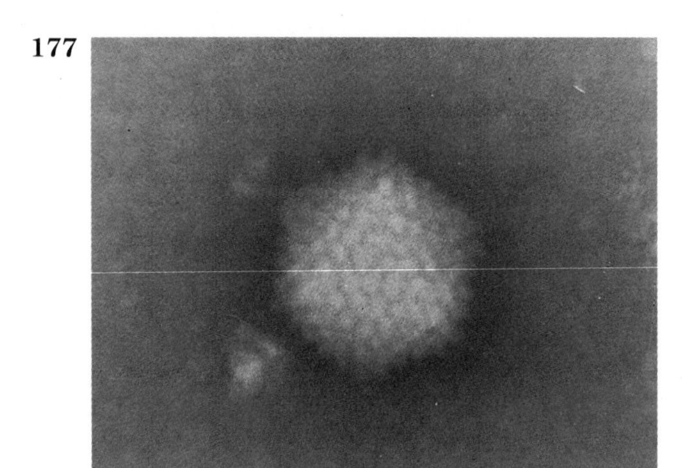

177 A negative-stain electron micrograph of adenovirus (× *120,000*).

178

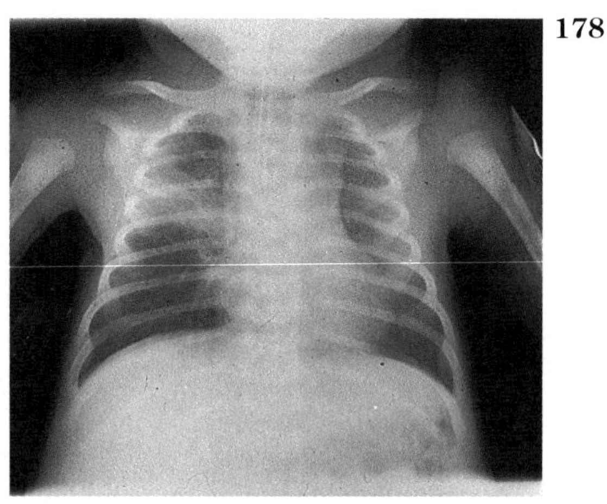

178 X-ray of a 6-month-old child with bronchiolitis, showing increased air trapping in both lungs and right midzone consolidation.

Bronchiolitis obliterans

Bronchiolitis may progress as a rare but fatal form called bronchiolitis obliterans. In most cases this form can be related to an infection from a variety of agents including measles, influenza, adenoviruses, *Mycoplasma pneumoniae* and pertussis. Symptoms similar to those of bronchiolitis may be noted, but progressive hypertranslucency with linear infiltration of the lung will be seen on X-ray (**179**). As the condition develops, there is increased respiratory difficulty which eventually leads to respiratory failure. The disease may be confirmed by lung biopsy (**180**). Histological examination shows fibrotic tissue and obliteration of the alveolar parenchyma.

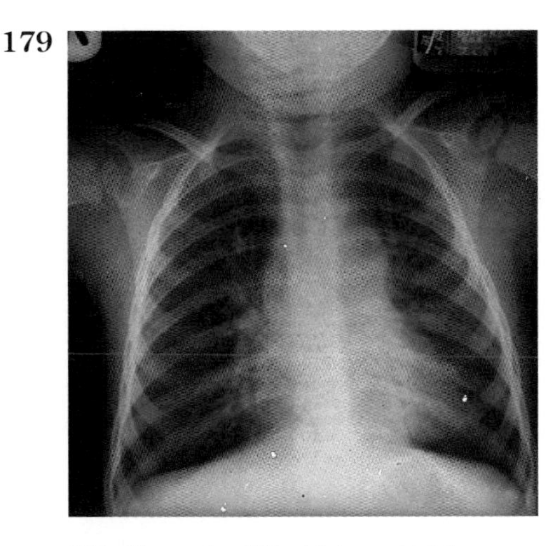

179 X-ray of a child with bronchiolitis obliterans, showing characteristic hypertranslucency of lungs and depression of the diaphragm due to progressive destruction of lung tissue and air trapping.

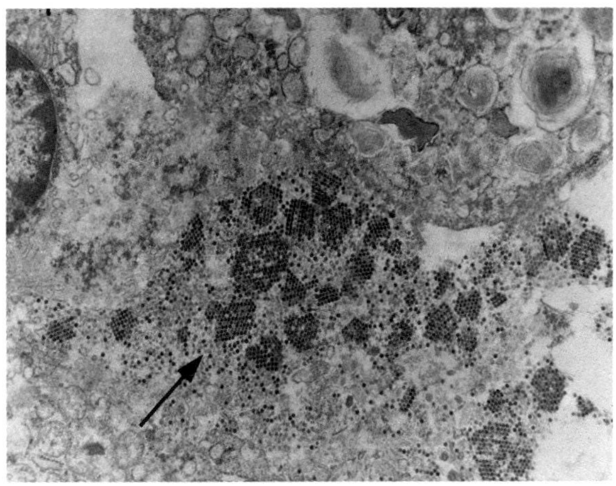

180 A negative-stain electron micrograph of adenovirus particles in a pneumatocyte in a lung biopsy taken from a child with bronchiolitis obliterans (× *2,000*).

Bacterial pneumonias

Bacterial pneumonias may be preceded by a viral infection. In infants and children involvement of the lung is usually more generalized and diffuse than in adults. The clinical presentation is essentially similar for each of the different bacteria causing pneumonia. There may be a history of a mild upper respiratory tract infection followed by an abrupt rise in temperature to 39°C or above, usually with tachypnoea and a cough. Auscultation of the chest may be normal or may demonstrate localized or generalized crepitations with dullness over the affected side. Because children do not readily provide sputum, the organism must be isolated from a throat swab, or from blood culture. A chest X-ray will reveal the site of the pneumonia.

Pneumococcal pneumonia

Streptococcus pneumoniae is still the most common bacterial pathogen responsible for childhood pneumonias (**181**). The pneumococcus produces an acute inflammatory reaction with an alveolar exudate that causes lobar consolidation (**182** & **183**). Sputum may contain red cells, giving it a rusty colour. However, children can seldom produce sputum because they tend to swallow it (**184**).

Infection is more common in winter and spring. Certain serotypes of *S.pneumoniae* (Types 1, 6, 14 and 19) are most often implicated. Infection from asymptomatic carriers in the general population is probably spread by droplet. The clinical presentation in the infant may be of a sick and toxic child with pallor, cyanosis and respiratory distress. The older

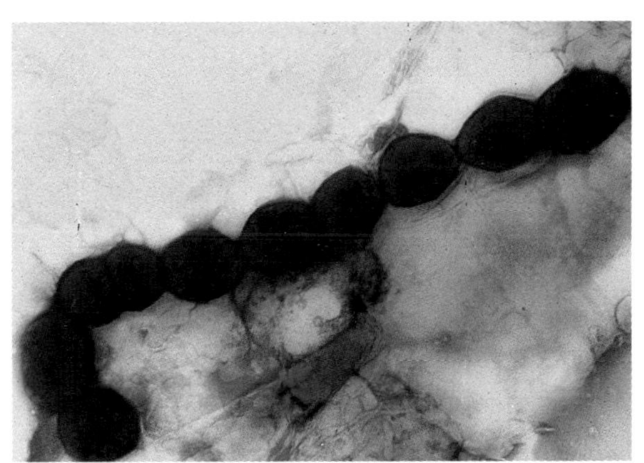

181 A negative-stain electron micrograph of *S. pneumoniae* (× *3,000*).

child may demonstrate rigors followed by a high temperature, cough, pleuritic pain and tachypnoea. On chest X-ray a pleural effusion may be present (**185**).

Occasionally, an empyema may develop (**186**), especially if the pneumonia is inappropriately or inadequately treated. Consolidation and partial or total collapse of the lung may be complications of acute pneumonia (**187**).

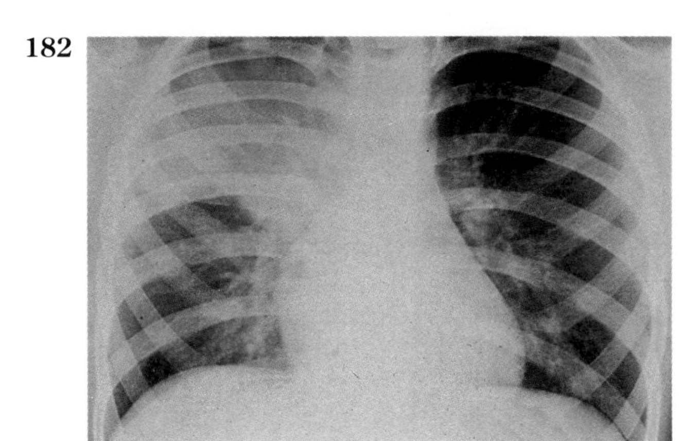

182 X-ray showing right upper lobe consolidation.

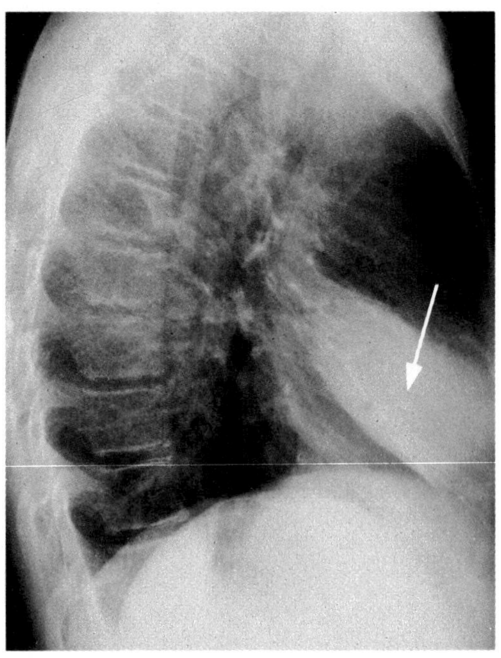

183 Right lateral chest X-ray showing right middle lobe consolidation.

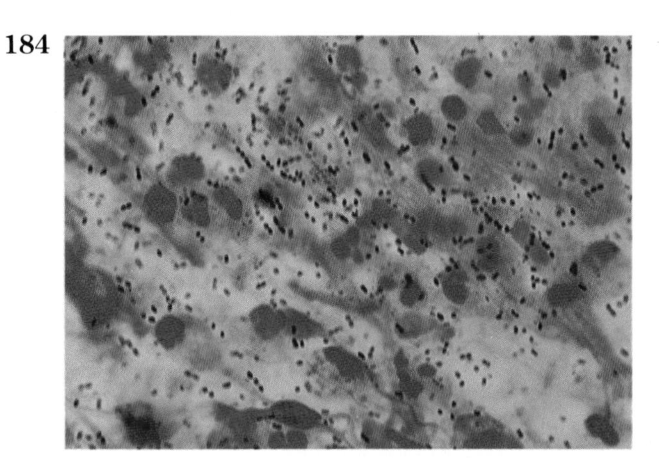

184 A gram-stain of sputum containing numerous *S. pneumoniae* organisms and white cells (× *1,000*).

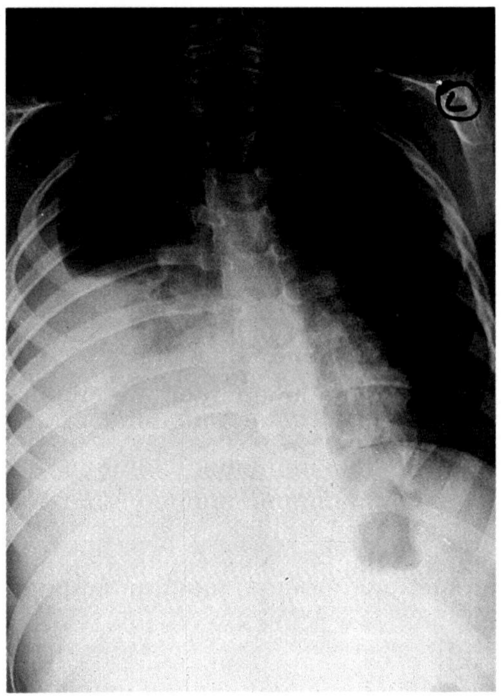

185 Chest X-ray showing a right pleural effusion.

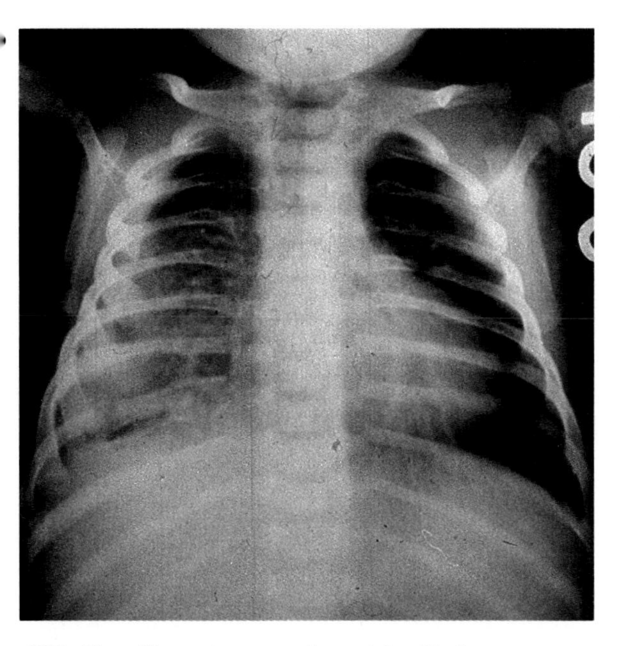

186 Chest X-ray demonstrating a right-sided empyema and pleural effusion.

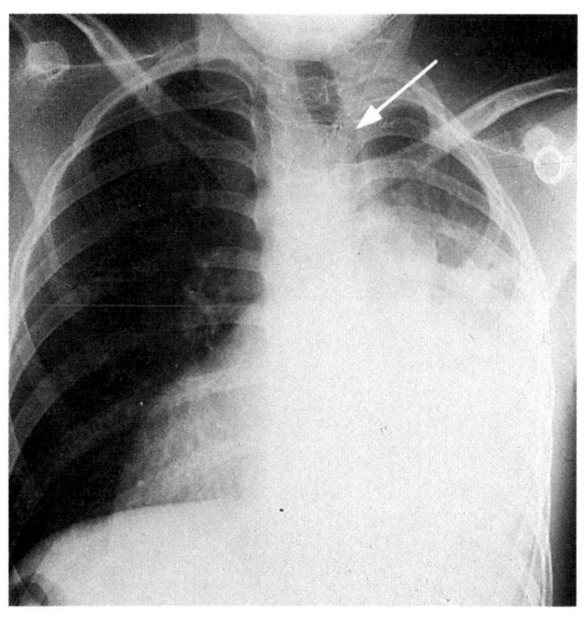

187 A chest X-ray showing left-sided consolidation and collapse, with deviation of the trachea to the left.

Staphylococcal pneumonia

Staphylococcus aureus infection occurs most frequently in children under one year of age and in those children who are debilitated and malnourished. *S.aureus* is to be found on the normal skin and 80% of neonates will become colonized soon after birth (**188** & **189**). Epidemics may occur in nurseries due to bacteria that are resistant to many antibiotics (methicillin-resistant *Staphylococcus aureus*: MRSA).

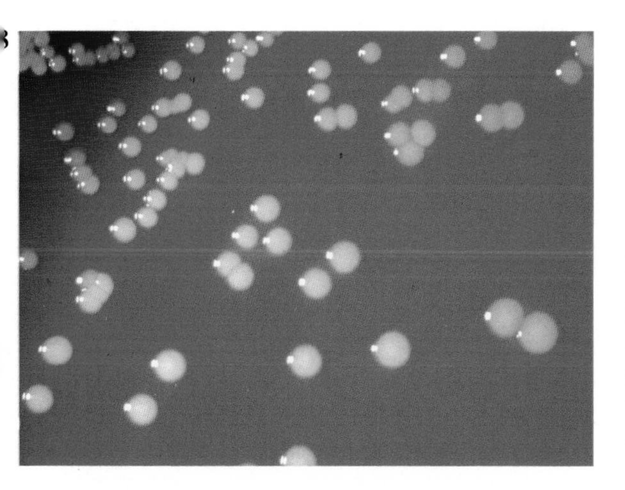

188 *S. aureus* after 18 hours of growth on blood agar.

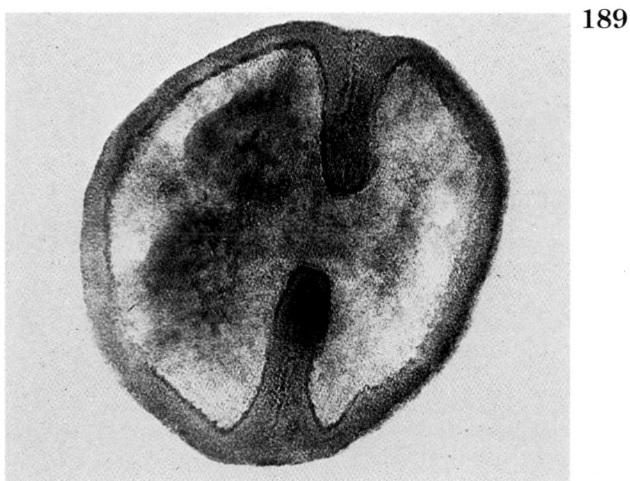

189 Thin-section electron micrograph of a dividing *S. aureus* (× *20,000*).

Staphylococcal pneumonia (**190**) may present with dramatic suddenness. If it is not treated vigorously, it carries a high mortality. *S. aureus* produces several different toxins and enzymes including haemolysin, leukocidin, staphylokinase and coagulase, the liberation of which causes a destructive pneumonia. Usually, one side of the lung is more affected than the other, although both may be involved, and there is a tendency toward multiple abscess formation (**191**). The abscesses may cavitate, and fluid levels from collections of pus are revealed on X-ray (**192** & **193**). On resolution the cavities may remain as air-filled sacs called pneumatocoels, which will disappear over several months (**194**).

A pleural effusion, which may progress to empyema, is not an uncommon complication. Urgent treatment with antistaphylococcal antibiotics, such as flucloxacillin, fucidic acid or a quinolone, should be given systemically to arrest infection.

190

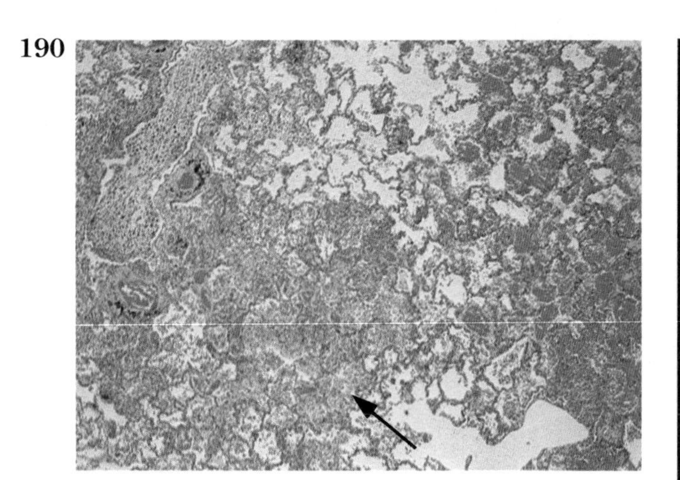

190 A gram-stain showing numerous staphylococci invading lung tissue (× *400*).

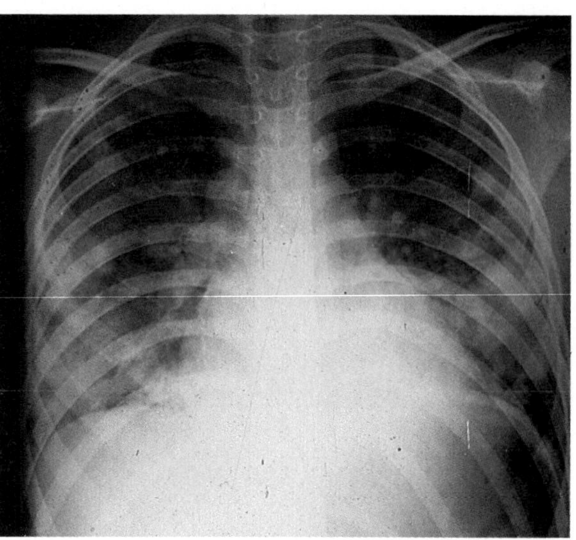

191 Chest X-ray of a child, demonstrating bilateral rounded opaque shadows caused by abscesses in staphylococcal pneumonia.

192

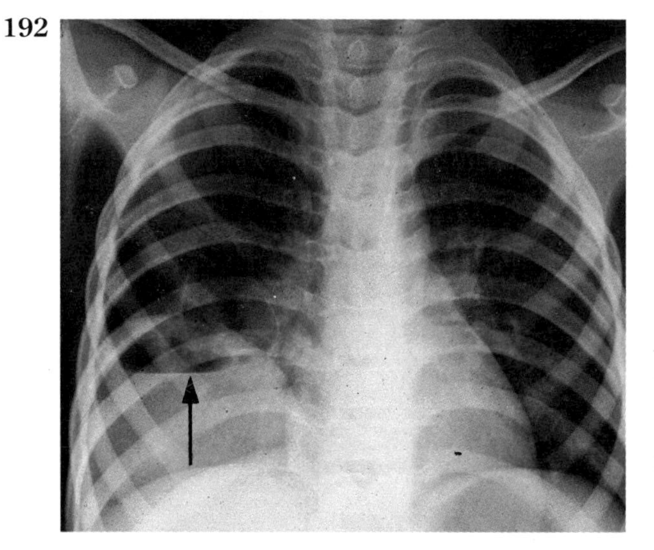

192 Chest X-ray of a right lower lobe staphylococcal abscess with a cavity and fluid level.

193

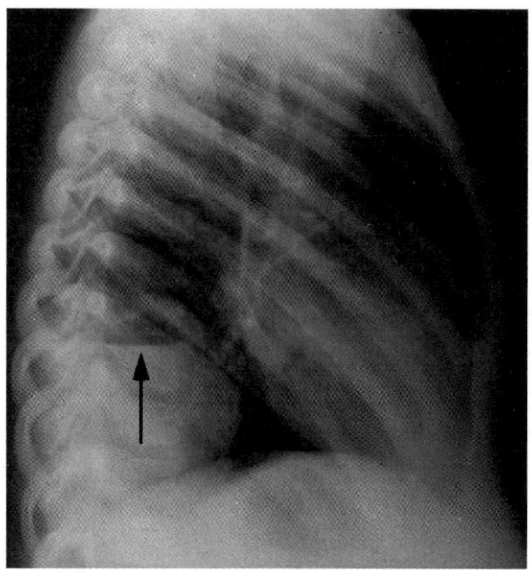

193 Lateral chest X-ray of the child shown in **192**.

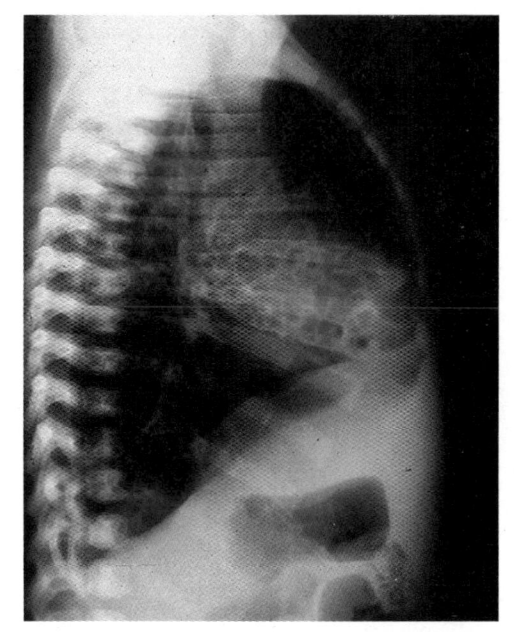

194 Right lateral chest X-ray showing numerous pneumatocoels in the right middle lobe in a case of resolving staphylococcal pneumonia.

Klebsiella pneumonia

Klebsiella pneumoniae may be recovered from the respiratory and gastrointestinal tracts in about 5% of normal children. However, *Klebsiella* pneumonia usually occurs in infants who are debilitated, who have had a preceding viral infection, or who suffer from some underlying abnormality, such as bronchiectasis or tuberculosis. The clinical presentation is similar to that of other types of pneumonia but it may be present as a destructive pneumonia with abscess formation (**195**).

Treatment with a cephalosporin and an aminoglycoside is effective in most cases.

Other less common causes of pneumonia in children include *Branhamella catarrhalis* (**196**) and *Streptococcus milleri*. Occasionally, organisms such as *Actinomyces israelii* may cause infection.

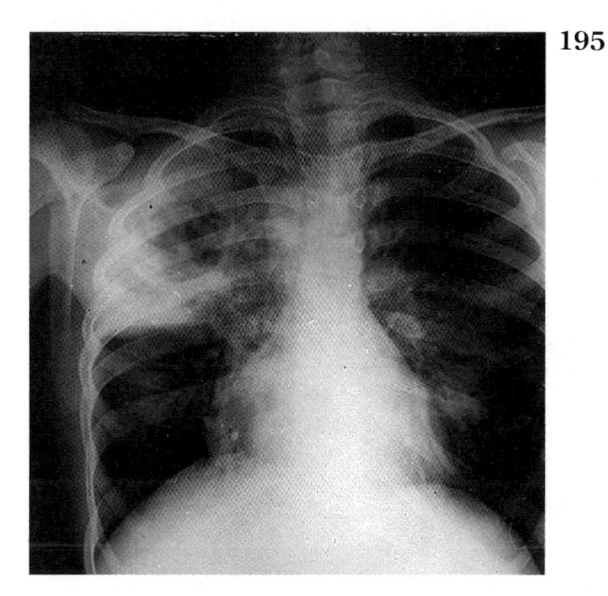

195 Chest X-ray of a right middle lobe cavitating *Klebsiella* pneumonia.

Haemophilus influenzae pneumonia

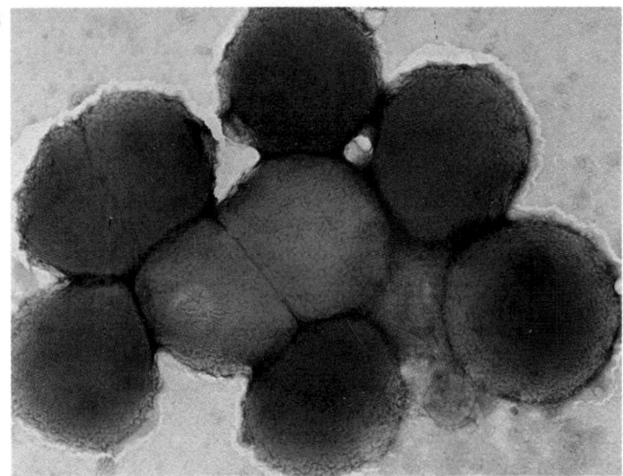

196 Negative-stain electron micrograph of *B. catarrhalis* (× *8,000*).

Haemophilus influenzae (type b) may cause pneumonia in children. It is a gram-negative coccobacillus with a surrounding polysaccharide capsule. *H.influenzae* pneumonia may present in a similar fashion to pneumococcal pneumonia with a lobar distribution. The onset, however, is usually less rapid and more insidious. The definitive diagnosis is made by culturing the organism from blood or, occasionally, from pleural fluid.

Pertussis (whooping cough)

Pertussis is caused by a gram-negative bacillus *Bordetella pertussis* (**197**). The bacillus is sheathed in a coat, with filaments extruding from the cell wall. These filaments, sometimes termed pili (fimbriae), are necessary for the organisms to adhere to the ciliated epithelium of the trachea and bronchus.

B.pertussis is spread by droplet and is not invasive. The characteristic symptoms of *B.pertussis* infection are caused by liberation of an exotoxin, pertussis toxin, which mediates the paroxysms of coughing. It is also responsible for certain factors such as histamine-sensitizing factor (HSF), lymphocytosis-promoting factor (LPF) and islet-activating protein (IAP). The incubation period for whooping cough is 7–10 days and the clinical course is traditionally divided into three stages: catarrhal, paroxysmal and convalescent (**198**).

In developing countries whooping cough is one of the principal causes of death from respiratory infection. The mortality is highest in children under one year of age because infants under 6 months may suddenly develop apnoea without necessarily having preceding characteristic coughing spasms (**199**). The coughing spasms tend to produce haemorrhages in the peri-orbital region and in the subconjunctiva (**200**), but they may also occur in the brain, where they are responsible for some of the serious neurological complications. Pertussis can lead to pneumonia. Chest X-ray may show bilateral hilar lymphadenopathy (**201**), which must be distinguished from lymph gland enlargement due to other causes, such as tuberculosis.

197 Negative-stain electron micrograph of *B. pertussis* (× *10,000*).

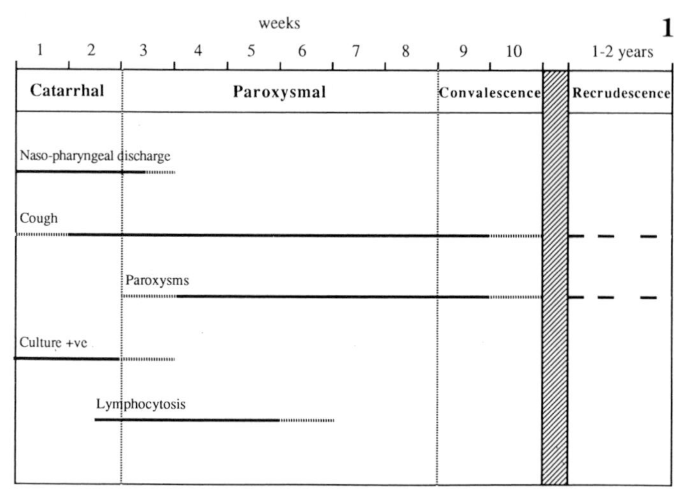

198 Clinical stages of whooping cough.

Whooping cough may cause an encephalopathy (**202**), which usually appears during the early paroxysmal phase. Hypoglycaemia may partly be responsible for some neurological symptoms since the pertussis toxin (IAP) causes stimulation of the islet cells in the pancreas. In older children paroxysms may cause a pneumothorax (**203**), or even interstitial and subcutaneous emphysema (**204**) following a leakage of air from ruptured alveolae into the pleural cavity or mediastinum. The severe coughing spasms may also cause prolapse of the rectum, especially in malnourished children, and tearing at the frenulum. Sometimes the tongue is bitten during the spasms (**205**).

The organism may only be isolated in the catarrhal and early paroxysmal phases. A special Bordet–Gengou medium is necessary for culture. A rapid diagnosis can be made using immunofluorescence on nasopharyngeal aspirates. A peripheral white cell count typically shows an absolute lymphocytosis.

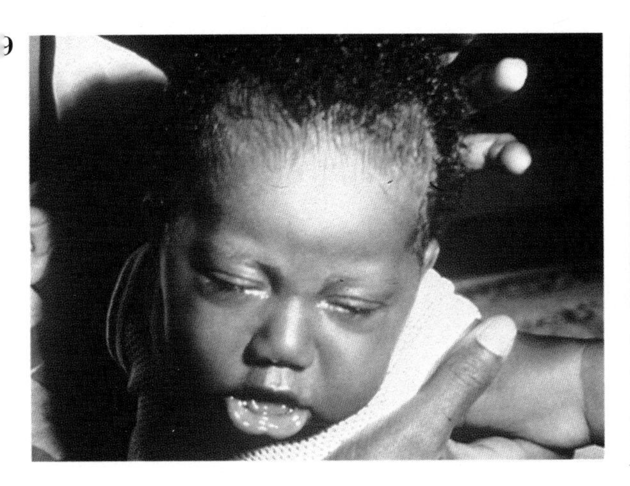

199 A child with whooping cough, experiencing a characteristic paroxysm of coughing.

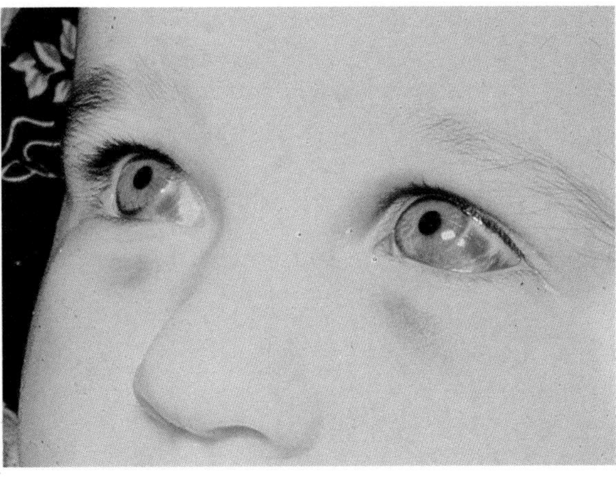

200 A child with whooping cough with bilateral periorbital and subconjunctival haemorrhages.

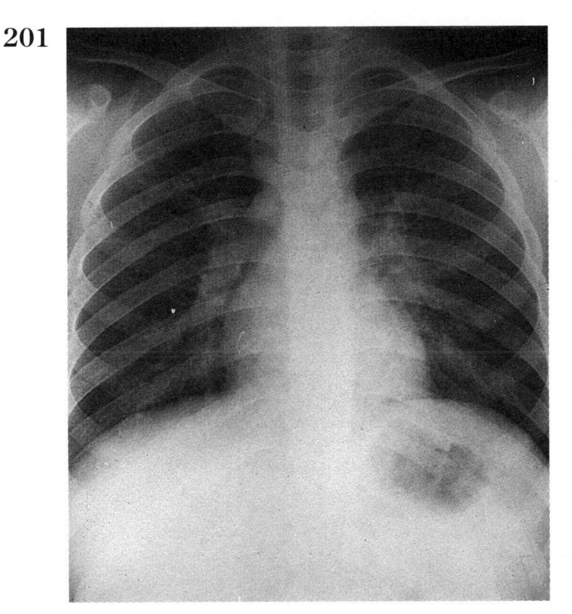

201 X-ray of a child with whooping cough, showing bilateral hilar lymph gland enlargement.

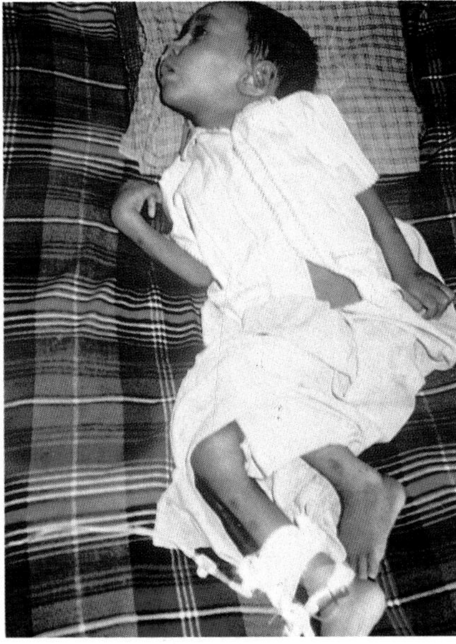

202 A Burmese child with acute encephalopathy due to whooping cough.

203

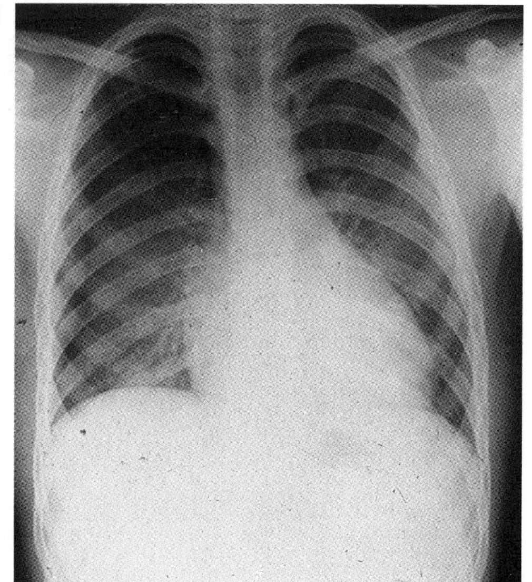

B.pertussis is sensitive to erythromycin, which has to be given early to modify the disease. Treatment is mainly supportive, with oxygen, the maintenance of hydration and nutrition, and prevention of aspiration pneumonia. Cough suppressants and antihistamines have not been found to modify the disease.

Vaccination with the whole cell pertussis vaccine should be given early in infancy. There is no evidence that the vaccine causes permanent neurological damage. An acellular vaccine is reported to produce fewer systemic and local adverse reactions.

203 X-ray of a right pneumothorax in a child with whooping cough.

204

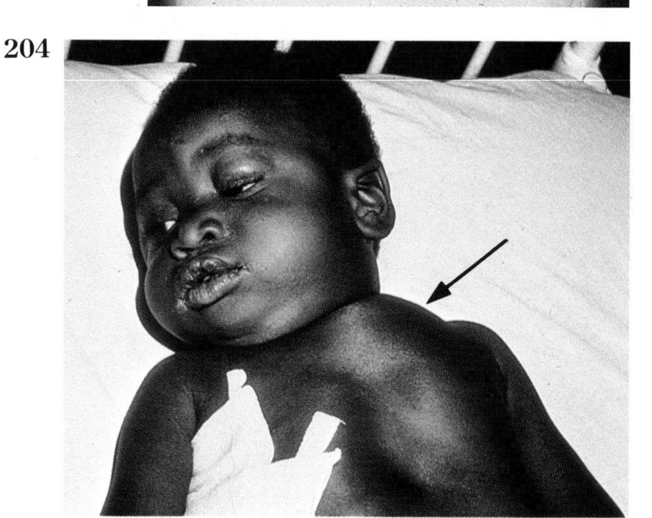

204 A boy with whooping cough, demonstrating subcutaneous emphysema.

2

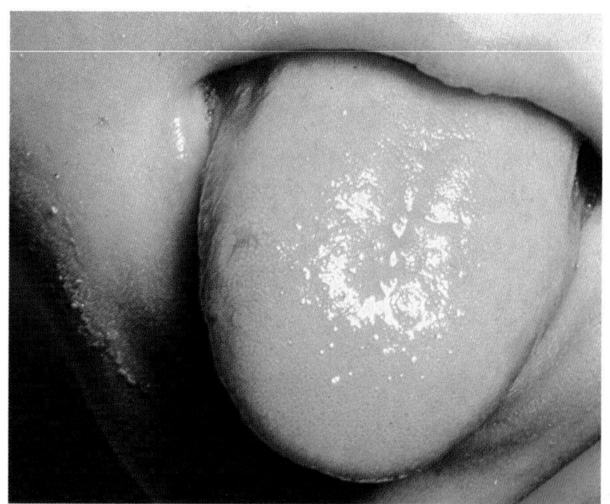

205 A tongue bitten during a coughing spasm in whooping cough.

Atypical pneumonias

Formerly, the term 'atypical pneumonia' was reserved for pneumonia caused by *Mycoplasma pneumoniae*, but it has now been extended to include pneumonias due to *Chlamydia trachomatis*, *C.pneumoniae*, *C.psittaci*, or *Legionella pneumophila*.

Mycoplasma pneumoniae pneumonia

Mycoplasma pneumoniae is a significant cause of pneumonia in older children and young adults. The incidence peaks between 10 and 15 years. Mycoplasmas have no cell wall but they can be grown on artificial media (**206**).

Mycoplasma pneumonia usually has a gradual clinical onset. There may be a history of headache, malaise and fever before the respiratory symptoms of cough and tachypnoea are present. There is usually bilateral pulmonary involvement (**207**). Extrapulmonary manifestations of mycoplasma infection may also be present. These include erythema nodosum, erythema multiforme (**208**) and Stevens–Johnson syndrome.

Culture of a throat swab or sputum on a special medium will demonstrate *M.pneumoniae*, but only in the early phase of the illness. Cold haemagglutinins may be present in the acute stage, and a rising titre of specific antibodies will confirm the diagnosis. Erythromycin, which should be taken for at least 10 days, is the treatment of choice.

206

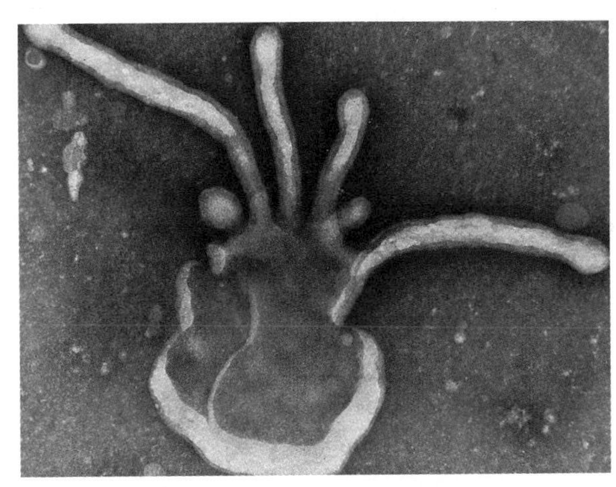

206 A negative-stain electron micrograph of *M. pneumoniae* (× *20,000*).

207

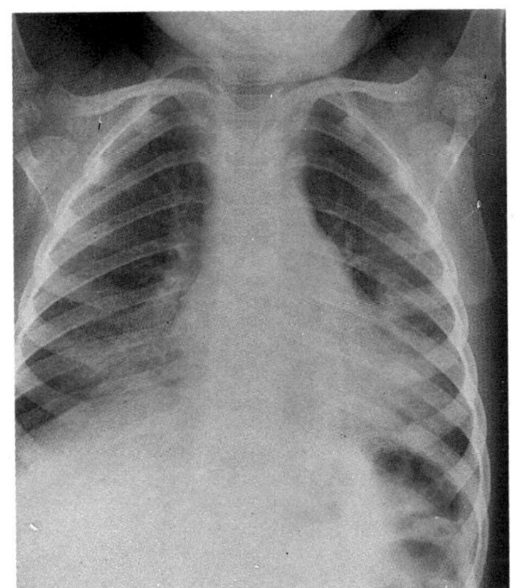

207 Chest X-ray of a child with *M. pneumoniae* pneumonia, showing bilateral lung involvement.

208

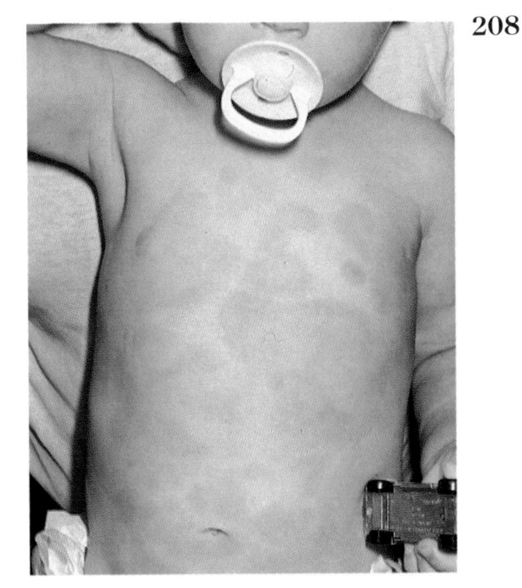

208 Erythema multiforme, a skin manifestation of *M. pneumoniae* infection.

Chlamydial pneumonia

Chlamydia trachomatis, C.pneumoniae and *C.psittaci* can all cause pneumonia in children. *C.trachomatis* is usually acquired by the neonate from the maternal birth canal (**209**). Infection may initially present with a purulent conjunctivitis (**210**) and later, within a few days, signs of pneumonia develop. Infection may be severe and can lead to respiratory failure.

C.psittaci is associated with birds (ornithosis). It

affects older children and adolescents. Constitutional symptoms of fever, myalgia, arthralgia and cough are common. An atypical pneumonia may develop. Chlamydial infections respond to erythromycin or tetracycline.

209

209 Chest X-ray of a neonate with *C. trachomatis* pneumonia, showing bilateral lung involvement.

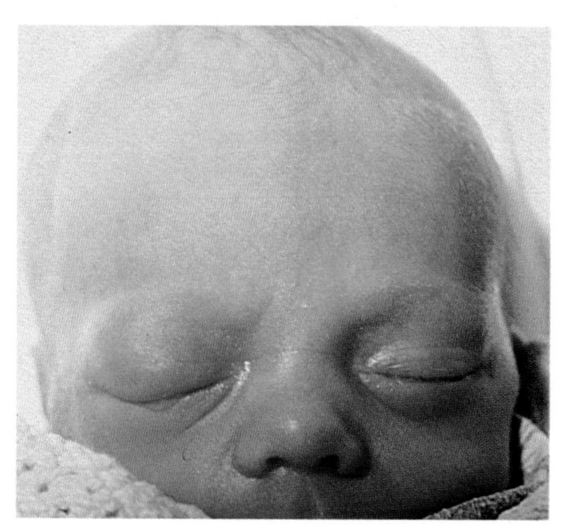

210 Chlamydial conjunctivitis in a neonate.

Tuberculosis

Tuberculosis (TB) is still an endemic disease in the UK, with approximately 5,000 notifications per year, 9% of which occur in children.

Pulmonary tuberculosis

211

211 A Ziehl–Neelsen stain of *M. tuberculosis* (× *1,000*).

In the UK, *Mycobacterium tuberculosis*, an acid- and alcohol-fast bacillus (**211**), is responsible for nearly all tuberculous infection. *M.bovis* is uncommon because of the pasteurization of milk and a national policy of keeping cattle tested for TB. Children under the age of 5 years are particularly vulnerable to infection because (a) they may be nursed by infective adults who pass on a heavy dose of the organism, (b) the immunity of infants and children is less well developed, limiting the host's response to the organism and (c) frequent intercurrent infection in childhood increases susceptibility. Measles is particularly likely to exacerbate TB.

The organism is spread by droplet infection. The incubation period is about 6 weeks, during which time a hypersensitivity reaction may occur, manifested as erythema nodosum (**212**), occasionally as a pleural effusion and, rarely, as phlyctenular conjunctivitis.

The bacillus first lodges in the lungs to form the primary focus (Ghon's focus), which in children is usually in the upper zone of the lung. This is followed by a primary complex, in which the lymph nodes on the affected side increase in size (**213** & **214**). At this stage, most infections tend to resolve, as the host mounts an immune response. However, some children will go on to develop local spread of infection with hilar enlargement, tuberculous bronchopneumonia (**215**) and cavitation. The lymph nodes may become so enlarged that they exert pressure on the bronchi, with obstruction leading to total or partial lung collapse. Lymph node pressure on the bronchi may also cause the development of obstruction and bronchiectasis. Haematogenous spread occurs in some children causing dissemination of infection throughout the body which results in miliary TB (**216**). Such a spread of *M.tuberculosis* may cause infection in any organ including the brain, bones, kidneys, adrenals and genitals.

M.tuberculosis is difficult to isolate. Since children swallow their sputum, it may be necessary to rely upon fresh early morning gastric washings to detect the organism. A Mantoux test at 1:1000 dilution usually gives a positive result (**217**) although in severe disseminated TB, measles infection and malnutrition, the result may be negative during active disease.

212

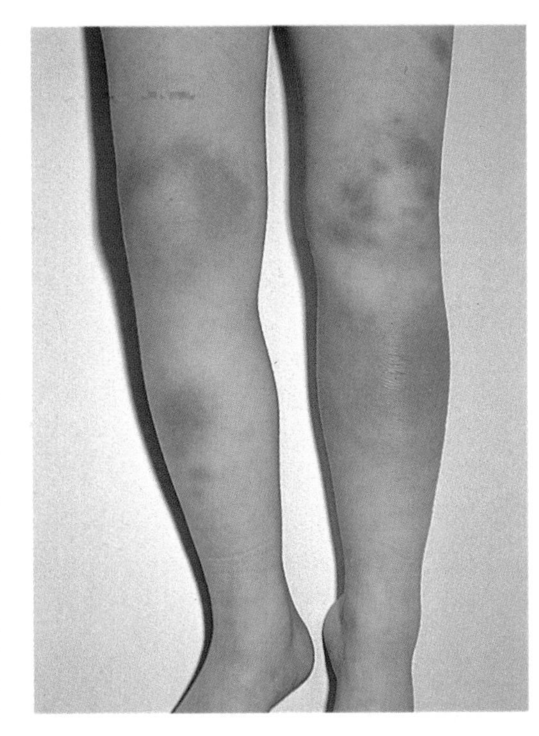

212 Erythema nodosum as a skin manifestation of primary tuberculosis.

3

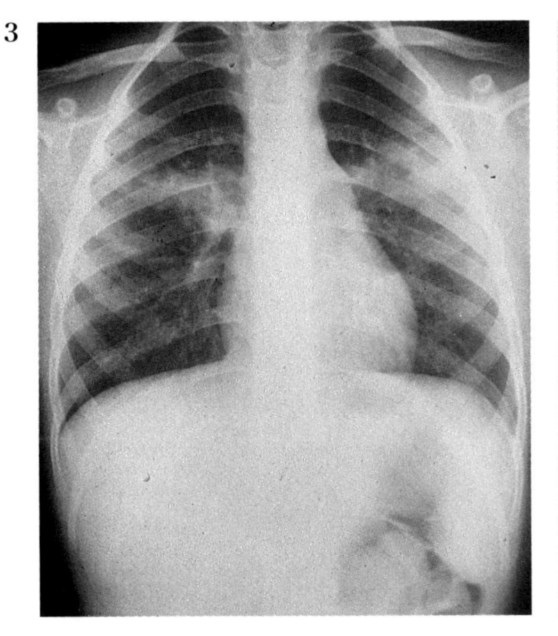

213 Chest X-ray of tuberculosis, showing a primary complex in the right lung, with hilar gland enlargement.

214

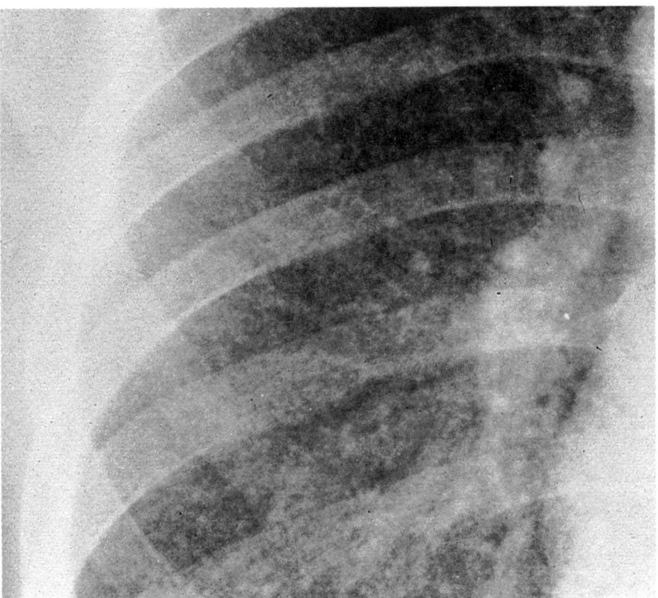

214 Close-up of an X-ray showing hilar gland enlargement.

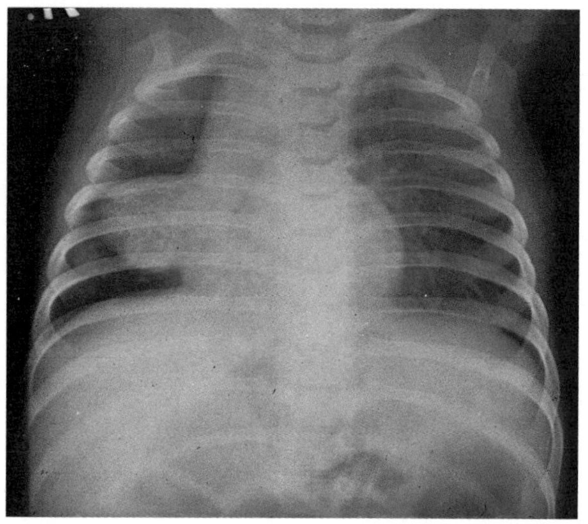

215 Chest X-ray showing a right middle lobe pneumonia due to primary tuberculosis.

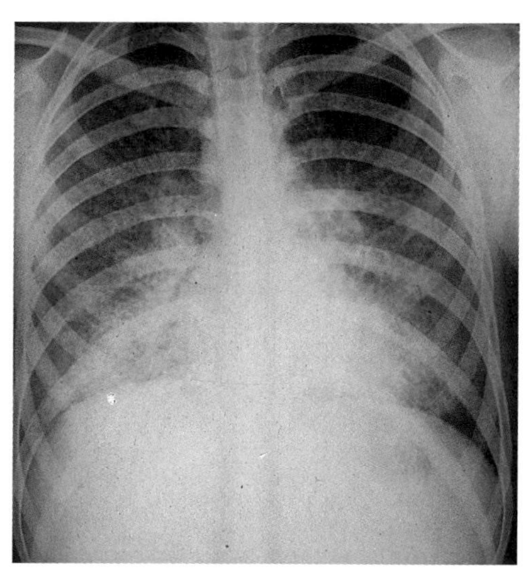

216 Chest X-ray showing bilateral lung involvement in miliary tuberculosis.

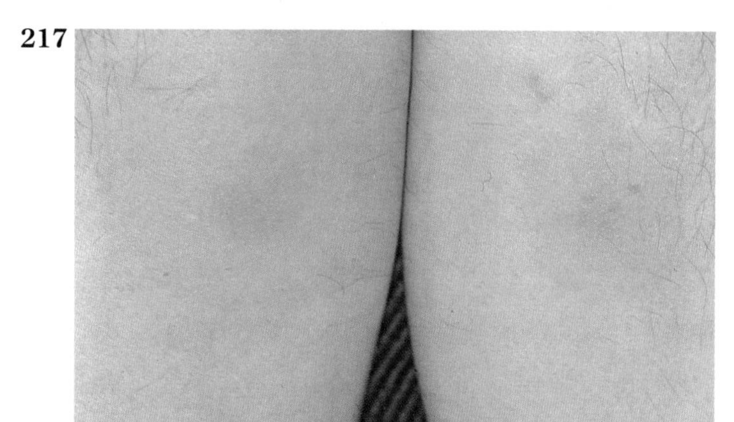

217 Positive Mantoux test (at 1:1,000 dilution) and Heaf test reactions in the same child.

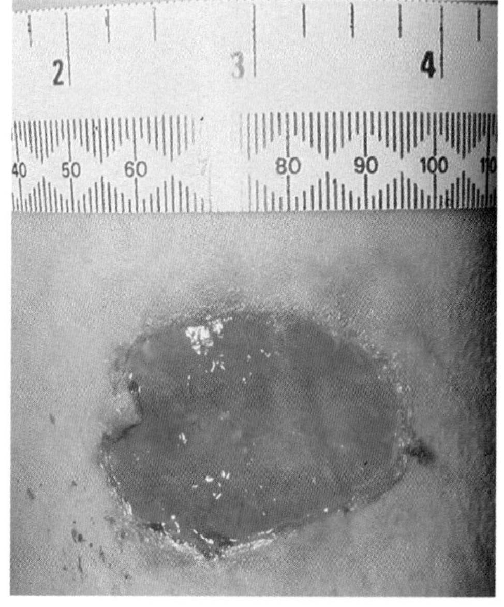

218 A BCG ulcer which appeared eight weeks after vaccination.

Treatment with multiple antituberculous drugs, which may include rifampicin, isoniazid and pyrazinamide, should continue for at least 6–9 months. Immunization with live Bacille Calmette-Guerin (B.C.G.) vaccine gives significant protection against severe disseminated tuberculosis but it does not provide complete protection. The vaccine is given intradermally. Occasionally, a severe reaction may occur 4–8 weeks after vaccination, with the possible complications of an ulcer (**218**), abscess or regional lymph node enlargement.

Bronchiectasis

Bronchiectasis is a chronic pulmonary condition that involves dilatation and infection of one or more bronchi. It is marked by a chronic cough and excessive sputum production. In the UK the most common cause of bronchiectasis is cystic fibrosis but in poor and underdeveloped countries bronchiectasis is usually secondary to partially treated or untreated infections. It occurs in association with measles, adenovirus infection, pertussis and tuberculosis. Bronchiectasis may either be localized to a single segment of lung or involve both lungs (**219**), as in cystic fibrosis.

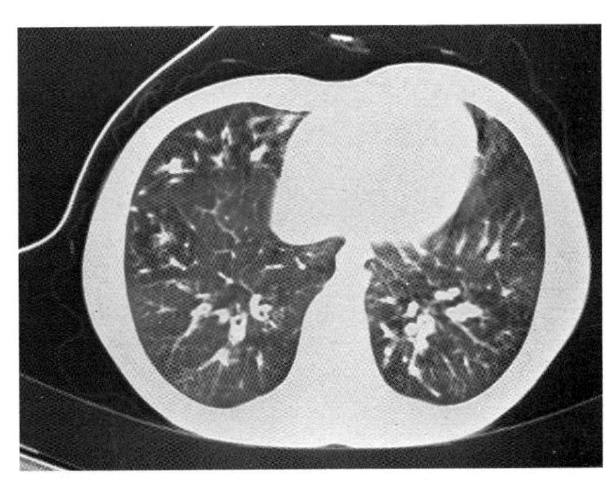

219 CT scan of a child with bilateral bronchiectasis, showing thickened and irregular bronchi.

Immotile cilia syndrome (Kartagener's syndrome)

Bronchiectasis is one complication of the immotile cilia syndrome, in which there is abnormal function of the cilia. The defect in cilia motility is due to a lack of ATPase-containing dynein, which is normally linked to the microtubules necessary for ciliary movement. The disease, which is autosomal recessive, has an incidence of fewer than one in 2,000 persons. The defect is associated with situs inversus or dextrocardia, chronic sinusitis, and chronic bronchitis which may lead to bronchiectasis (**220**).

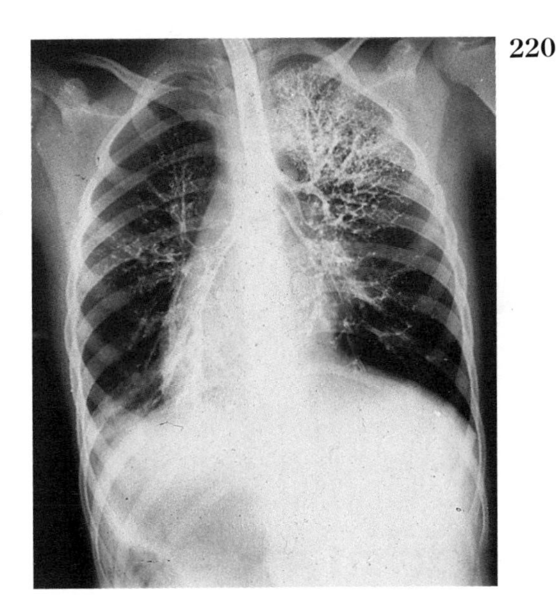

220 Chest X-ray and bronchogram of Kartagener's syndrome, showing bronchiectasis, situs inversus and dextrocardia.

Cystic fibrosis

Cystic fibrosis is the main cause of bronchiectasis in the UK. It is an autosomal recessive condition in which the asymptomatic heterozygote exists in about 1 in 25 people. The abnormal gene, which exists in the long arm of chromosome 7, gives rise to a defective transport protein, which facilitates chloride ion transport in exocrine glands.

Although the lungs are normal at birth, they are particularly susceptible to repeated infection because of the production of thick mucous. Progressive destruction of the lung occurs (**221–225**). Initially, the most marked changes may be noted in the upper zones of the lungs. However, because of the progressive damage due to infections, all zones will eventually be affected.

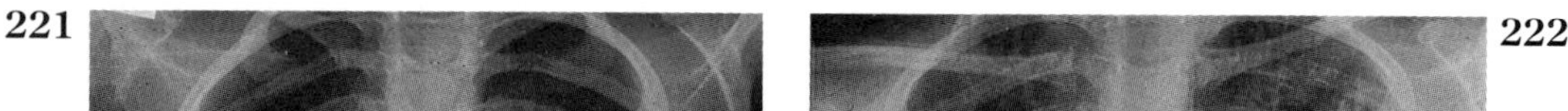
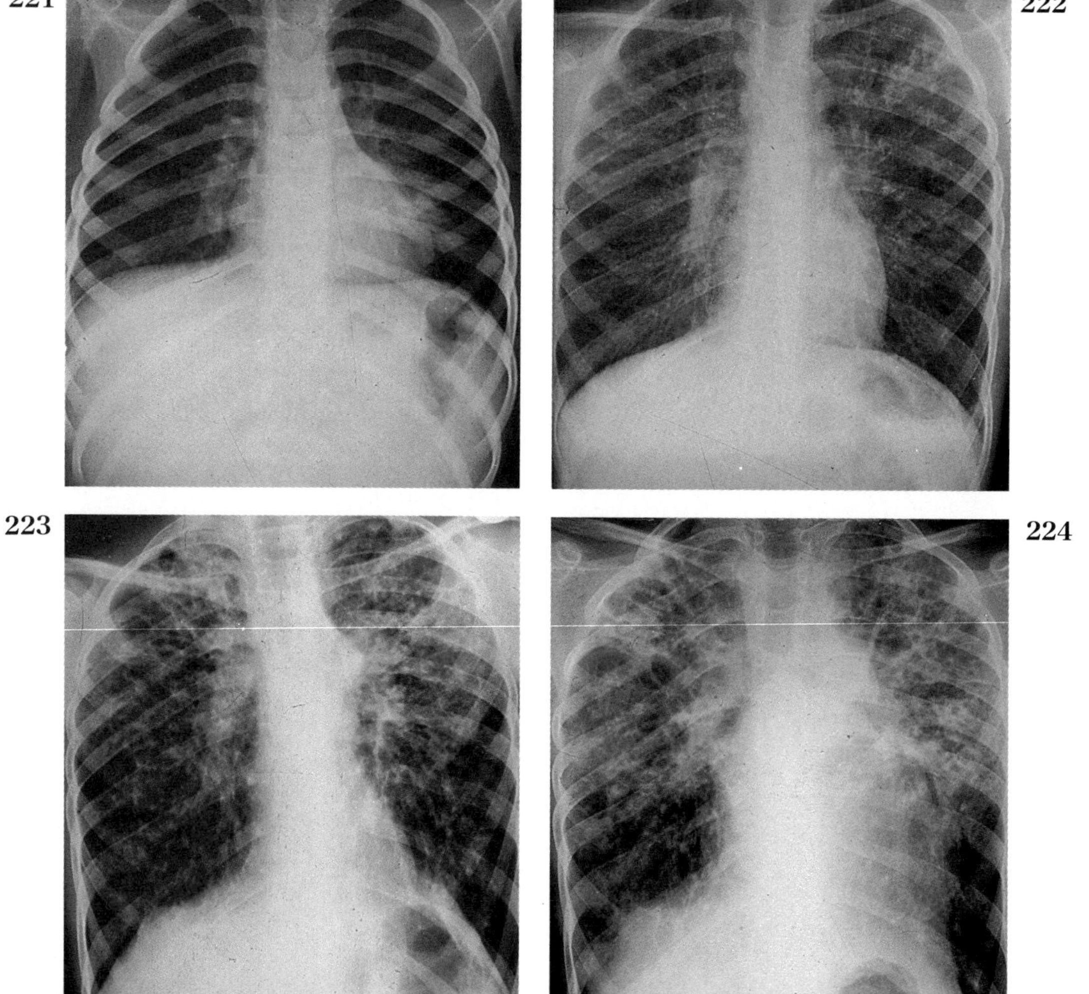

221–224 A series of chest X-rays of a child with cystic fibrosis showing the progression of disease from 1 year of age (**221**). **222** shows the child at 5 years of age, **223** was taken at 9 years of age, and **224** shows the child at 13 years of age.

In the first few months of life staphylococcal infections are common but thereafter *Pseudomonas aeruginosa* and *P.cepacia* (**226**) become the most intractable organisms responsible for progressive lung destruction. As more and more lung tissue is destroyed and alveolar fibrosis takes place, pulmonary hypertension may result (**227**).

Cystic fibrosis affects all the exocrine glands of the body. It may present in the neonatal period, occurring in 10% of affected children with acute obstruction due to meconium ileus. The sweat glands are affected and produce excessive loss of salt. The definitive diagnosis of the disease is made by estimating the concentration of salt in the sweat: concentrations of >40 mmol of sodium or chloride suggest cystic fibrosis. Pancreatic function is impaired (**228**) resulting in malabsorption of food and in a failure to thrive. Children with advanced disease often become wasted and develop a pulmonary osteodystrophy (**229**) as a result of chronic pulmonary lung disease.

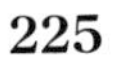

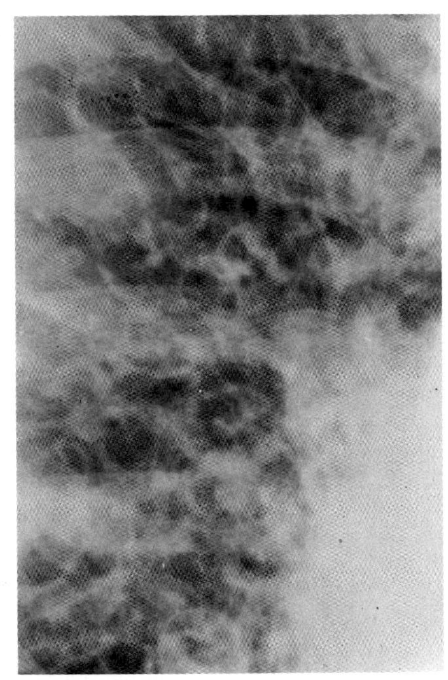

225 Segment of a chest X-ray in cystic fibrosis, showing peribronchial thickening in advanced disease.

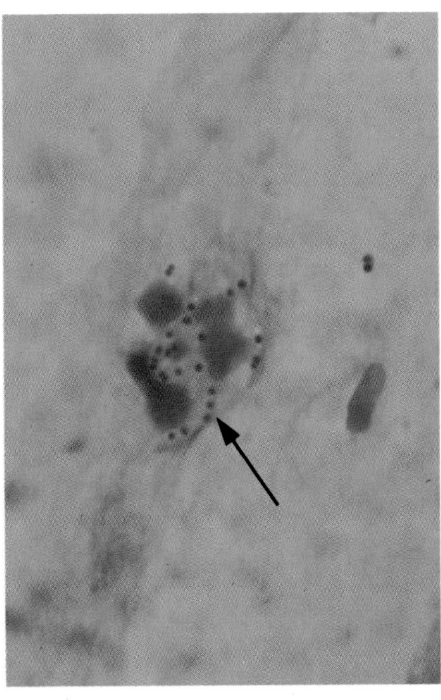

226 A gram stain showing a neutrophil engulfing short gram-negative rods of *P. cepacia* (× *1,000*).

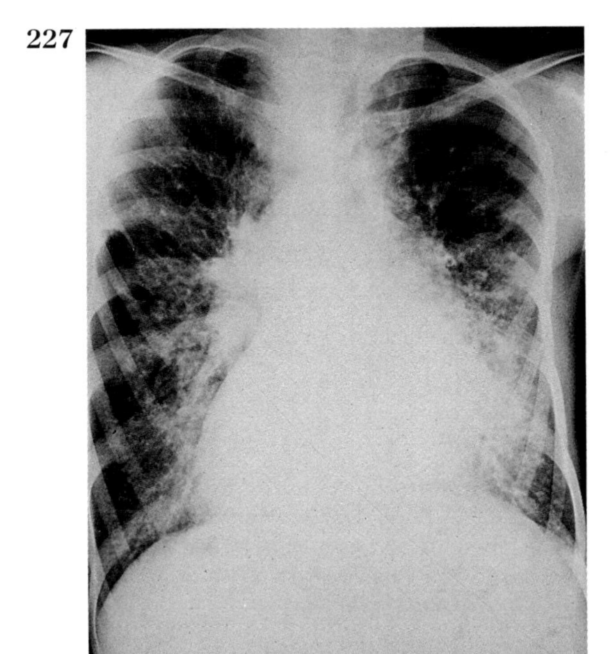

227 Chest X-ray showing advanced cystic fibrosis with complicating pulmonary hypertension.

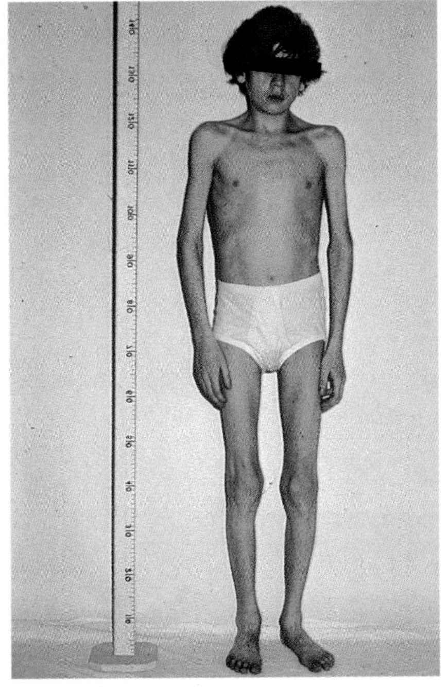

228 A boy with cystic fibrosis. Chest deformity from chronic pulmonary infection, together with generalized muscle wasting from poor pancreatic function, is visible.

Better treatment has improved the prognosis for most children with cystic fibrosis. Prevention of chest infections includes frequent and regular physiotherapy. Infection is treated with intensive courses of antibiotics against pathogens, particularly *P.aeruginosa* and *P.cepacia*, using systemic or nebulized antibiotics. Optimal nutrition can be achieved by using efficient supplements of pancreatic extract and, occasionally, short periods of total parenteral nutrition. The long-term complications of cystic fibrosis are shown in **Table 16**.

Now that the specific gene for cystic fibrosis has been isolated, early antenatal diagnosis is possible. In the future, treatment aimed at correction of the abnormal protein transport defect may be possible.

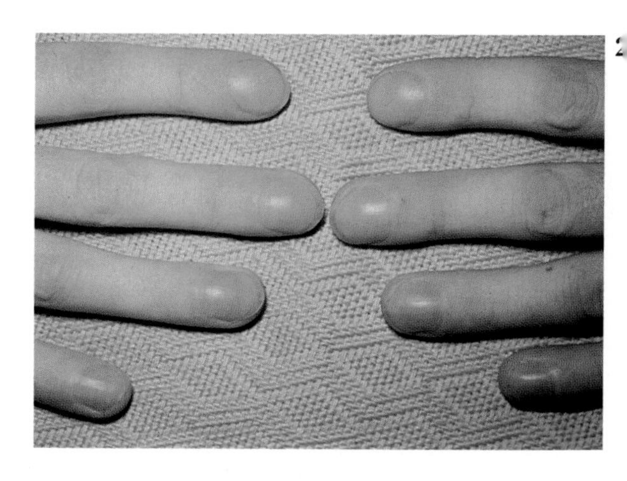

229 Pulmonary osteodystrophy manifested as finger clubbing.

Table 16. Complications and Sequelae of Cystic Fibrosis.

Cardiopulmonary	*Gastrointestinal*	*Other complications*
Pneumothorax	Meconium ileus	Salt depletion
Pulmonary abscess	Chronic diarrhoea and failure to thrive	Male sterility
Aspergillosis	Intussusception	
Haemoptysis	Acute meconium ileus equivalent	
Empyema	Rectal prolapse	
Nasal polyps	Pancreatitis	
Sinusitis	Diabetes mellitus	
Pulmonary hypertension	Liver cirrhosis	
Cor pulmonale	Portal hypertension	

5 Infections of the cardiovascular system

The heart and cardiovascular system may be infected directly by bacteria, as in subacute bacterial endocarditis (SBE); indirectly through immune mechanisms, as in rheumatic fever; or by toxins, such as the diphtheria toxin.

Infective endocarditis

Transient bacteraemia is common even in normal healthy people. It may occur during any bacterial infection, after dental treatment and even as a result of vigorous brushing of the teeth. In healthy children it seldom causes colonization or infection of the cardiovascular system unless there is some pre-existing abnormality. Worldwide, the most common cause of acquired valvular abnormality is rheumatic fever. This predisposes to subacute bacterial endocarditis, now rare in developed countries. In the UK, bacterial endocarditis in children is mainly associated with congenital abnormalities (**Table 17**).

Although *Streptococcus viridans* (**230** & **231**) is the most common bacterium associated with endocarditis,

Table 17. Groups of Children at Risk of SBE.

- Children with congenital heart disease, especially those with aorticopulmonary shunts, left-sided outflow obstruction, and ventricular septal defects
- Children with immune deficiencies
- Children with chronic central venous catheters
- Children with prosthetic valves
- Neonates with chronic indwelling lines for nutrition and monitoring
- Children with valves damaged by previous rheumatic fever

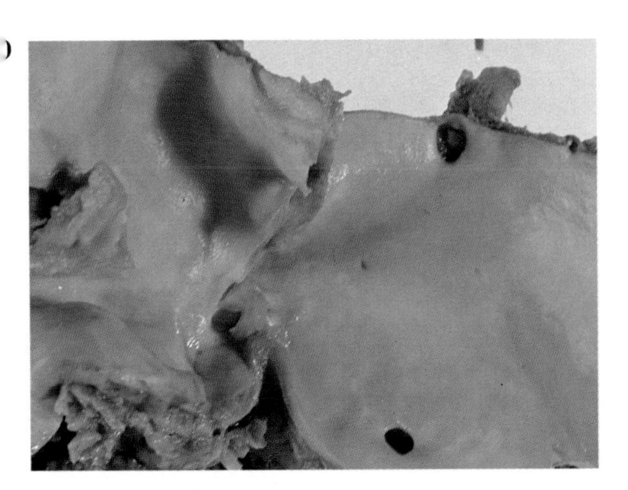

230 Coarctation of the aorta showing bacterial vegetations which grew *S. viridans*.

231

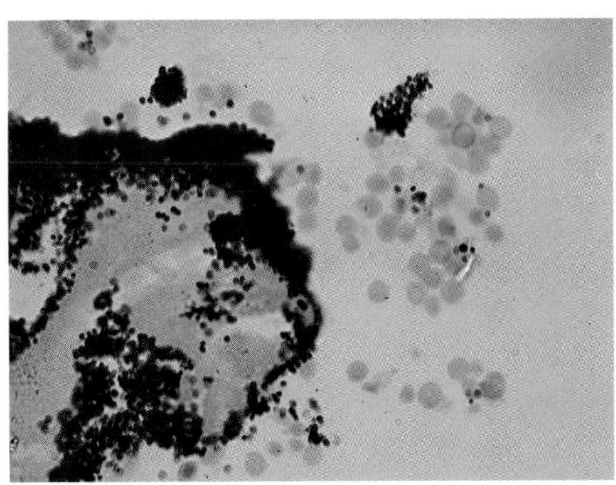

231 Gram-stain of bacterial vegetations on a valve showing gram-positive *S. viridans* infection (× *400*).

232

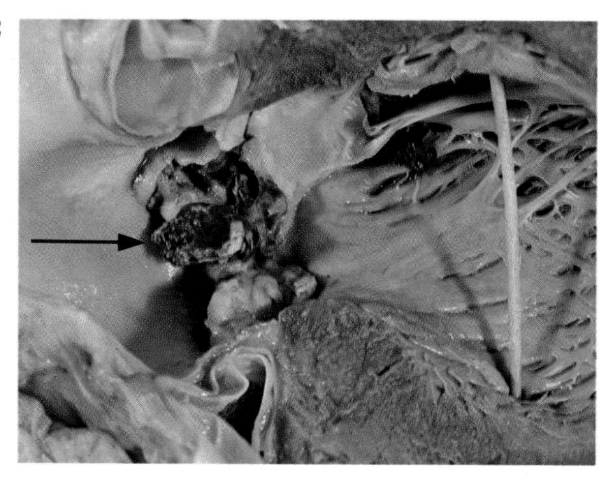

232 An aortic valve with vegetations growing on the valve cusps.

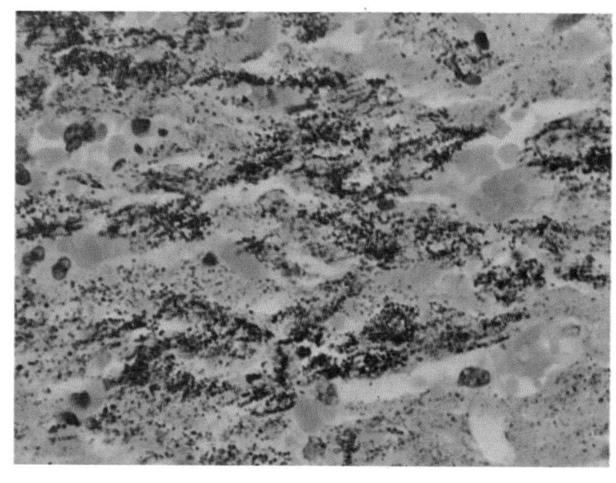

233 Gram-stain demonstrating *S. aureus* invading the myocardium (× *400*).

Table 18. Organisms Commonly Associated with SBE.

- *Streptococcus viridans*
- Coagulase-negative staphylococci
- *Haemophilus aphrophilus*
- *Enterococcus* spp.
- *Candida albicans*
- *Aspergillus* spp.

234

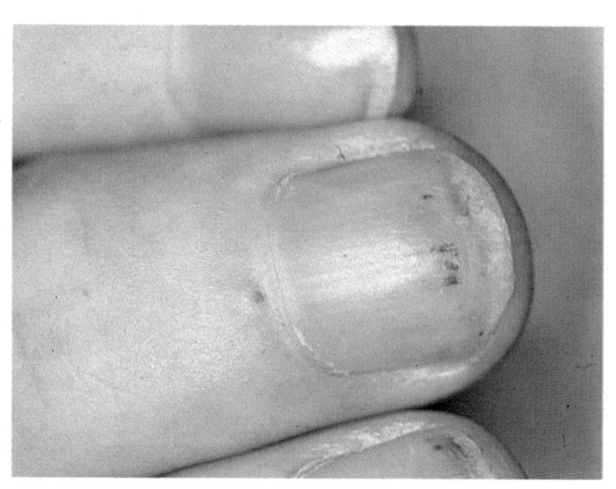

234 Splinter haemorrhages under the fingernail in a case of SBE.

many other organisms have been implicated (**232** & **233**), especially in relation to invasive procedures, prosthetic valves and in the immune-compromised child (**Table 18**).

The signs and symptoms of SBE may be very non-specific. There may be intermittent fever with weight loss, malaise and anaemia. Petechiae and splenomegaly may occur and infected microemboli may cause cerebral abscesses, mycotic aneurisms and haemorrhage. The classic skin manifestations, thought to be mediated by immune complexes, tend to develop late in the disease. They include splinter haemorrhages (**234**), which are found beneath the nails, and Osler's nodes, which are small, tender, intradermal nodules found on the tips of the fingers and toes. Such features are rare in children.

In suspected cases of SBE, a series of at least three separate blood cultures should be taken. The infective organism can be recovered in over 90% of cases. Echocardiography may be used to detect vegetations on abnormal valves (**235**), congenital anomalies or prosthetic valves (**236**). It may also be used to detect pericardial effusion, which may be of a purulent nature (**237**). An electrocardiogram and a plain chest X-ray (**238**) may also aid diagnosis. The ECG will show low voltage complexes across all standard chest leads (**239**).

A combination of antibiotics is always indicated. Penicillin G combined with an aminoglycocide is recommended. In cases of staphylococcal endocarditis, flucloxacillin and vancomycin may be substituted. Treatment should continue for at least 4–6 weeks. Serum bacteriocidal levels of antibiotics should be determined during the initial stages of treatment.

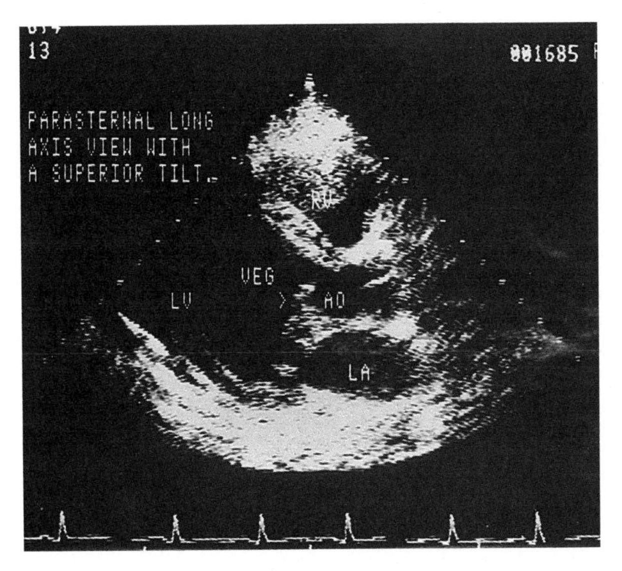

235 Echocardiogram showing bacterial vegetations on an aortic valve.

236

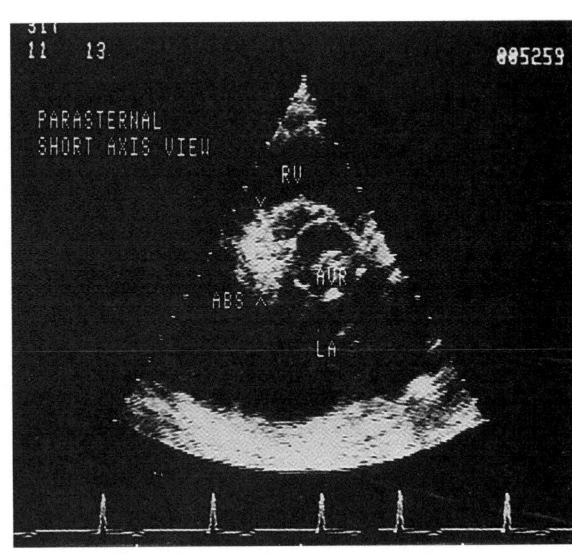

236 Echocardiogram showing bacterial vegetations on a prosthetic aortic valve.

237

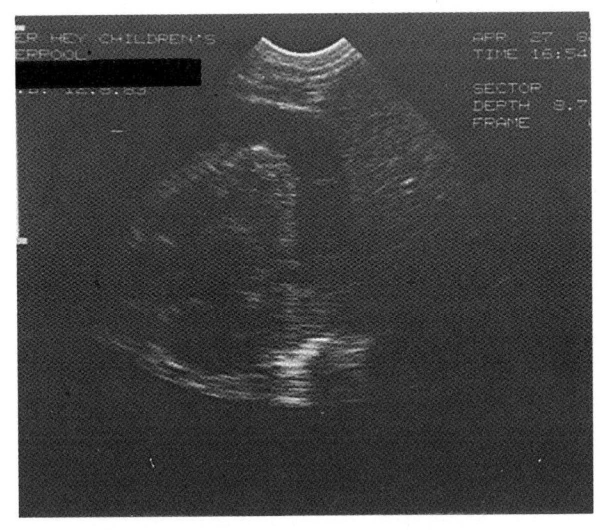

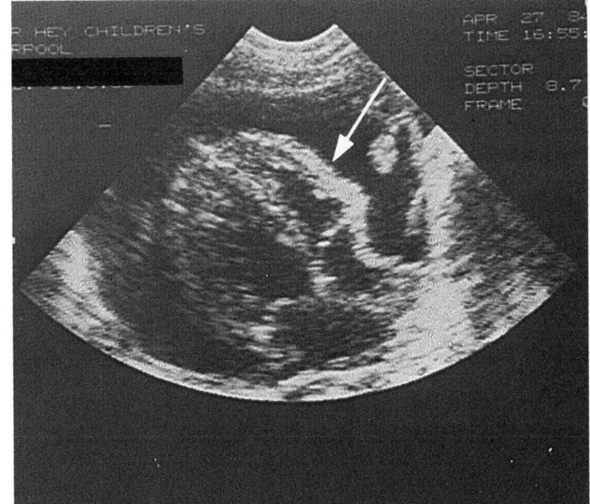

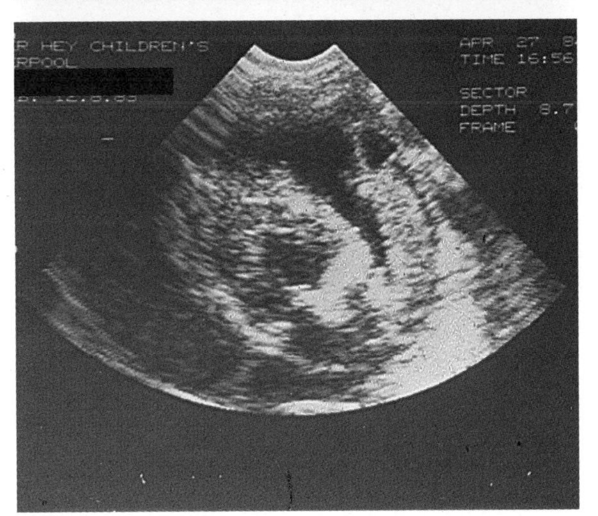

237 Echocardiogram of a pericardial effusion, clearly showing the heart surrounded by an effusion.

238

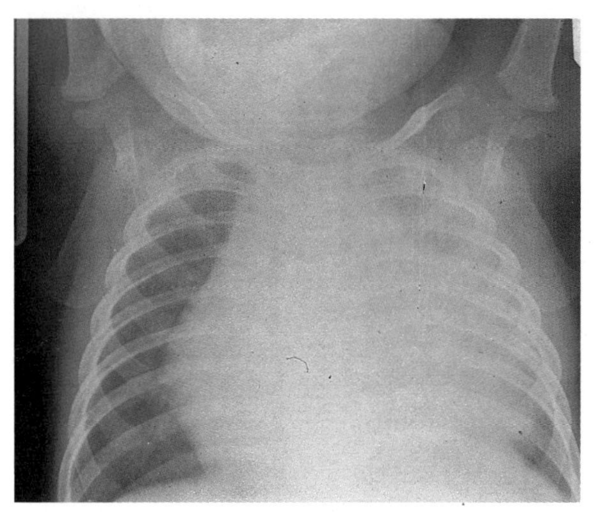

238 X-ray of a child with a purulent pericardial effusion.

239

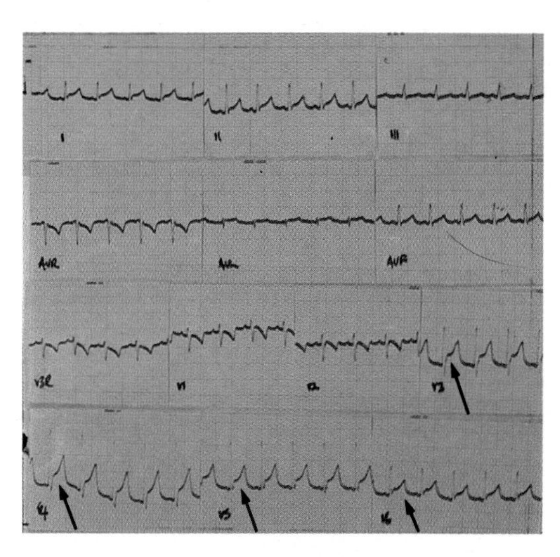

239 ECG of a child with purulent pericardial effusion, showing low-voltage complexes across all standard leads, and ST elevation.

Pericarditis

Pericarditis in children is usually a manifestation of a more generalized infection. It is an acute event, presenting clinically as an effusion of fluid in the pericardial cavity. Cardiac tamponade may occur due to the excess fluid (**240**).

Purulent pericarditis is usually a complication of secondary infection elsewhere, which may not be obvious. The organisms most commonly responsible are *Streptococcus pneumoniae*, *S. pyogenes* and *Staphylococcus aureus*. Occasionally, *Escherichia coli* and *Haemophilus influenzae* may cause infection. If cardiac tamponade occurs, surgical intervention with wide resection of the pericardium may be necessary (**241** & **242**).

240

241

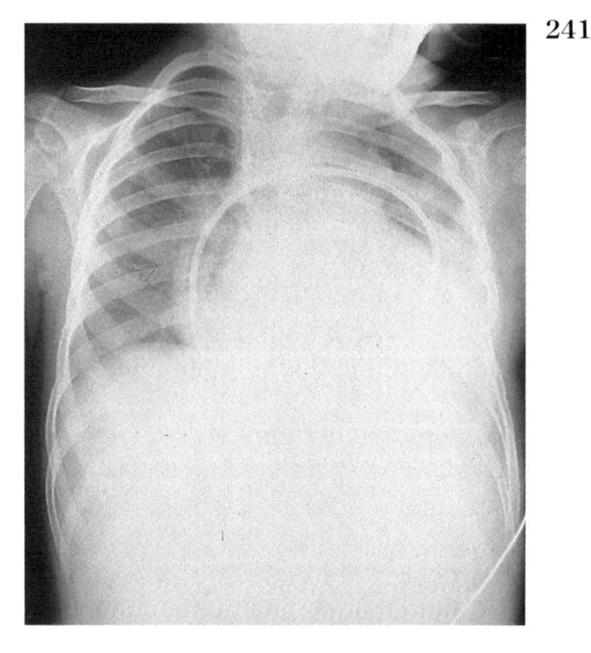

240 Echocardiogram showing cardiac tamponade with atrial collapse.

241 Chest X-ray of a child, demonstrating a pneumopericardium following aspiration of the purulent pericardial effusion.

242

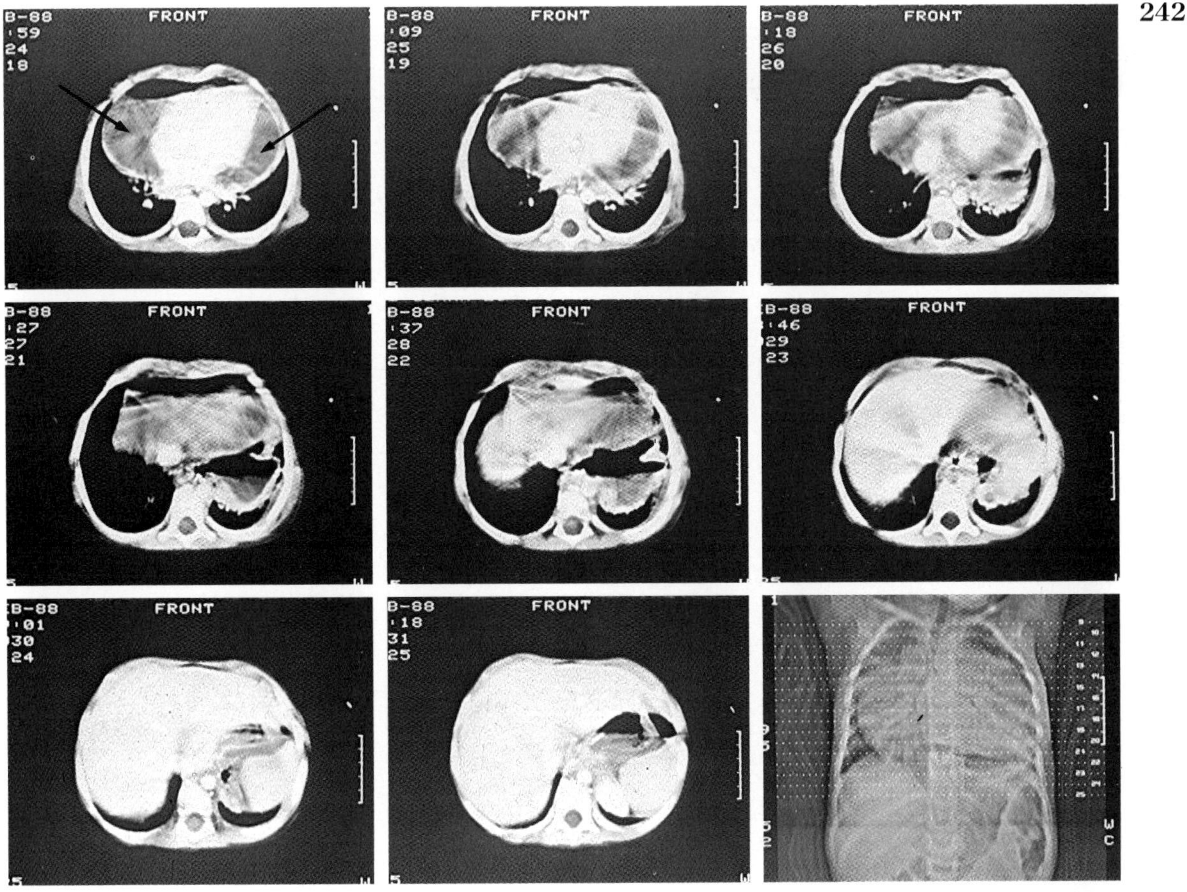

242 CT scan of the child shown in **241**, demonstrating gross purulent pericardial effusion following surgery for a hiatus hernia.

Viral pericarditis

Viral pericarditis is uncommon in children, but it can present in the neonatal period. It may be caused by enteroviruses including Coxsackie virus B4. Viral pericarditis usually takes a benign course but cardiac tamponade may occur.

A pericardial effusion may be seen on chest X-ray. An electrocardiogram may also be useful in diagnosis and it will usually show a raised ST segment concave upwards which is most obvious in the inferior leads (**243**).

243

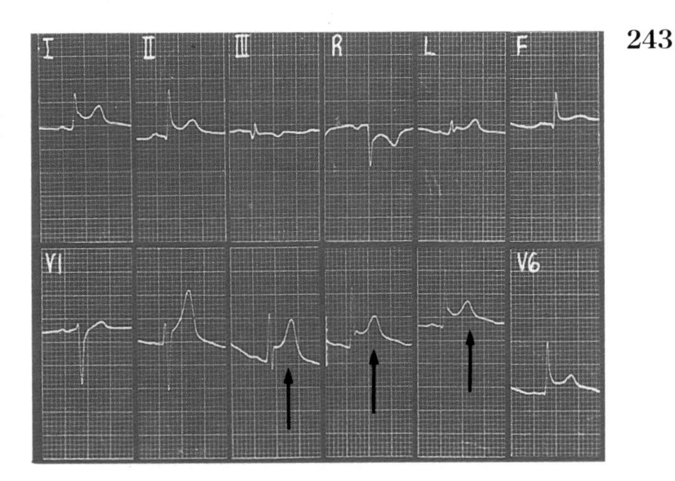

243 ECG of a child with pericarditis, demonstrating a raised ST segment concave upwards in the chest leads.

Myocarditis

Many infectious agents may cause myocarditis. These include bacteria, viruses, rickettsia and parasites.

Viral myocarditis

244

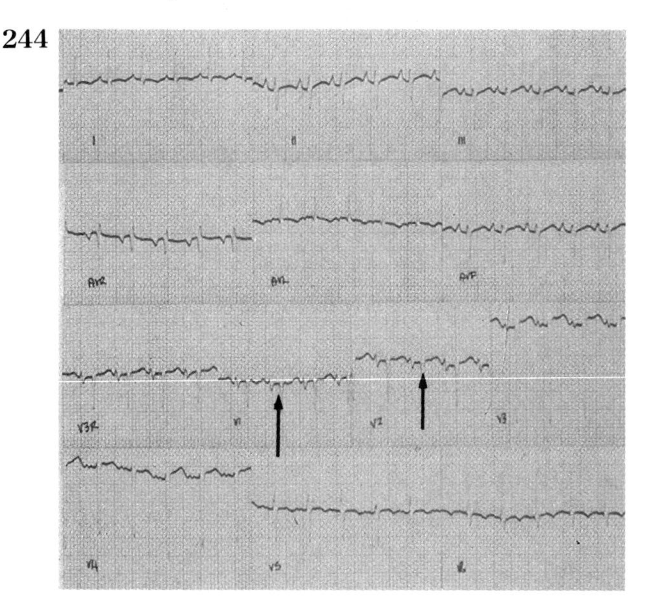

Several viruses have been shown to cause acute myocarditis. The enteroviruses Coxsackie virus A and B and ECHO virus have all been implicated in neonatal infections, which may be rapidly fatal. An electrocardiogram may be helpful in diagnosis. Typically, it will show T-wave inversion in chest leads associated with occasional ectopic beats (**244**).

244 ECG of a child with myocarditis, demonstrating T-wave inversion in chest leads.

Diphtheria and diphtheritic myocarditis

Diphtheria, which can damage the heart and peripheral nerves, together with the adrenals, kidneys and liver, is caused by an exotoxin liberated by the gram-positive bacillus, *Corynebacterium diphtheriae* (**245**). The bacterium usually colonizes the upper respiratory tract, but it occasionally infects the skin or the middle ear.

245

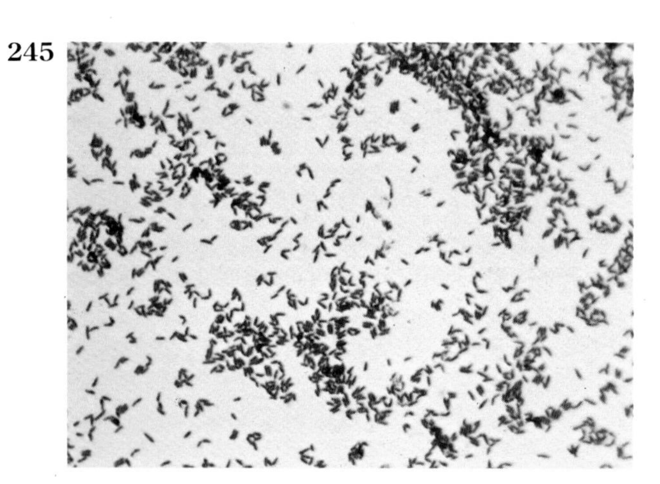

The exotoxin inactivates the peptide elongation factor, thus preventing protein synthesis, and has a direct action on the heart muscles, causing degeneration and necrosis.

The signs and symptoms of myocarditis often present in the second or third week following infection of the upper airways. The disease is characterized by a rapid pulse of low volume which may lead to congestive heart failure (**246**). Mortality can be as high as 40%. The toxin may also affect the Schwann cells, causing a polyneuritis which manifests as an upper motor neurone paralysis. It presents initially with nasal regurgitation of fluids, voice changes and a descending paralysis (**247** & **248**). If respiration can be maintained, the prognosis is ultimately good.

In order to identify those contacts who are susceptible to diphtheria a Schick test may be performed. The result will be positive in those without immunity.

245 Gram stain of *C. diphtheriae*. The characteristic pattern of 'chinese lettering' is clearly visible (× *1,000*).

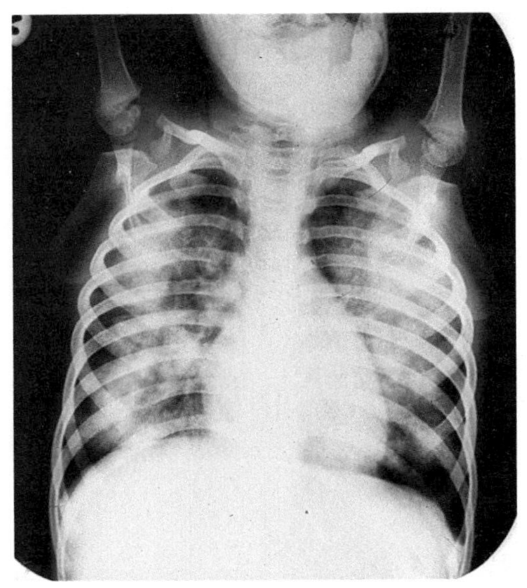

246 Chest X-ray showing pulmonary oedema due to diphtheritic myocarditis.

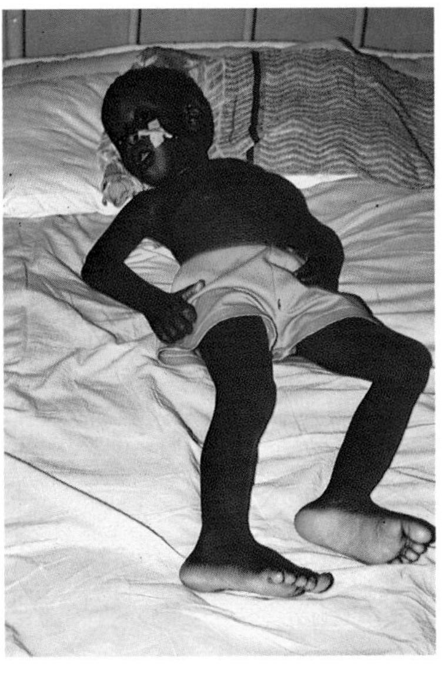

247 Diphtheritic polyneuritis in a Sudanese boy with a characteristic expressionless face and flaccid paralysis.

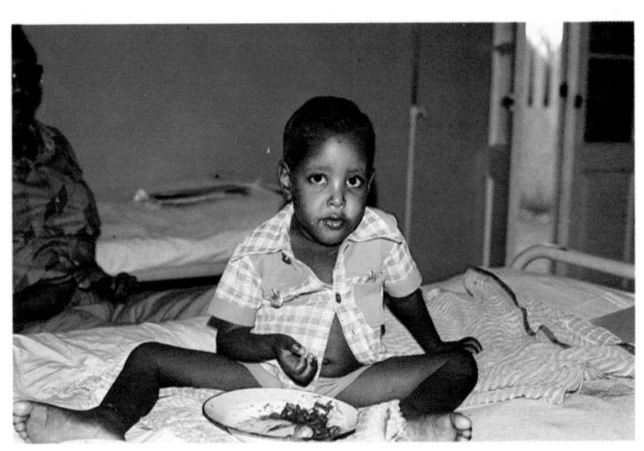

248 The same boy as shown in **247**, having recovered two weeks later.

Rheumatic fever

Rheumatic fever remains the most common infective cause of heart disease in children worldwide, although it is now rare in developed countries. Approximately 15% of the population have a genetically predisposed susceptibility to rheumatic fever. Infection with a group A β-haemolytic streptococcus (**249**) appears to sensitize the lymphocytes, which then form antibodies that crossreact with antigens on cardiac muscle. The signs and symptoms of rheumatic fever appear 3–4 weeks after a streptococcal pharyngitis, which may be inapparent.

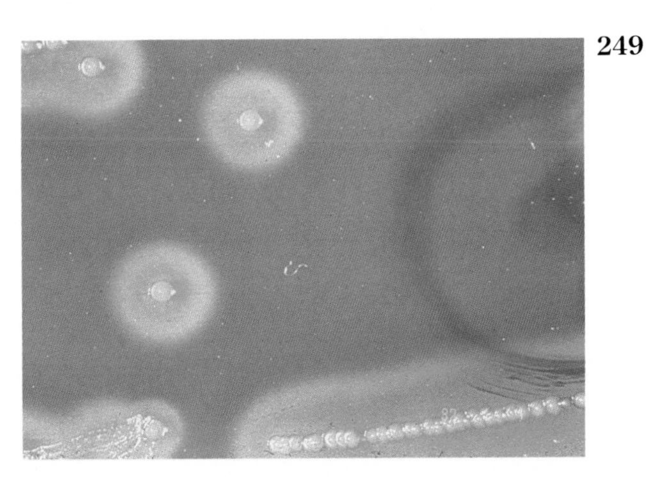

249 β-haemolytic streptococci demonstrating a zone of haemolysis on a blood agar culture plate.

250

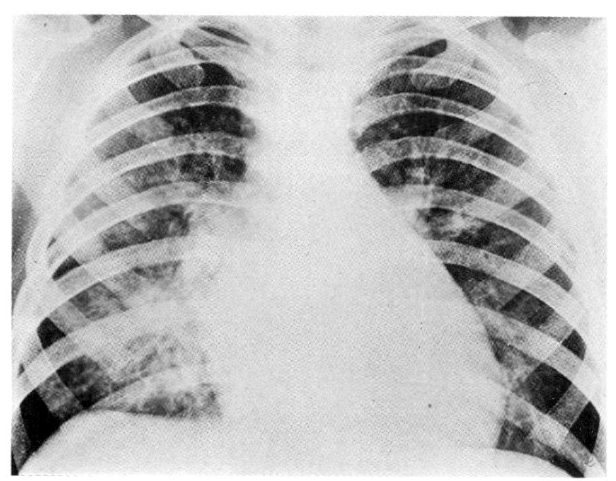

250 Chest X-ray showing cardiomegaly and pulmonary oedema due to rheumatic myocarditis.

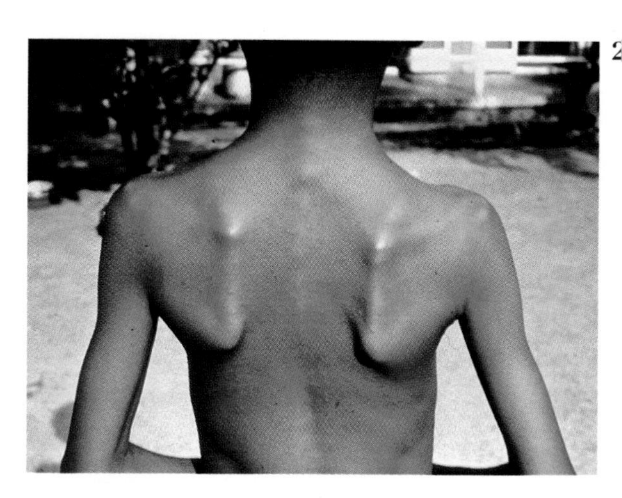

251 Rheumatic fever demonstrating rheumatic nodules over the scapula.

Because rheumatic fever may be confused with other causes of arthritis and fever, the modified Jones criteria are used to aid diagnosis (**Table 19**). Two major or one major and two minor criteria with supporting clinical evidence of infection should indicate rheumatic fever.

Although the clinical signs may be non-specific and subtle, the child may present with cardiomegaly (**250**), evidence of mitral or aortic incompetence, pericardial effusion or friction rub, and with heart failure. A painful arthritis may also occur. Usually more than one joint is affected, with the arthritis tending to migrate or 'flit' from joint to joint. The large joints, such as those of the ankles, hips and elbows, are most commonly affected. Subcutaneous nodules may be seen over the joints, on the back of the scalp, and down the spine (**251** & **252**). Erythema marginatum is a rare rash that usually appears on the trunk and limbs, sparing the face (**253**). Sydenham's chorea frequently occurs 2–3 weeks after the acute illness and may persist for several months. Involuntary movements (**254**) may be accompanied by emotional lability.

The mainstays of treatment for acute rheumatic fever are penicillin to eradicate any remaining streptococci, bedrest to avoid unnecessary heart strain, and salicylates to inhibit inflammation. At least 75 mg/kg of salicylates should be given daily in divided doses. Administration of the drugs should be continued for as long as is necessary or until the ESR becomes normal. Prednisolone may be used where there is active carditis or heart failure. There is no evidence that steroids reduce the risk of permanent damage to heart valves but they may shorten the patient's hospital stay.

Table 19. Major and Minor Clinical Manifestations of Rheumatic Fever According to the Modified Jones Criteria.*

Major manifestations	*Minor manifestations*
Polyarthritis (75%)	Fever
Carditis (40–50%)	Arthralgia
Sydenham's chorea (10%)	Previous history of rheumatic fever
Erythema marginatum (5%)	Raised erythrocyte sedimentation rate (ESR) or C-reactive protein
Subcutaneous nodules (1%)	Leucocytosis
	ECG changes
	Raised anti-streptolysin O titre
	Positive throat swab for group A β-haemolytic streptococcus

*It is usually accepted that a diagnosis can be made when two major, or one major and two minor criteria are fulfilled.

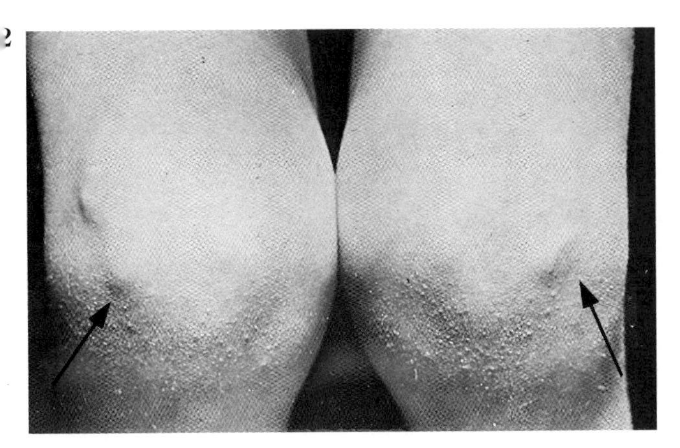

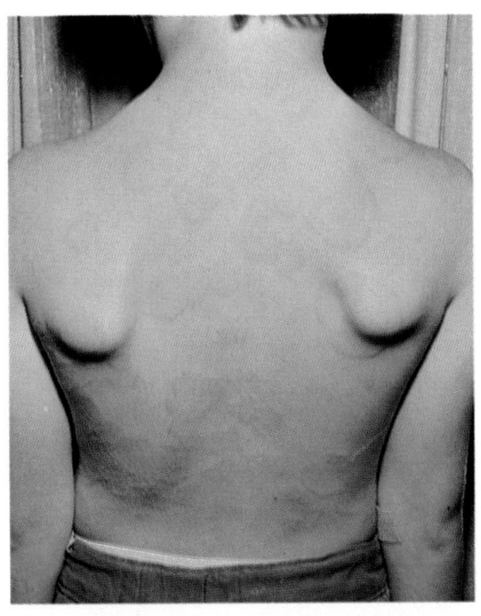

252 Rheumatic fever demonstrating rheumatic nodules over both knees.

253 Rheumatic fever with the characteristic rash of erythema marginatum.

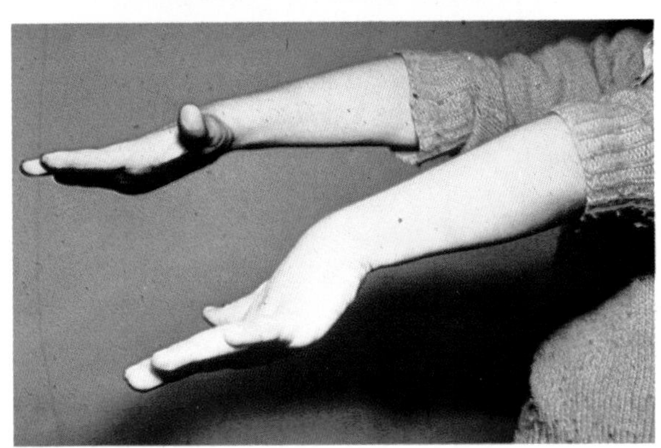

254 Rheumatic fever with Sydenham's chorea. The patient was unable to maintain extension of the arms and hands due to involuntary movements caused by the chorea.

Kawasaki disease (mucocutaneous lymph node syndrome)

Although no particular causative organism has been identified for Kawasaki disease, it has many of the epidemiological features of an infectious disease. Kawasaki disease is serious because it mainly affects children and, if untreated, more than 20% of cases will develop cardiac abnormalities. It has a fatality rate of about 1%. Approximately 80% of those affected are under 5 years of age, and boys are slightly more at risk than girls (in a ratio of 1.4:1). There is a greater risk for siblings, among whom the incidence is 2%, than for the general population and the incidence among Asians, especially those from Japan, is also markedly higher. Symptoms recur in 4% of children.

Several infectious agents have been suggested as causes of Kawasaki disease, for example Rickettsia spp., *Proprionabacterium acnes* and, more recently, retroviruses, but none has been conclusively implicated.

Table 20. Diagnostic Clinical Criteria for Kawasaki Disease.

- Presence of fever for >5 days
- Mucosal inflammation including sore/cracked lips, injected pharynx, or strawberry tongue
- Lymphadenopathy
- Polymorphic rash
- Bilateral conjunctivitis
- Characteristic changes in the peripheries: erythema of the palms and soles, desquamation of the fingers and toes, and peripheral non-pitting oedema

255

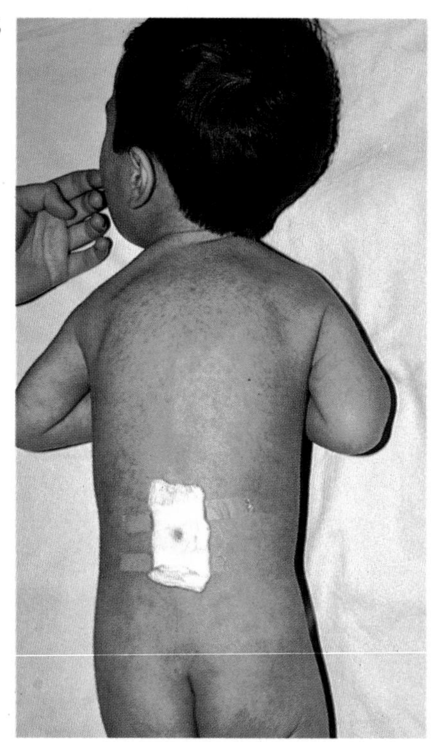

255 Kawasaki disease demonstrating the morbilliform rash that may simulate measles. A lumbar puncture was performed in this child and the CSF revealed features of aseptic meningitis.

Clinically, Kawasaki disease may present like measles. As a result criteria have been devised to differentiate the two diseases (**Table 20**). Kawasaki disease usually starts with a prodromal period of fever and irritability. A rash may then appear over the face, trunk and limbs. This may simulate a morbilliform rash and can be varied (**255** & **256**). A non-purulent conjunctivitis may also be apparent, another feature reminiscent of measles. Other characteristic clinical signs include a magenta colour of the lips, accompanied by fissuring of the angle of the mouth (**257**), and erythema of the palms of the hands and the soles of the feet, with dorsal oedema. The skin of the tips of fingers and toes peels during the convalescent phase (**258**). Other less common clinical manifestations may include those listed in **Table 21**.

Kawasaki disease is essentially a vasculitis that affects arteries including the coronary arteries. If left untreated, cardiac abnormalities may develop, the most serious of which are coronary aneurisms and myocardial infarction. Echocardiography is the most sensitive and specific investigation for detecting early abnormalities (**259**).

A thrombocytosis may occur, rising above $900,000 \times 10^9/l$. Treatment should be instituted as early as possible. Intravenous immunoglobulins are given in combination with initial high dose salicylates, which will significantly shorten the course of the disease and reduce the risk of cardiac damage.

256

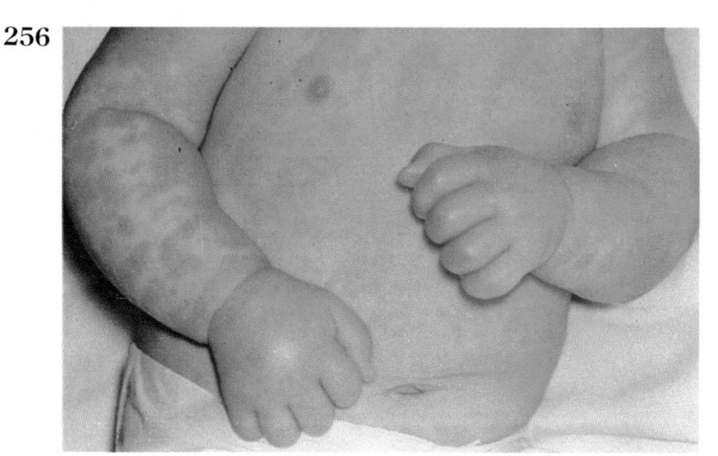

256 Kawasaki rash and oedema on the dorsal aspect of the hands.

2

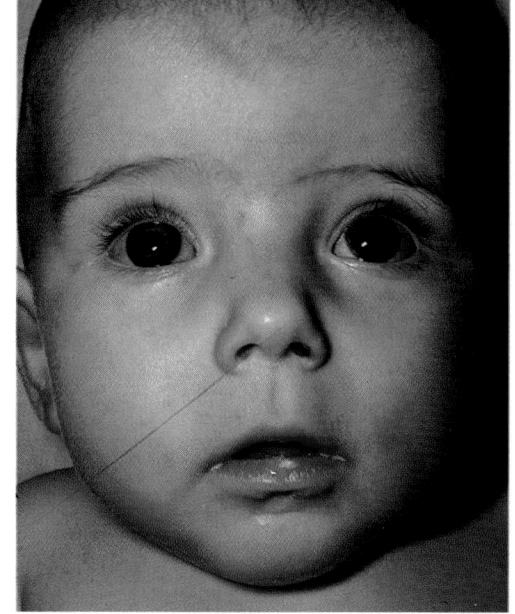

257 Kawasaki disease demonstrating erythema of the lips, with angular fissuring and a non-purulent conjunctivitis.

Table 21. Clinical Features Associated with Kawasaki Disease.

Cardiovascular	Coronary aneurysm Thrombosis of coronary arteries Pericardial effusion Myocarditis
Gastrointestinal	Diarrhoea Abdominal pain Hydrops of gall bladder Hepatitis (mild jaundice)
Respiratory	Cough Coryza X-ray changes
CNS	Aseptic meningitis Convulsions and coma VII cranial nerve palsy
Joint	Arthritis
Blood	Thrombocytosis Leukocytosis
Urine	Proteinuria Dysuria

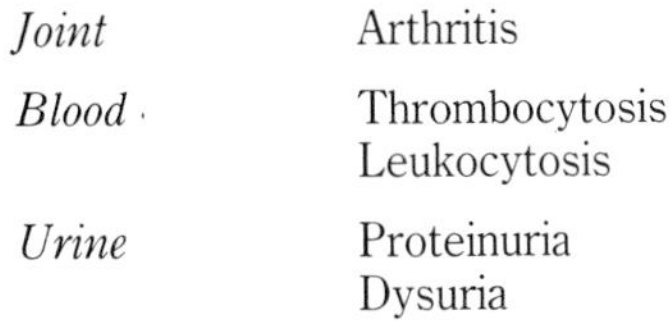

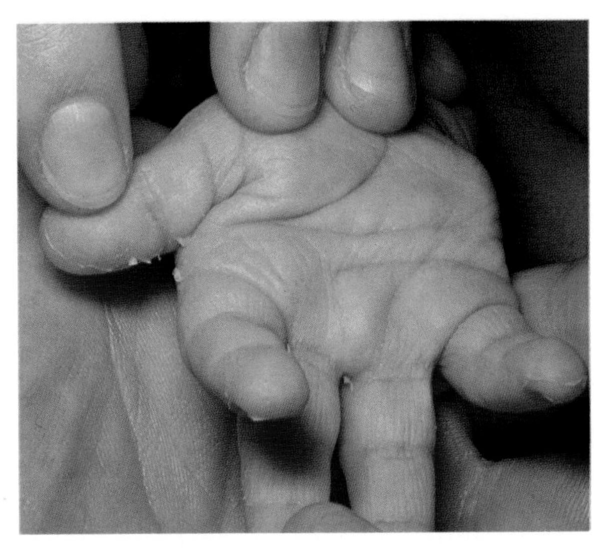

258 Kawasaki disease demonstrating peeling of skin from the tips of the fingers.

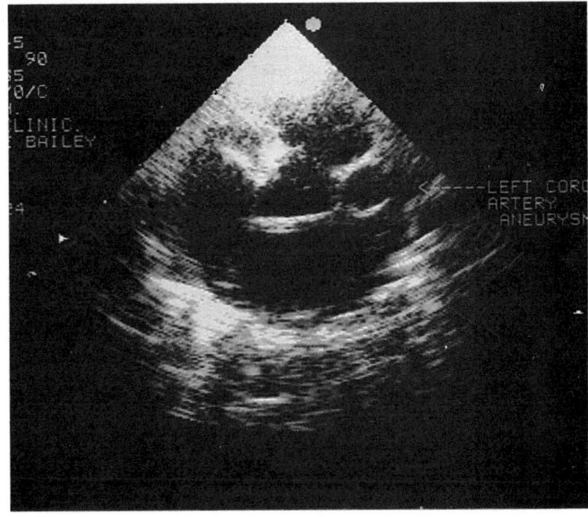

259 Echocardiogram showing a coronary artery aneurysm in the third week of Kawasaki disease.

Mediastinitis

Mediastinitis rarely occurs in the absence of traumatic injury to the oesophagus, trachea or a main bronchus. It may arise as a complication of endoscopy, surgery or an attempted tracheal intubation. Rupture may also occur as a result of removal of an impacted foreign body from the oesophagus (**260**).

The initial symptoms may be vague but they are usually marked by increasing discomfort and difficulty when swallowing or breathing. Occasionally, obstruction of the venous return may cause neck vein engorgement.

A chest X-ray will show a widening of the mediastinum (**261**). The trachea and oesophagus are displaced forward, and mediastinal emphysema may be noted. A pleural effusion or pyopneumothorax may occur.

Urgent treatment with parenteral broad-spectrum antibiotics is essential because rapid clinical deterioration is likely. If a mediastinal abscess forms, surgical drainage may be necessary.

260

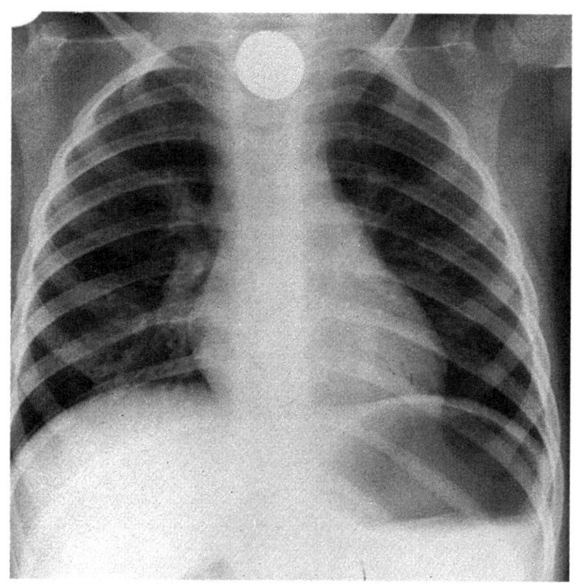

260 Chest X-ray showing a coin lodged in the oesophagus.

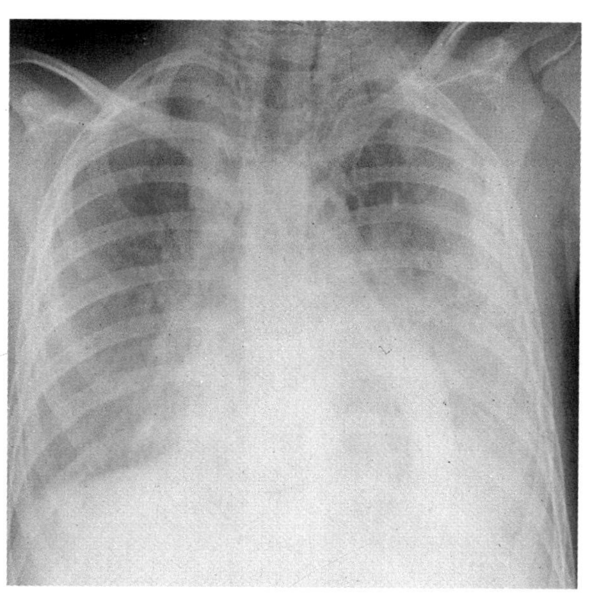

261 Chest X-ray of mediastinitis following oesophagoscopy, demonstrating widening and air in the mediastinum.

6 Infections of the nervous system

Central nervous system

Acute purulent meningitis

Although several different micro-organisms can produce purulent meningitis in neonates (**Table 22**), three bacteria, *Neisseria meningitidis*, *Haemophilus influenzae* and *Streptococcus pneumoniae*, are responsible for most cases outside the neonatal period. Infection causes inflammation of the meninges (principally the pia mater and arachnoid) leading to an inflammatory exudate in the CSF.

The pathogenesis of infection by the three bacteria is similar and in each case the bacteria are part of the normal nasopharyngeal flora. Rates of colonization with these pathogens vary with age, sex, geography and socioeconomic conditions. Bacteria translocate from the mucosa into the bloodstream. How and why is not clear but there is possibly a link with concurrent infection with upper respiratory tract viruses. The bacteraemia may then resolve spontaneously or may lead to organisms lodging in the meninges, thereby initiating an inflammatory response which is amplified by bacterial breakdown products such as peptidoglycan, teichoic acid, endotoxin and capsular polysaccharide, and by host factors such as tumour necrosis factor, interleukins 1 and 6, eicosanoids and platelet-activating factors.

The clinical features of meningitis include those of infection (e.g. fever, rigors) and of meningism (neck stiffness (**262**), Kernig's sign and photophobia). However, such features may not always be present and a high index of suspicion is required. Prior to attempting to obtain CSF by lumbar puncture, it is advisable to determine whether there is significantly raised intracranial pressure (**263**), since taking CSF under such circumstances can lead to coning. Signs of raised intracranial pressure include a bulging fontanelle, papilloedema, bradycardia and an altered state of consciousness.

Table 22. Pathogens in Meningitis.

	Purulent	*Lymphocytic*
Neonates	Group B streptococci *Listeria monocytogenes* *Eschericia coli* and other coliforms *Pseudomonas aeruginosa* *Candida albicans*	Herpes simplex Enteroviruses
Older Children	*Neisseria meningitidis* *Haemophilus influenzae* *Streptococcus pneumoniae* *L. monocytogenes* *Naegleria fowleri*	*Mycobacterium tuberculosis* *Leptospira* spp. *Treponema pallidum* *Borrelia* spp. Enteroviruses Mumps virus Anthropod-borne togaviruses Adenovirus Lymphocytic choriomeningitis virus Human immunodeficiency virus

262 A child with meningitis and neck stiffness.

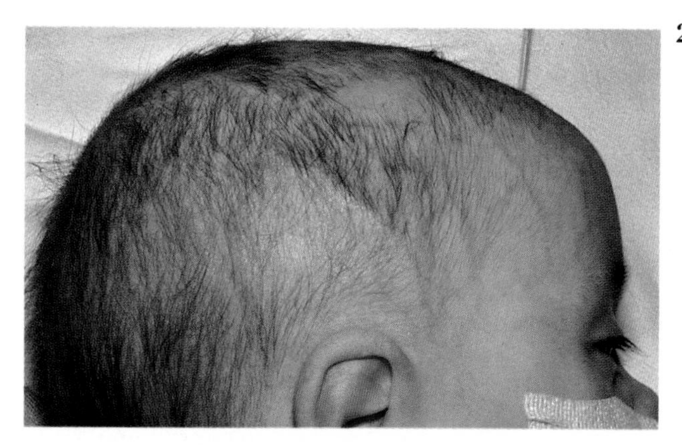

263 A child with meningitis. The bulging fontanelle is indicative of raised intracranial pressure.

Neisseria meningitidis

A gram-negative diplococcus, *Neisseria meningitidis* is the major cause of bacterial meningitis outside the neonatal period in England and Wales. The bacterium adheres to the nasopharyngeal mucosa using pili (**264**). In addition to pili, meningococci possess a polysaccharide capsule which renders the bacteria relatively insusceptible to phagocytosis. Epidemiologically, meningococci are subdivided into 8 different capsular serogroups (A,B,C,W135,X,Y,Z and 29E), and further subtyped according to their respective outer membrane proteins. Group A meningococci are responsible for the large spreading epidemics of disease that are seen particularly in sub-Saharan Africa, whereas Group B meningococci are responsible for the sporadic cases seen in the UK.

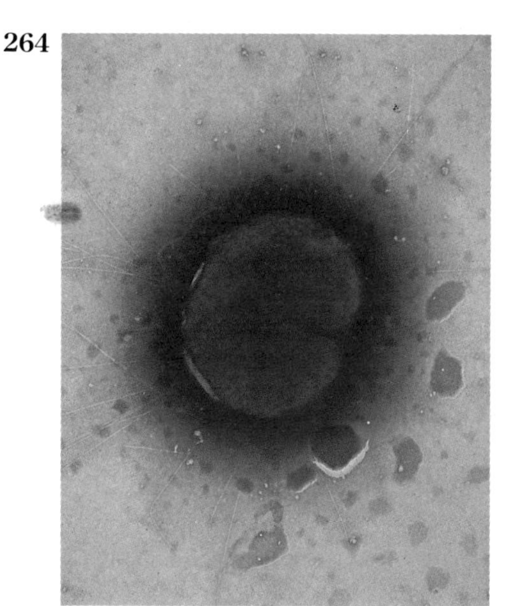

264 Negative-stain electron micrograph of *N. meningitidis* demonstrating pili (× *9,000*).

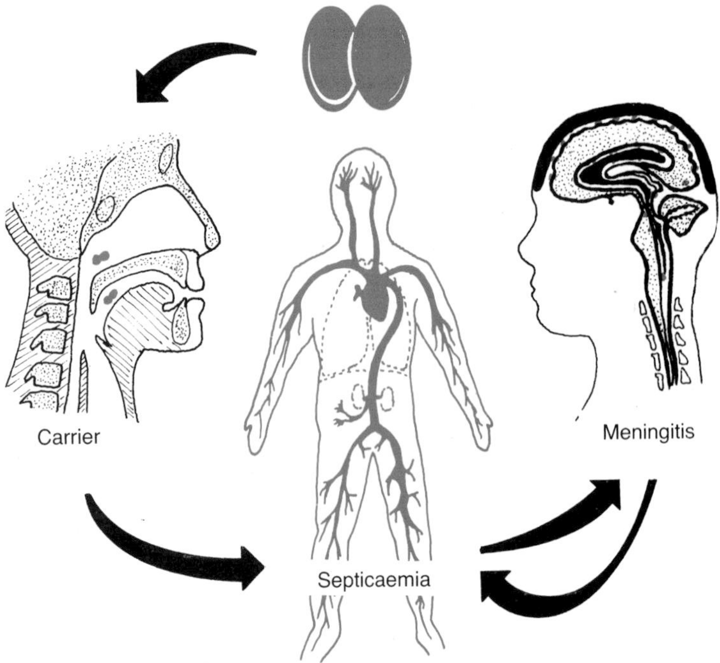

265 The pathogenesis of meningococcal disease.

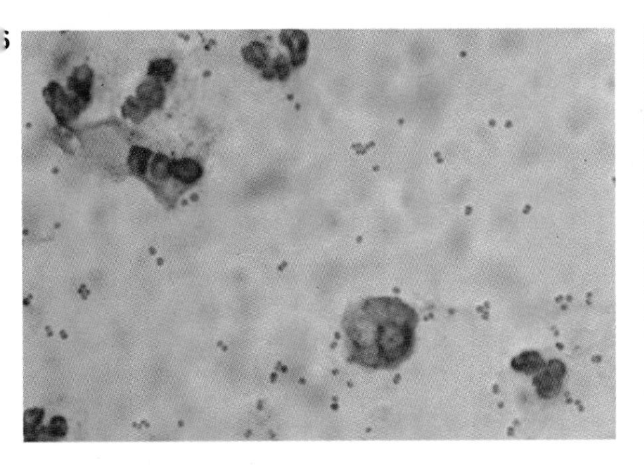

266 Gram-stained film of CSF from a child with meningococcal meningitis, demonstrating gram-negative cocci, pus cells and some intracellular meningococci (× *1,000*).

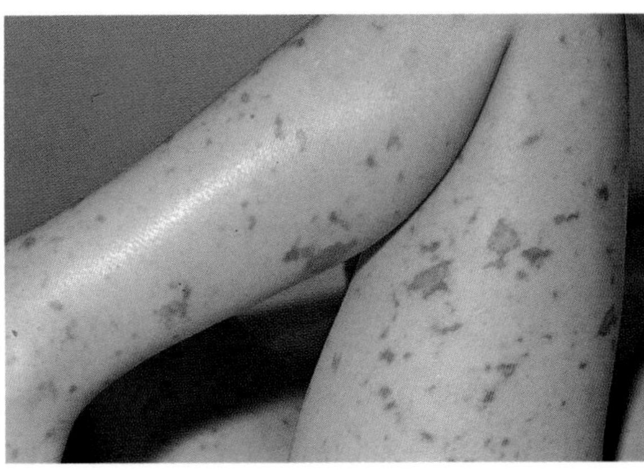

267 A child with a petechial rash and meningococcal septicaemia.

Between 5% and 40% of the population carry meningococci in the nasopharynx, from which the organisms translocate to produce a primary bacteraemia (**265**). This may then seed to the meninges to produce meningococcal meningitis (MM), in which there will be a purulent exudate, together with gram-negative diplococci both inside neutrophils and extracellularly (**266**). MM generally has a good prognosis with a mortality rate of less than 1%.

In certain patients the primary bacteraemia leads to fulminant meningococcal septicaemia. In such cases, there are rarely signs of meningitis, the CSF is usually not purulent and bacteria are not present. Patients present with a petechial (**267**) or maculopapular (**268**) rash which can evolve over a very short period of time to become purpuric (**269**) and ecchymotic (**270**). The rash is due to haemorrhage from capillaries and occurs throughout the body, affecting mucous membranes (**271**) and the adrenals (**272**), and producing the Waterhouse–Friderichsen syndrome. Its pathogenesis

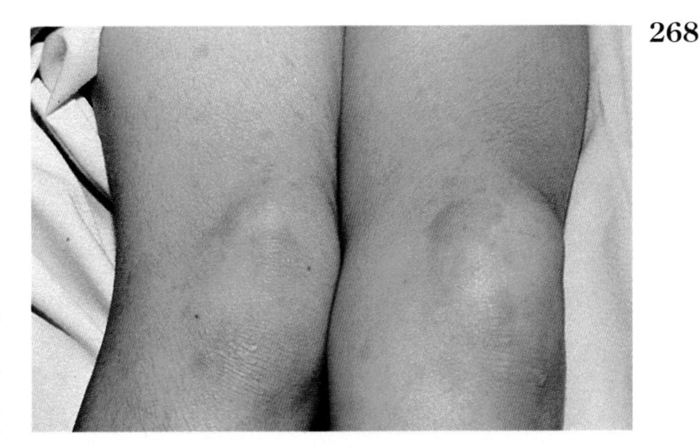

268 Maculopapular rash in a child with meningococcal disease.

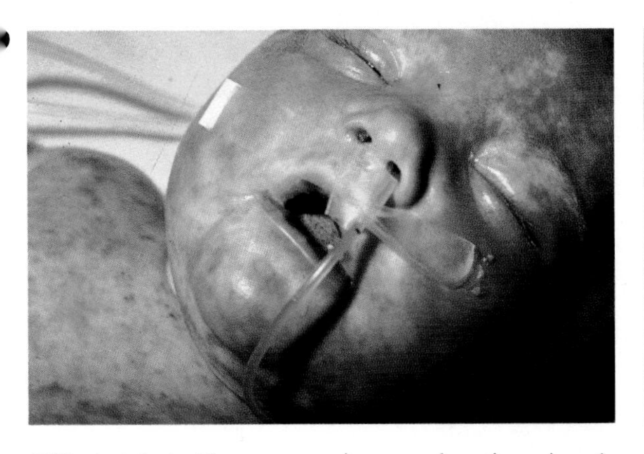

269 An infant with severe meningococcal septicaemia and a widespread purpuric rash.

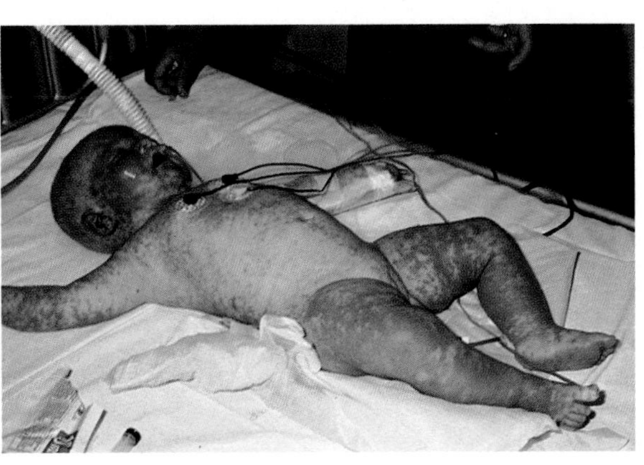

270 An infant with severe meningococcal septicaemia and extensive ecchymoses on both legs.

depends upon both the host and bacterial factors. Patients with defects in the final components of the complement cascade (C6,7,8) and in properdin are at greater risk of developing the disease.

Fulminant meningococcal septicaemia is apparently caused by the release of endotoxin. The outer membrane of all gram-negative bacteria has a high content of lipopolysaccharide or endotoxin, and certain bacteria, such as the meningococci, continually 'bleb' part of their outer membrane (**273**). Thus, large amounts of endotoxin are released into the circulation. Endotoxin then initiates a whole series of activities including capillary endothelial damage, activation of Hageman factor, disseminated intravascular coagulation, secretion of tumour necrosis factor, and shock.

The mortality from fulminant meningococcal septicaemia can be as high as 70%, and affected patients will require transfer to an intensive care unit and ventilatory support. In addition, a proportion of patients who develop MM may get a secondary bacteraemia (from the meninges) which precipitates meningococcal septicaemia. These patients are also at great risk of fatal disease.

Among the complications of meningitis are the development of hydrocephalus, neurological problems including ataxia and paralysis, and visual problems. Persistent hearing deficit is a major complication and it has been shown that endotoxin has a direct effect upon labyrinthine cells. Arthritis may develop before, during or after the illness. However, it most frequently occurs afterwards due, it is thought, to an immune phenomenon since the fluid is invariably sterile. Those who survive fulminant meningococcal septicaemia may develop gangrene of the skin (**274**) or even of the limbs.

The treatment of meningitis involves the use of bactericidal antibiotics that can cross into the CSF in therapeutic concentrations. Currently, most meningococci are sensitive to penicillin, chloramphenicol and cefotaxime, all of which achieve therapeutic levels in CSF. Some low-level resistance to penicillin has been reported from several countries.

Close family contacts of patients with meningococcal disease are 400–700 times more likely to develop meningococcal infection than the rest of the population. Thus chemoprophylaxis with rifampicin (or tetracycline or ciprofloxacin in adults) is indicated.

Polysaccharide vaccines are available for prevention of infection due to Group A and C meningococci. Unfortunately, Group B capsule (a homopolymer of N-acetyl neuraminic acid) is a self antigen (on neuronal tissue) and no vaccine is available.

271

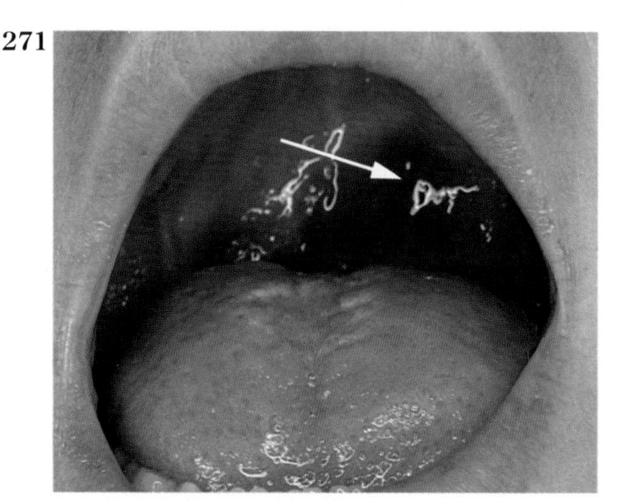

271 Large palatal haemorrhage in a child with meningococcal septicaemia.

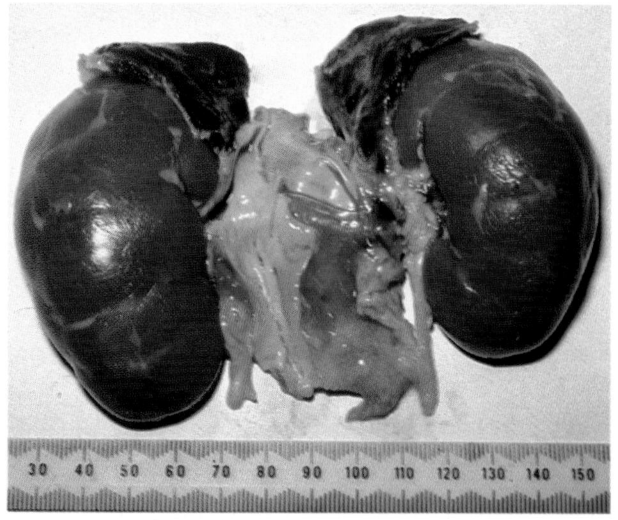

272 The kidneys and adrenals of a child who died from meningococcal septicaemia. The adrenals show gross haemorrhage.

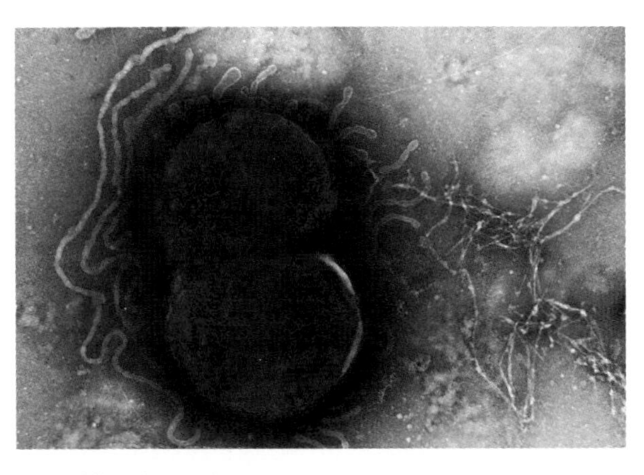

273 Negative-stain electron micrograph of *N. meningitidis*, showing the release of outer membrane containing large amounts of endotoxin (× *10,000*).

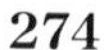

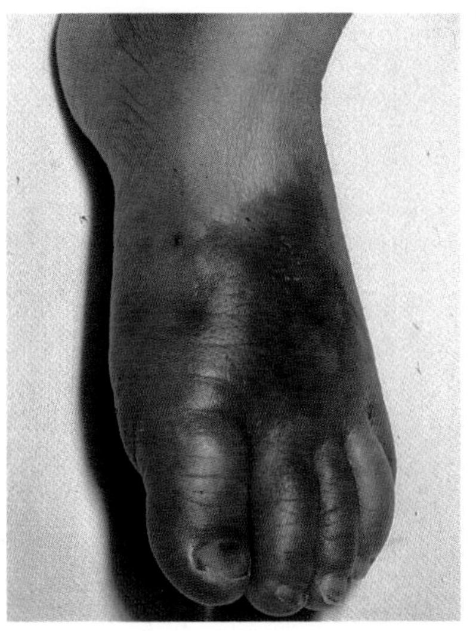

274 Early gangrene of the skin of the foot in a child who had recovered from meningococcal septicaemia.

Haemophilus influenzae

Haemophilus influenzae, a pleomorphic gram-negative coccobacillus (**275**), is the second most common cause of bacterial meningitis in children in the UK. In certain countries, e.g. the USA and Australia, it is the most common cause. The most pathogenic isolates are capsulate. There are six capsular serotypes (a–f) but type b is the major invasive pathogen. Invasive infection in children over 7 years of age is rare. The presentation of *H. influenzae* meningitis is similar to that of meningitis due to other agents. Although a disease similar to meningococcal septicaemia can occur with *H. influenzae*, it is uncommon. The mortality from *H. influenzae* meningitis (up to 12%) is higher than that for MM and up to 29% of survivors have severe to significant handicap.

Treatment can pose problems. Up to 10% of *H. influenzae* isolates are resistant to ampicillin, 5% to chloramphenicol, and some are resistant to both. However, to date, all isolates are sensitive to cefotaxime. The course of infection can be eventful. By day 4 or 5 a proportion of those infected develop pyrexia which, in some, is due to subdural effusions (**276**). As with meningococcal disease, chemoprophylaxis for family contacts is indicated for *H. influenzae* meningitis. A capsular polysaccharide (polyribitol)–protein conjugate vaccine has proved effective in preventing disease.

275

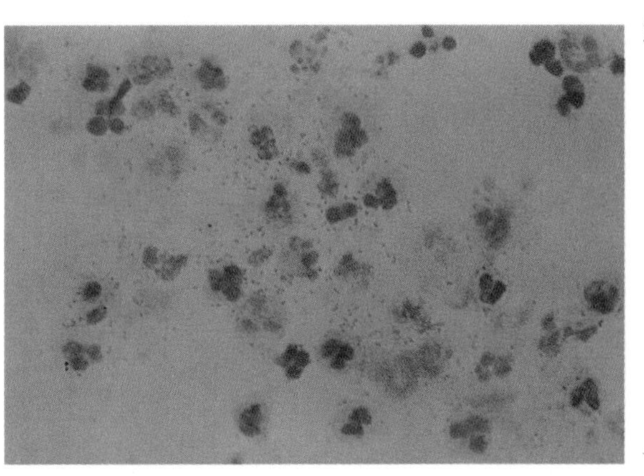

275 Gram-stained film of CSF showing *H. influenzae* (small pleomorphic gram-negative coccobacilli) and pus cells (× *1,000*).

276

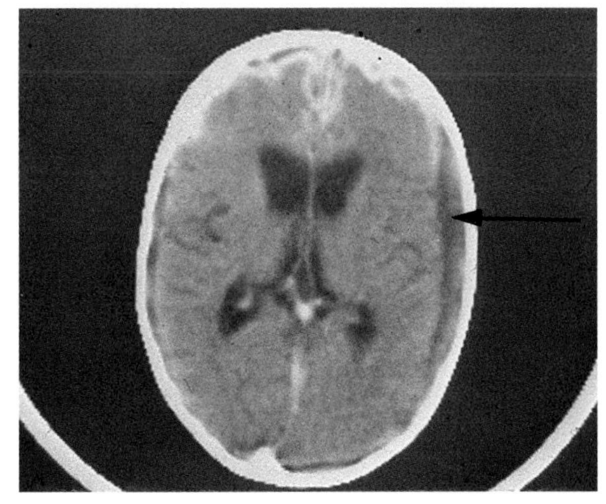

276 CT scan of the skull of a child with *H. influenzae* meningitis, showing a subdural effusion.

Streptococcus pneumoniae

Streptococcus pneumoniae, a capsulate gram-positive diplococcus (**277**), is not a common cause of meningitis in children in developed countries but is very common in developing countries. The pathogenesis is as for *N. meningitidis* and *H. influenzae*. However, recurrent pneumococcal meningitis can occur in association with cryptic fractures of the base of the skull (**278**), which allow nasopharyngeal flora direct access to the subarachnoid space. Most pneumococci are sensitive to penicillin, although there does seem to be a gradual increase in resistance. All are sensitive to cefotaxime. Chemoprophylaxis in close contacts is not indicated. There are over 80 different pneumococcal capsular serotypes, but certain serotypes (e.g. 1,3,6,7) are more often implicated in invasive disease. A vaccine incorporating the 23 most commonly occurring serotypes has been produced.

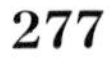

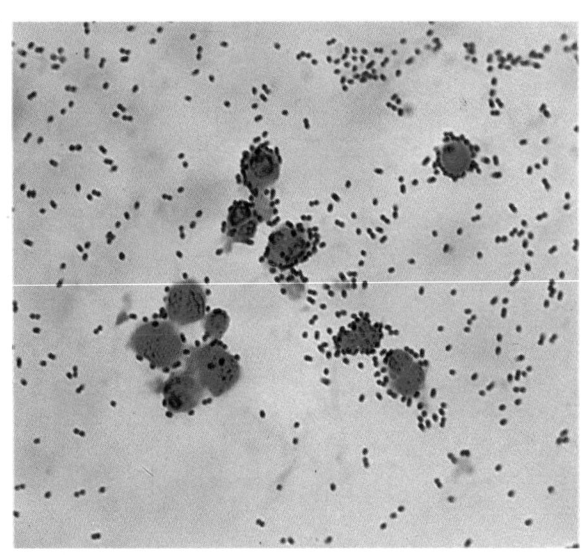

277 Gram-stained film of CSF from a child with pneumococcal meningitis, showing pus cells and gram-positive diplococci (× *1,000*).

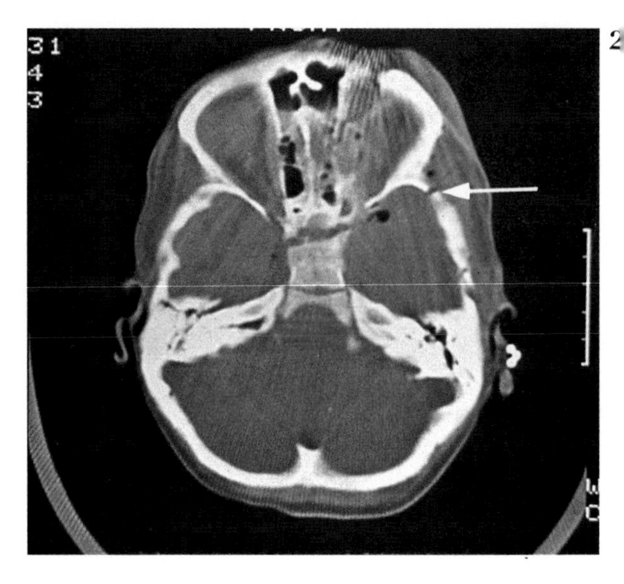

278 CT scan of a skull with a fracture of the base.

Rapid diagnosis of bacterial meningitis

279

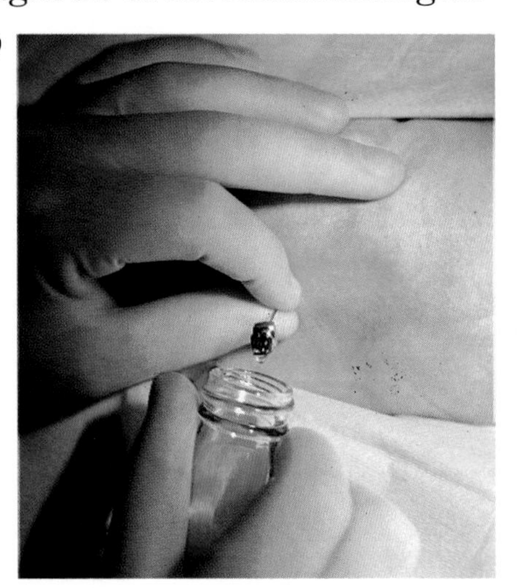

279 Lumbar puncture being performed.

Although it is possible to detect bacteria or their antigens in blood, the definitive aetiological diagnosis of bacterial meningitis depends upon examination of CSF. If intracranial pressure is not significantly raised, CSF is usually obtained by lumbar puncture (**279**). The fluid is then examined for the changes described in **Table 23**. Gram film will give an aetiological diagnosis in up to 80% of cases. Countercurrent immunoelectrophoresis (CIE) (**280**) and latex particle agglutination (**281**) are sensitive, specific and rapid adjuncts to diagnosis.

Table 23. Cerebrospinal Fluid.

	Normal	*Purulent meningitis*	*Aseptic meningitis*
Volume	40–120 ml		
Appearance	Clear	Turbid	Clear to opalescent
Pressure	<180–200 mmH_2O	Raised	Normal
Protein	0.15–0.4 g/l	0.5–6.0 g/l	0.5–1.0 g/l[b]
Mononuclear cells	0–5×10^6/l	Can be raised	15–500×10^6/l
Neutrophils	0	100–3,000×10^6/l	Occasional
Glucose[a]	2.2–3.3 mmol	0–2.2 mmol	2.2–3.3 mmol

[a] Must be compared with blood glucose (about 60% blood glucose level in CSF normally).
[b] In tuberculous meningitis the protein concentration is usually high.

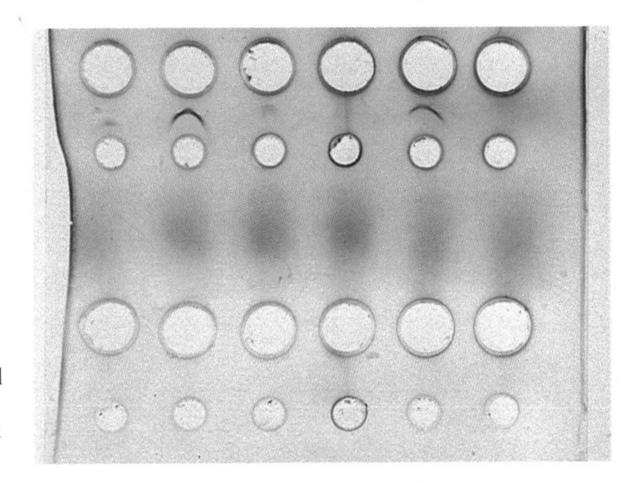

280 The results of countercurrent immunoelectrophoresis. The blue bands between the small and large wells are precipitin lines. These indicate that antigens reactive with the specific antiserum are present in CSF.

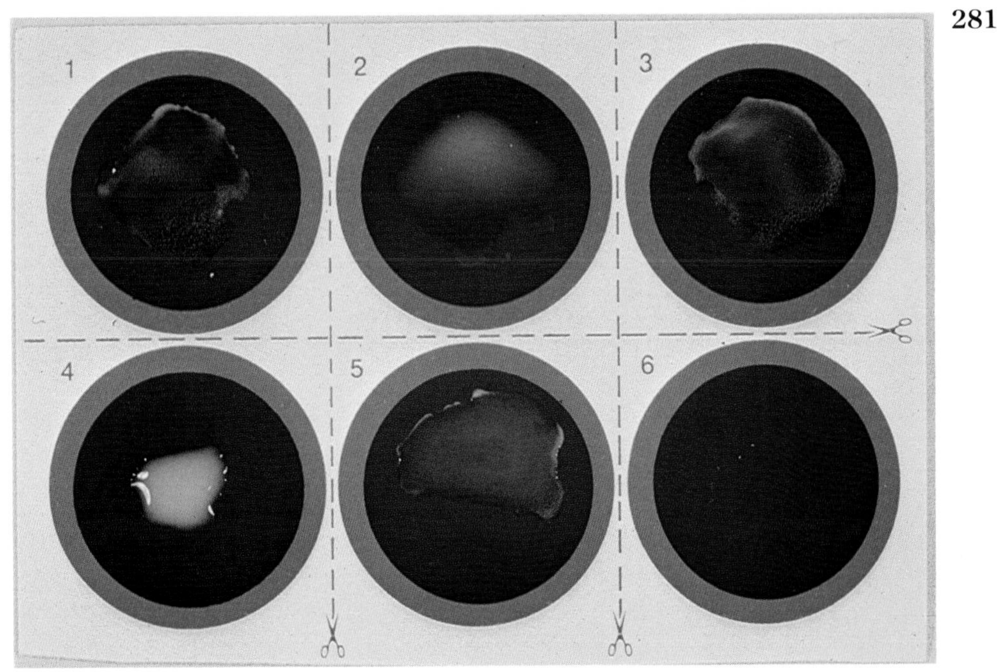

281 A latex particle agglutination test. Samples 1, 3 and 5 are positive.

Acute lymphocytic meningitis

No accurate figures are available for the incidence of viral meningitis. The spectrum of infection ranges from mild, transient headaches, in which cases patients are unlikely to visit their doctor, through to full-blown meningitis. The CSF of affected patients is clear to opalescent (**Table 23**) and contains an excess of lymphocytes ($100–500 \times 10^6/l$), although in early infection there may also be low numbers of polymorphs. CSF glucose is normal (since it is not being utilized by neutrophils), as is the protein level. The two major pathogens involved are enteroviruses (in summer) and mumps virus (in winter).

Enteroviruses

Enteroviruses comprise a large group of small (25–30 nm) unenveloped cuboidal RNA viruses. Infection with echoviruses (e.g. Echo 7 or 30) and Coxsackie viruses (e.g. A9 or B2) is associated with meningitis, meningoencephalitis and encephalitis. They account for up to 85% of cases. Transmission is faeco-oral, with virus replicating initially in the pharynx and intestinal tract. It is the exception rather than the rule for meningitis to occur. Meningitis can occur in association with specific enteroviral syndromes, such as herpangina, but this is also exceptional. There is no specific therapy nor is a vaccine available for prevention of infection.

Mumps virus

282

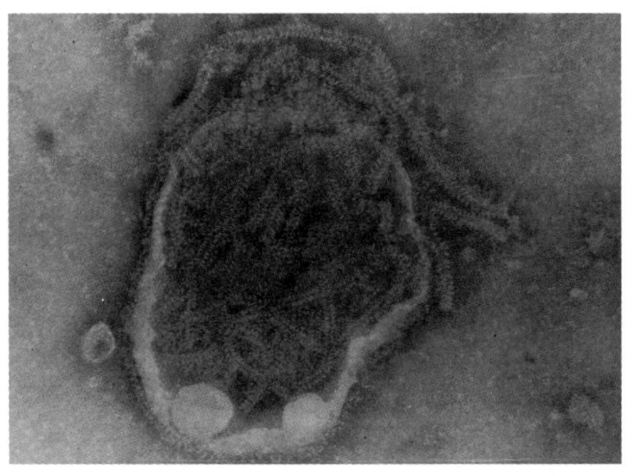

282 Negative-stain electron micrograph of mumps virus, demonstrating the herringbone-like RNA nucleocapsid (× *25,000*).

The childhood disease of mumps is caused by an enveloped RNA virus (**282**). Estimates of the proportion of cases of mumps infection in which meningitis occurs vary from 1–50%. 1–10% of patients with parotitis develop meningitis but 35–50% of those with mumps meningitis do not have parotitis. Meningeal infection occurs far more commonly in boys than in girls. Meningeal signs may precede or follow parotitis. There is no specific therapy but live attenuated virus is included in measles, mumps and rubella (MMR) cover given at one year of age. The prognosis is good, with unilateral deafness occurring in one in 20,000 cases of mumps meningitis.

Lymphocytic choriomeningitis

Lymphocytic choriomeningitis virus (an arenavirus) is a rare cause of meningitis. It is an enveloped RNA virus (110–130nm) which contains ribosomal particles (**283**), giving it a granular appearance (*arena* is Latin for sand). An inapparent persistent pathogen in mice and hamsters, it is excreted in urine and may be accidentally transmitted to humans. The disease is apparently immune mediated, involving cytotoxic T cells and natural killer (NK) cells. Person-to-person spread has not been documented.

283

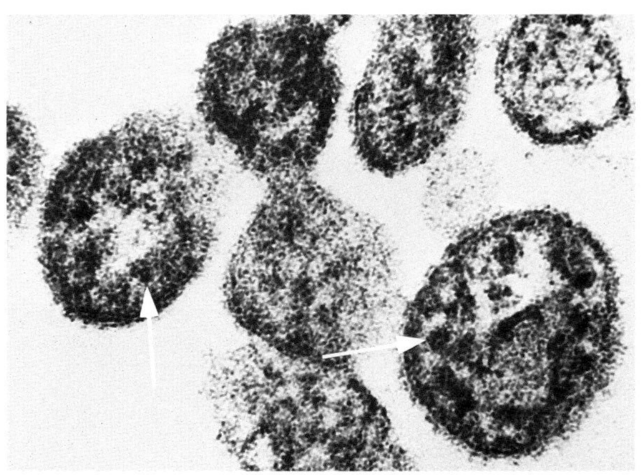

283 Thin-section transmission electron micrograph of an arenavirus, demonstrating ribosomal particles inside its lipid envelope (× *200,000*).

Other agents

The spirochaetes (**284**) *Treponema pallidum* (syphilis) and *Borrelia burgdorferi* (Lyme disease) are both causes of acute lymphocytic meningitis. In the case of syphilis, meningitis generally occurs in the secondary stage. Lyme disease is transmitted by ticks. Although meningeal irritation is common in the early stages, infection is uncommon in children. Penicillin is the treatment of choice.

Leptospira spp., which are also finely coiled spirochaete bacteria, 6–20μm long (**285**), can also be responsible for acute aseptic meningitis. The organisms are excreted in animal urine (e.g. *L. icterohaemorrhagiae* from rats, *L. hardjo* from cattle, and *L. canicola* from dogs). Infection in children generally follows recreational exposure to contaminated water (e.g. fishing, canoeing). The disease occurs in two phases. In the initial phase bacteraemia develops 7–12 days after infection, presenting with high fever, muscle and abdominal pains, and chills. *Leptospira* can be cultured from CSF but there are usually no signs of meningism. The disease then shows clinical improvement, but relapses 2–3 days later with meningitis and, if severe, with hepatic (Weil's disease) and renal involvement. This second phase is apparently immune mediated. It is unlikely that *Leptospira* spp. will be cultivated from CSF at this stage but diagnosis can be made using urine culture and measurement of antibody levels. Treatment with penicillin is of value only in the initial septicaemic phase, not in the meningitic phase.

It must be remembered that partially treated bacterial meningitis may present as an aseptic meningitis. Antigen detection plays a central role in the diagnosis of this condition (**280** & **281**).

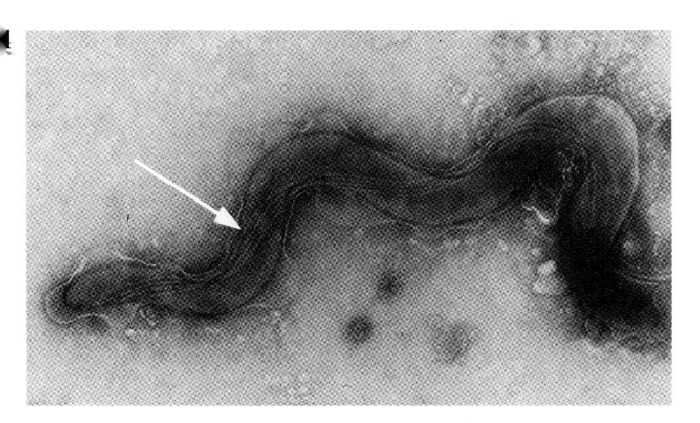

284 Negative-stain electron micrograph of *T. pallidum*, demonstrating flagellae (× *3,000*).

285

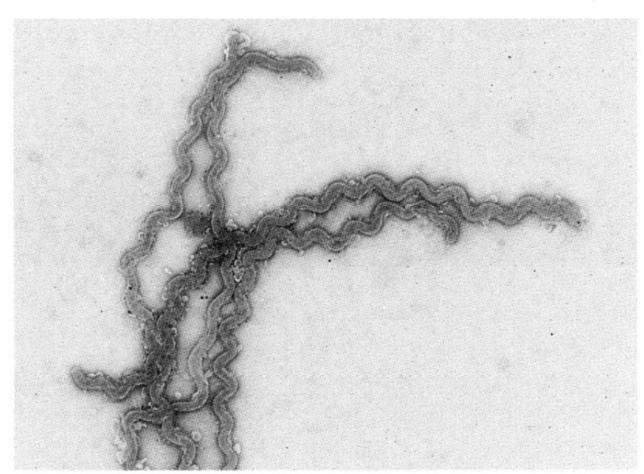

285 Negative-stain electron micrograph of *L. canicola* (× *1,000*).

Chronic meningitis

The aetiology of chronic meningitis is shown in **Table 24**. Typically, the disease develops over a period of 1–2 weeks and the features persist and progress. In certain cases the disease is linked to some form of immune deficit (e.g. *Cryptococcus neoformans* in AIDS), but in others it is due to a primary pathogen, for example *Mycobacterium tuberculosis* or *Brucella abortus*.

Table 24. Pathogens in Chronic Meningitis.

Bacteria	*Fungi*	*Parasites*
Mycobacterium tuberculosis	*Cryptococcus neoformans*	*Toxoplasma gondii*
Brucella spp.	*Candida albicans*	Cystocercosis
Treponema pallidum		
Borrelia burgdorferi		

Tuberculosis

Of the causes listed in **Table 24**, the most important are *Mycobacterium tuberculosis* and *M. bovis*. Tuberculosis (TB) is a relatively common cause of meningitis in tropical countries, but it is now rare in the UK. Consequently, it is a diagnosis that is easily missed in developed countries, and, as a result of delayed treatment, it may have dire consequences. Untreated, it is inevitably fatal, having a relentless progression over 3–6 weeks.

286

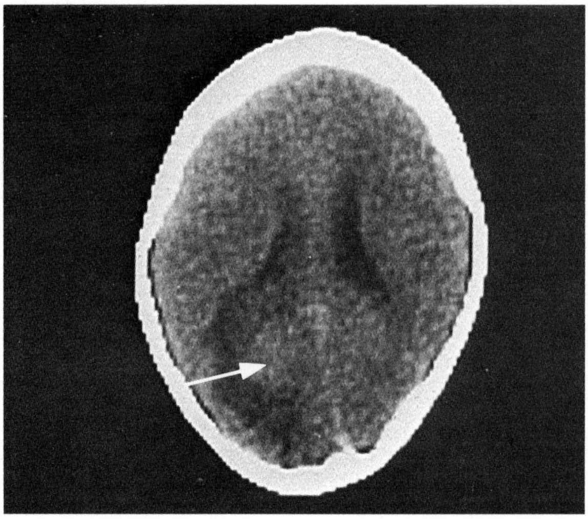

286 CT scan of a skull with tuberculoma.

M. tuberculosis is an acid–alcohol fast bacillus that is slow growing. Disease may arise from the spread of adjacent caseous foci into the meninges, producing an acute inflammatory caseous meningitis that affects, in particular, the basal leptomeninges. The child may have prodromal features of anorexia, irritability, restlessness, nausea and abdominal pain. Signs of meningitis then appear but in up to 20% of cases there may not be a pyrexia. In some children (generally those under 10 years of age), signs of infection mimic those of a brain tumour or abscess. This results from the formation of a tuberculoma (**286**), often located at the base of the brain around the cerebellum.

Diagnosis depends firstly upon considering the possibility of TB meningitis, and secondly upon obtaining CSF. Typically, CSF is under increased pressure, appearing slightly turbid, and containing up to 500×10^6 cells/l (lymphocytes and monocytes). The protein is usually raised, and on occasion the CSF forms a 'spider's web' clot when left to stand. Mycobacteria are demonstrable by Ziehl–Neelsen or auramine phenol stains, but only when concentrations are above 10^4–10^5 bacteria/ml. Adjuncts to diagnosis include detection of mycobacterial antigens or of tuberculostearic acid in CSF, and identification of specific antibody in serum. Culture takes up to 6 weeks.

Treatment is with a combination of isoniazid, rifampicin and pyrazinamide (with or without ethambutol) for 6–12 months. Clinical response usually occurs within 2 weeks. Live attenuated BCG vaccine has a variable efficacy in prevention.

Brucellosis

Brucella spp. (*melitensis*, *abortus* and *suis*) are small gram-negative coccobacilli (**287**). They primarily cause infection in animals, and infection in man occurs by ingestion (in milk) or inhalation of infective material. Brucellosis usually presents as a pyrexia of unknown origin (see Chapter 10), but it may also present as meningitis or encephalitis late in the infection. Diagnosis is made by isolation of the bacterium from blood or other infected tissues and by demonstration of an IgM anti-brucella response. Treatment includes cotrimoxazole and rifampicin.

287

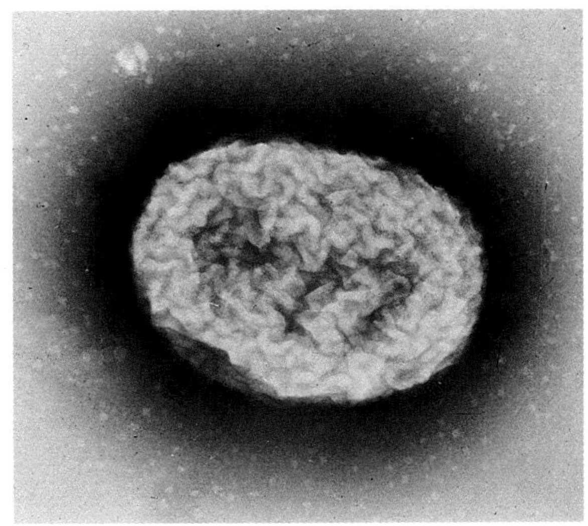

287 Negative-stain electron micrograph of *B. abortus* (× *10,000*).

Lyme disease

Caused by the spirochaete *Borrelia burgdorferi*, this recently described infection is transmitted to man from animals via ticks such as *Ixodes ricinus*. It is more common in the summer months, beginning as a flu-like or meningitis-like illness accompanied by erythema chronicum migrans. Weeks to months later, some patients develop cardiac, CNS and musculoskeletal signs and symptoms, with intermittent attacks of arthritis. The organism can be seen in or isolated from the infected sites. However, the most practical diagnostic test is demonstration of IgM and IgG antibodies to *B. burgdorferi* antigens, in particular flagellar and outer membrane proteins, using an enzyme-linked immunosorbent assay (ELISA). For antimicrobial chemotherapy, penicillin or tetracycline are the drugs of choice. Penicillin G at high doses (up to 20 million units/day) for 10 days is often effective in chronic meningitis.

Cryptococcus neoformans

Cryptococcus neoformans is a dimorphic yeast with a thick capsule. It can cause acute, subacute or chronic meningitis. Infection follows inhalation of spores from the environment. Usually, infection occurs in immune-compromised hosts (e.g. leukaemics, AIDS patients), and the disease frequently has an insidious onset with a picture similar to that of TB meningitis. Diagnosis is reached by demonstration of capsulate yeasts in CSF (**288**) and by culture of cryptococcus on Sabouraud's agar or other media. A latex particle agglutination test is also available to aid diagnosis. Treatment is with antifungal agents, such as amphotericin B or fluconazole, and should be continued for at least 6 weeks.

288

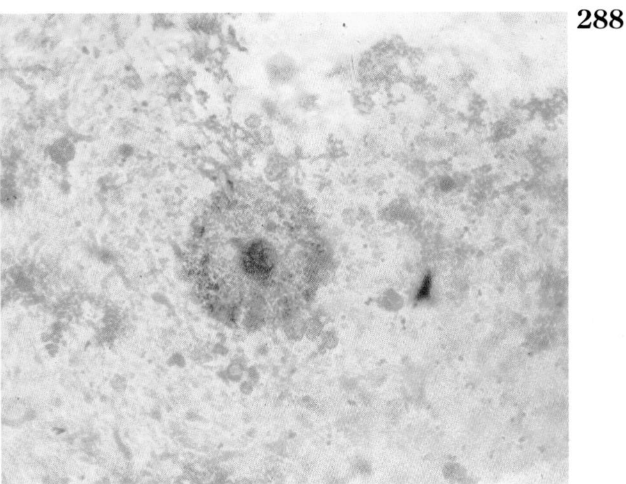

288 Capsulate *C. neoformans* in CSF (× *1,000*).

Focal suppuration

Cases of focal suppuration include brain abscesses, subdural empyema, epidural abscess and central venous thrombophlebitis. All such cases are relatively rare, and arise either by haematogenous or local spread.

Brain abscess

289

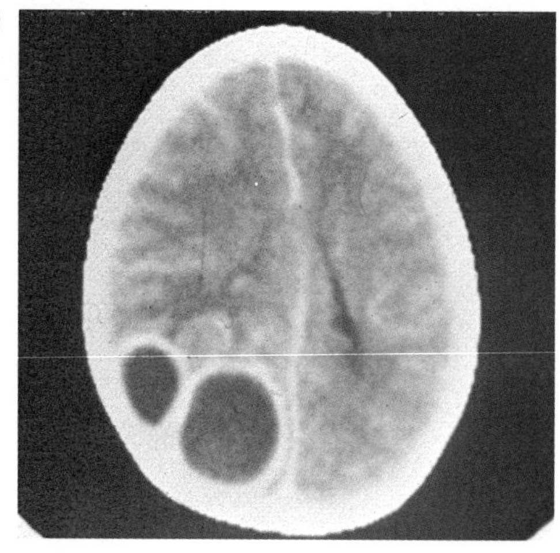

289 CT scan of a skull with a loculated brain abscess.

The presentation of a brain abscess often depends upon its site and size. There may be signs of infection, but until the abscess is sufficiently large, focal signs will not be apparent. For example, patients with a frontal lobe abscess may take weeks or months to develop focal signs, whereas abscesses near the motor or visual cortex will be rapidly apparent. In addition, there may be signs of raised intracranial pressure. CSF is usually sterile, with a moderate pleocytosis (about 4×10^6 cells/l). Radiographs and CT scans (**289**) of the skull will localize the abscess.

The causative micro-organisms differ according to whether it is haematogenous or local spread that has led to the development of the abscess. Local spread (for example, from a dental abscess or chronic sinusitis) is often polymicrobial, with a strong anaerobic component (e.g. *Bacteroides melaninogenicus*). With haematogenous spread, *Staphylococcus aureus* plays a major role. Other important pathogens include *Streptococcus milleri*, *Streptococcus pneumoniae* and coliforms. The mainstay of treatment comprises aspiration and drainage of the abscess, together with appropriate antimicrobial chemotherapy. Initial therapy should include cover for anaerobes and *S. aureus*.

Subdural empyema

290

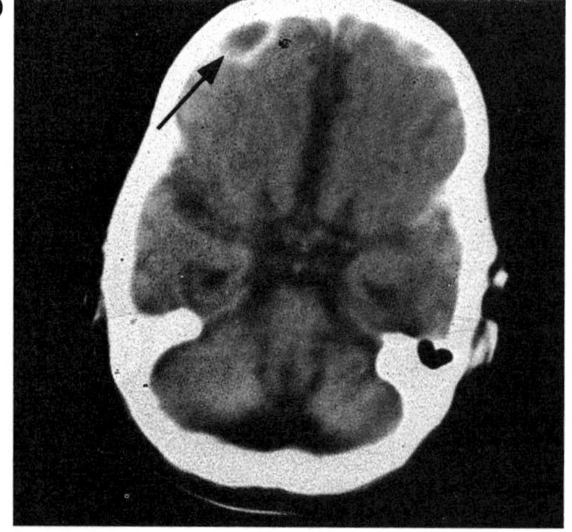

Bacteria may reach the subdural spaces following meningitis as a result of contiguous infection (sinusitis, otitis media), or via haematogenous spread. The most frequently involved pathogens are *H. influenzae*, *S. pneumoniae* and coliforms. Signs of infection include headache, rising fever, meningeal irritation, and increasing neurological deficit from pressure on the cortex. Diagnosis requires radiological investigations, especially CT scanning (**290**). Antimicrobial chemotherapy, including penicillin, chloramphenicol and metronidazole, should cover all potential pathogens. Drainage through burr holes is also of benefit.

290 CT scan of a skull with a subdural empyema.

Encephalitis

Encephalitis, that is inflammation of the brain, can occur either alone or with meningitis (meningoencephalitis). It may arise due either to direct invasion of the brain by micro-organisms or to an immune response to particular pathogens (postinfectious encephalitis). The agents responsible for infective encephalitis are shown in **Table 25**, and those for postinfective encephalitis in **Table 26**.

The manifestations of encephalitis include headache, fever, meningism, and cerebral dysfunction. Cerebral dysfunction includes alterations in the conscious state, varying from lethargy to coma and abnormalities of thought processes, speech and personality. In addition there may be focal signs including fits, hallucinations and behavioural disorders.

The specific diagnosis of encephalitis can be difficult and a definitive diagnosis usually requires brain biopsy. CSF will show pleocytosis (about 200×10^6 cells/l) and, occasionally, the infective agent can be grown. Detection of local antibody (i.e. in CSF) production and of viral genome, together with EEG can be useful adjuncts to diagnosis.

Treatment includes management of the unconscious patient, anticonvulsants, and the monitoring and relief of raised intracranial pressure. Specific therapy is available for only a few of the aetiological agents.

Table 25. Agents Responsible for Infective Encephalitis.

Viruses	*Bacteria*	*Protozoa*
Herpes simplex	*Treponema pallidum*	*Toxoplasma gondii*
Enteroviruses	*Brucella* spp.	*Naegleria fowleri*
Measles virus	*Chlamydia psittaci*	*Plasmodium* spp.
Mumps virus	*Borrelia burgdorferi*	*Trypanosoma* spp.
Varicella-zoster	*Rickettsia* spp.	
HIV		
Rubella		
Adenovirus		
Lymphocytic choriomeningitis virus		
EBV		
Cytomegalovirus		
Influenza virus		
Arthropod-borne togaviruses		
Rabies		

Table 26. Agents Responsible for Post-infection or Post-immunization Encephalitis.

Viruses	*Bacteria*
Measles (v[a], i[b])	*Bordetella pertussis* (v)
Mumps (v, i)	*Mycoplasma pneumoniae* (i)
Rubella (v, i)	*Clostridium tetani* (v)
Rabies (v)	*Legionella pneumophila* (i)
Varicella-zoster (i)	
EBV (i)	
Influenza (v)	
Hepatitis A (i)	

(a) v = vaccine.
(b) i = infection.

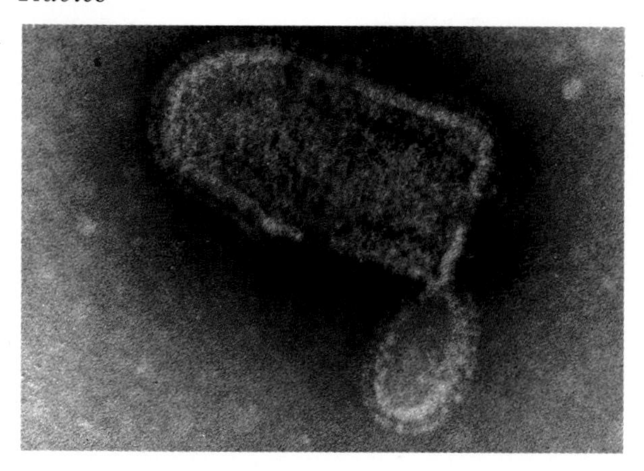

291 Negative-stain electron micrograph of rabies virus (× *60,000*).

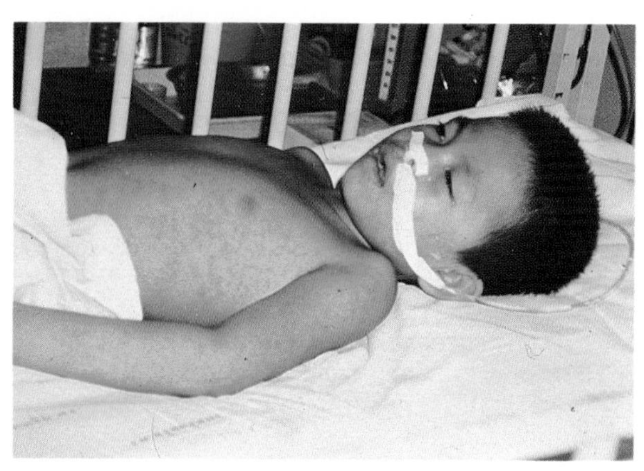

292 A Thai child with rabies and a maculopapular rash.

Rabies is caused by an enveloped RNA virus with a characteristic bullet shape (**291**). Predominantly a disease of animals, it is transmitted to man accidentally. In Europe, wild animals, such as foxes, comprise the predominant reservoir. However, in Asia and Africa, dogs and cats are more important reservoirs. Infected animals have the rhabdovirus in their saliva and it is transmitted to man by bites or by licking of cuts and grazes. Infection by inhalation of aerosols (e.g. in caves occupied by bat colonies) can occur but it is rare.

Virus moves to the CNS along the peripheral nerves by axonoplasmic transport. The length of the incubation period is directly related to the distance from the site of inoculation to the brain. The spread up the spinal cord and throughout the brain is rapid. Very long incubation periods (2 years) have been described but the average length of time is 20–90 days.

Illness begins insidiously with anxiety or depression. Furious (**292**) and paralytic (dumb) forms of rabies can occur. Furious rabies is characterized by agitation, hyperexcitability, bizarre behaviour, and hoarseness due to laryngeal spasm. Hydrophobia is caused by the painful laryngeal and pharyngeal spasms that occur on attempting to swallow. Flaccid paralysis without hydrophobia occurs in up to 20% of infected patients. Diagnosis depends upon demonstration of virus in saliva, CSF or urine, of viral antigens in cerebral or corneal epithelial cells, or upon demonstration of inclusion bodies in the brain (Negri bodies, **293**). Unfortunately it is not possible to demonstrate that infection has occurred until the illness has developed.

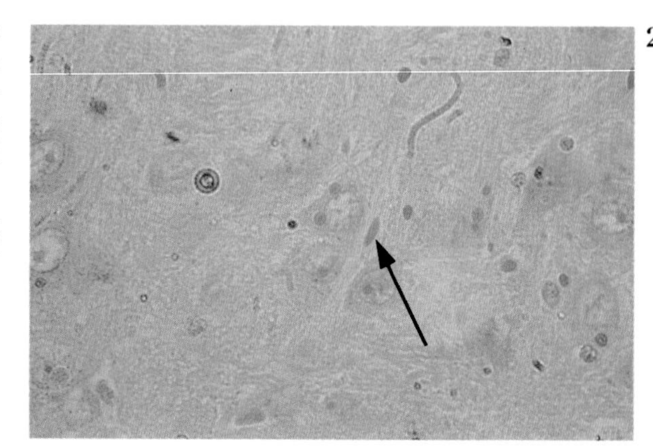

293 A section of brain from a patient with rabies, demonstrating Negri bodies (× *400*).

Treatment and prophylaxis include the use of vigorous wound toilet, human rabies immunoglobulin, and the human diploid cell vaccine. Vaccines derived from brain tissue should be avoided since they offer poor protection and may produce allergic encephalitis.

Other viruses

Enteroviruses are the most common cause of encephalitis, with Coxsackie viruses and Echoviruses being equally important. Outside the neonatal period, HSV-1 is a cause of focal encephalitis. Measles and mumps, which used to be important causes of encephalitis, are now rare ($0.7/10^3$ cases of measles; $3/10^3$ cases of mumps).

Reye's syndrome

Reye's syndrome usually presents following a mild viral infection. It consists of a postinfectious encephalopathy, fatty degeneration in the liver, and a rise in serum transaminase. There is little evidence of inflammation in the liver or brain at postmortem. The disease can progress from deep coma to death in a very short period of time.

The disease is rare after 18 years of age and is less common in metropolitan areas ($0.4/10^5$) than in towns or rural areas ($1.8/10^5$). Many cases are reported after influenza B infection, but several other viruses have been implicated. An epidemiological link between Reye's syndrome and prior salicylate ingestion has been described. Management requires admission to an intensive care unit in order to maintain open airways and control cerebral oedema, but the prognosis is not good.

Toxoplasma gondii

Encephalitis is not a common occurrence in toxoplasmosis and is most likely to occur in the immune-compromised individual or in congenital infection. In most cases, focal lesions are produced in the brain (**294**). Treatment is with spiramycin or pyrimethamine plus sulphadiazine.

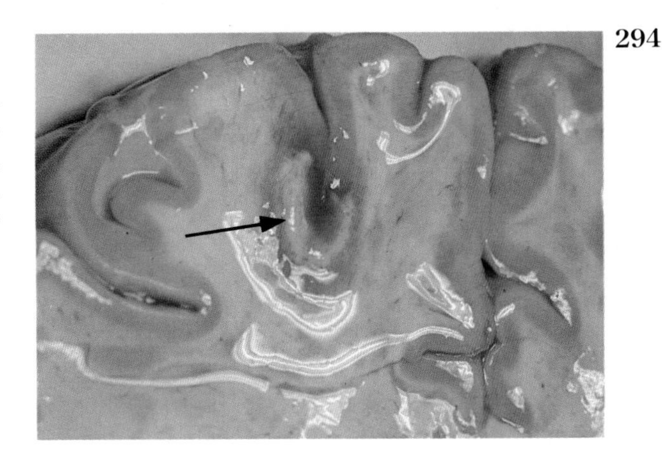

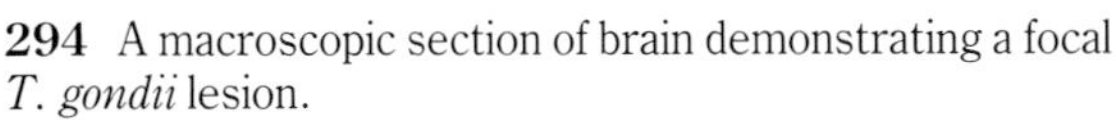

294 A macroscopic section of brain demonstrating a focal *T. gondii* lesion.

Encephalopathic illnesses

Encephalopathic illnesses are also called 'slow virus' infections and, as the latter name suggests, all have a long incubation period.

Progressive multifocal leukoencephalopathy

Progressive multifocal leukoencephalopathy (PMFLE) is a rare and fatal condition that occurs in immune-compromised individuals. It is caused by infection with the polyomavirus J–C (**295**).

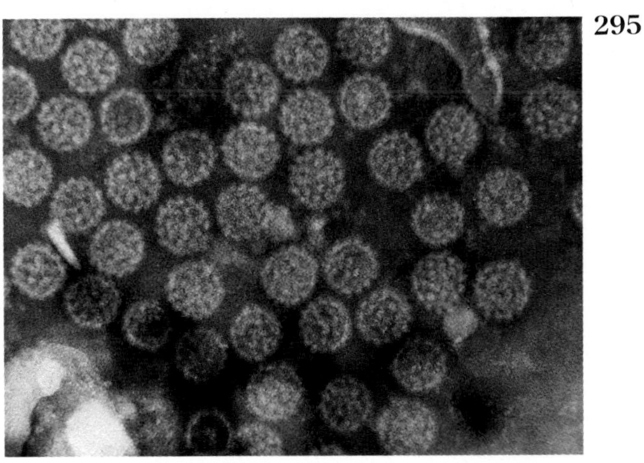

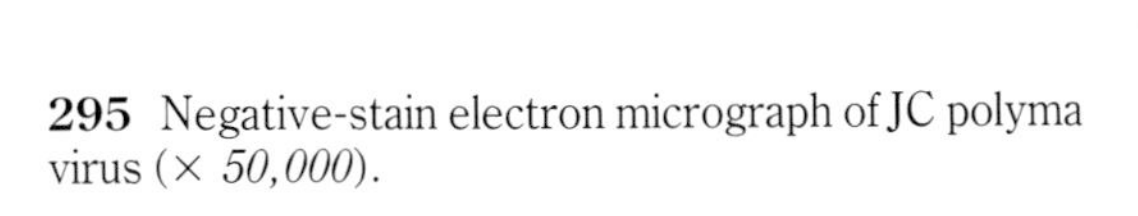

295 Negative-stain electron micrograph of JC polyma virus (× *50,000*).

Subacute sclerosing panencephalitis

Subacute sclerosing panencephalitis (SSPE) is a rare and late sequelae of measles ($1/10^6$ cases of measles). It occurs 2–10 years after the acute attack (mean = 7 years) and is apparently due to incomplete replication of measles virus in neuronal cells. Virus antigens are expressed on the surface of cells, and nucleocapsid can be seen within them (**296**). The antigens are recognized by the immune system, resulting in the death of the infected cells. SSPE has an insidious onset with lethargy, forgetfulness and alterations in behaviour. The patient gradually loses higher mental function and has epileptic seizures, finally lapsing into coma. Diagnosis is dependent upon demonstrating a characteristic EEG pattern in the early stages of disease (**297**), detection of virus on brain biopsy, and detection of relatively high levels of anti-measles virus antibody (but not anti-measles M protein) in CSF. There is no effective therapy, but the incidence of SSPE is decreasing in countries with good measles immunization programmes.

296

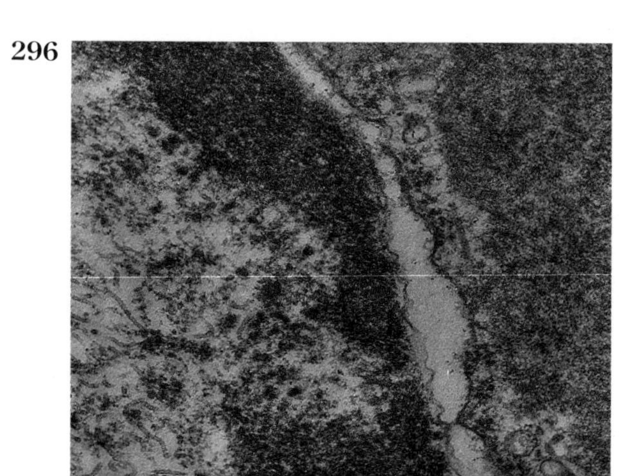

296 Thin-section electron micrograph of the brain of a child with SSPE. Intracytoplasmic measles nucleocapsids are visible (× *20,000*).

297

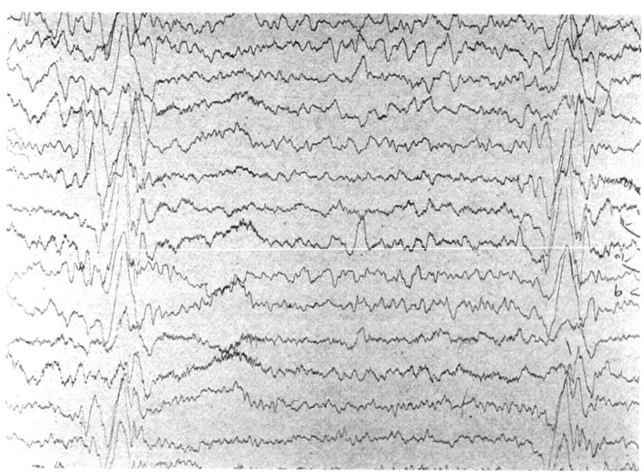

297 Typical electroencephalogram pattern in SSPE.

Creutzfeldt–Jakob disease

298

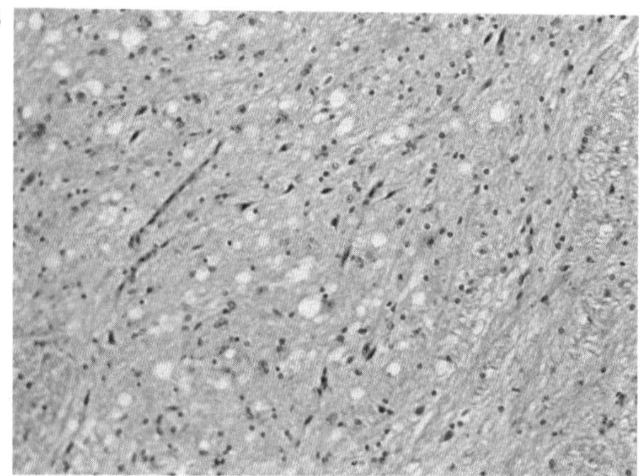

298 A section of brain showing vacuoles in neuronal cells and neutrophils typical of a spongieform encephalopathy (× *200*).

Creutzfeldt–Jakob disease (CJD) is just one example from a group of spongieform encephalopathies which includes kuru in man, scrapie in sheep and bovine spongieform encephalopathy in cattle. These encephalopathies are due to so-called 'prions' (proteinaceous infectious agents), which are apparently self-replicating proteins. Infection, which presents as an incurable presenile dementia, is extremely rare in children, but has occurred following the use of a human growth hormone preparation contaminated with CJD agent. The disease progresses rapidly with the onset of spasticity, mycoclonic jerks, rigidity and tremor. This is followed by epileptic fits and, eventually, by complete mental and physical disintegration. Diagnosis is reached with the help of clinical features and characteristic EEG (repetitive triphasic complexes), but it is usually only definitive at postmortem. The brain shows generalized atrophy and marked spongieform changes in the deep cortical layers (**298**), which are due to cytoplasmic vacuoles. Detergent extraction of cerebral tissue and treatment with protease will reveal typical prion fibrils (**299**). Prions are highly resistant to disinfectants and boiling, and there is no specific treatment.

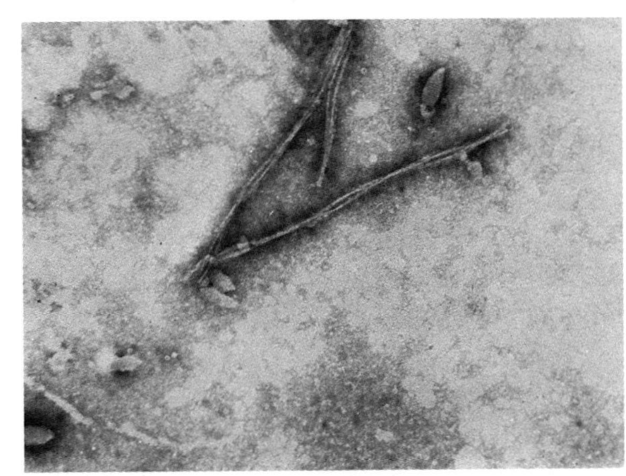

299 Negative-stain electron micrograph of fibrils in an extract of fresh brain tissue (basal nuclei) from a cow with bovine spongieform encephalitis (× *24,000*). (Crown Copyright.)

Poliomyelitis

Although poliomyelitis is rare in developed countries, it is a major problem in developing countries, and in temperate areas, infection peaks in late summer. The disease is due to infection with the picornavirus, poliovirus, which has three antigenic types (1,2,3). Recently, a poliomyelitis-like disease has been reported following infection with Enteroviruses 70 and 71.

The virus is excreted in the faeces of infected individuals and is spread faeco-orally. The ingested virus infects the lymphoid tissue of the nasopharynx and intestine. Paralytic polio occurs in only 1–2% of those infected, and in approximately 5% meningoencephalitis. The remainder are infected asymptomatically. All will continue to excrete virus in faeces for weeks or months. The infectivity within households is high (100% attack rate), and the infective dose is low. It has been estimated that 1g of faeces contains enough virus to infect 100 monkeys. The incubation period for the paralytic disease is 6–20 days. The risk of developing paralytic disease is greater the older the child and if the tonsils have been removed or if there has been a recent intramuscular injection. Prodromal features, which include anorexia, headache, sore throat and signs of meningism, last for 1–7 days. Weakness and flaccid paralysis develop in the lower limbs, usually asymmetrically, and muscle pain and fasciculation are apparent. In less than 15% of cases, various cranial nerves and brainstem centres (including the respiratory centre) may be affected. The majority (80%) of those with initial paralysis will have significant long-term paralysis (**300**), which may (**301**) or may not restrict mobility. Although some recovery can be expected, most improvement (60%) will occur in the first 3 months, and as much as can ever be expected by 3 years postinfection.

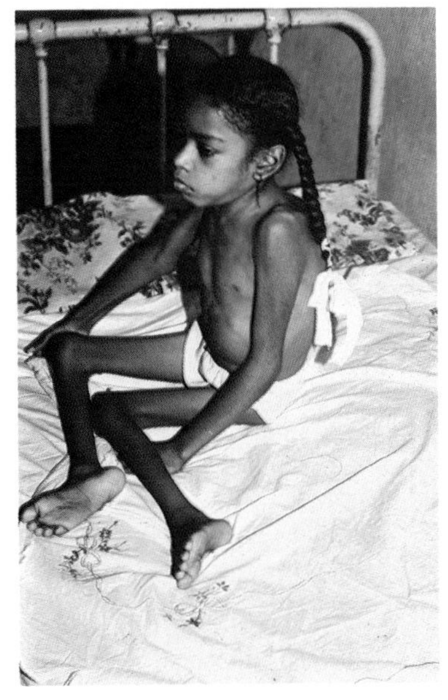

300 A child with flaccid paralysis and wasting of both legs following poliomyelitis.

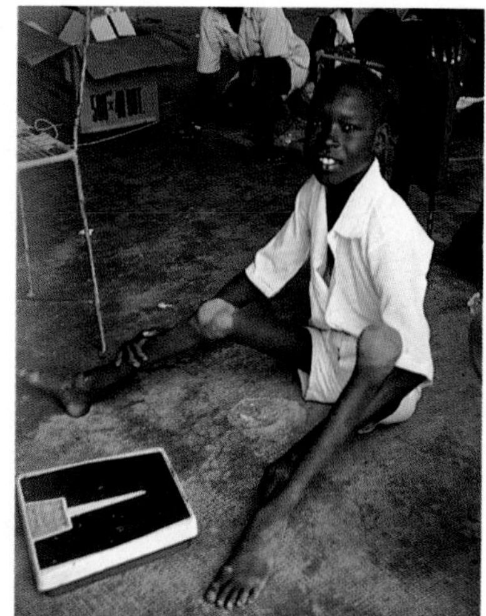

Diagnosis is made by observation of the characteristic clinical features and by isolation of virus from CSF, faeces or the throat and/or demonstration of a rising poliovirus antibody titre. There is no specific treatment. Prevention entails using either a live attenuated vaccine (Sabin) given orally (OPV), or killed virus (Salk) given by injection (IPV). OPV should not be given to immune-compromised individuals since it can produce poliomyelitis, especially type 3.

301 A child with paralytic polio. Note the calluses of both knees, a reaction to their being dragged during movement.

Infections affecting peripheral nerves

Guillain–Barré syndrome

Guillain–Barré syndrome (GBS) is an acute demyelinating disease that affects the peripheral nervous system. It presents as a progressive motor paralysis, with diminished reflexes and minor sensory disorders, such as paraesthesiae. Generally, CSF has a low cell count and raised protein. Diagnosis can be difficult and the pathogenesis of the disease is unclear. It is now, however, the most common cause of acute paralytic disease in developed countries where poliomyelitis has been eradicated. Typically GBS follows days or weeks after a non-specific viral infection. The incidence of disease varies from 0.6–1.9/100,000, rising with increasing age. There is evidence strongly linking GBS with prior cytomegalovirus, Epstein–Barr virus, Coxsackie A virus, *Campylobacter jejuni* and *Mycoplasma pneumoniae* infections, and with influenza virus (A/Jersey) vaccine. No specific treatment exists and most patients recover spontaneously, although up to 25% experience some residual disability and 2–5% die.

Leprosy

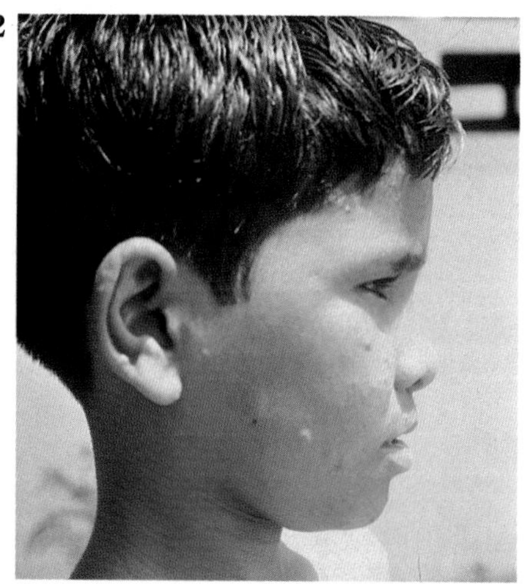

Hansen's disease or leprosy is caused by the acid-fast *Mycobacterium leprae*. Prolonged exposure to bacteria shed by an infective case is necessary for disease to spread, and the incubation period varies from 1 to 5 years. Spread is thought to be by droplets from nasopharyngeal mucosa. The course of the disease depends upon the host's immune response to infection. It appears that subclinical infection, which is associated with a strong cellular immune response, is common. If the cellular immune response is one of delayed hypersensitivity, tuberculoid leprosy (TL) occurs (**302**) with granulomas and tissue damage. If there is a poor cellular immune response, lepromatous leprosy (LL)

302 A child with tuberculoid leprosy. Note lesions on ear and cheek.

arises (**303**) with bacterial multiplication in the skin, peripheral nerves and the reticuloendothelial system. The bacterium, whose initial target is the Schwann cells of subcutaneous peripheral nerves (**304**), prefers cooler parts of the body. TL affects principally the ulnar nerve at the elbow, the lateral popliteal at the knee, the median at the wrist, and the posterior tibial nerve at the ankle. The nerves become palpable as hard, stiff cords and the patient will complain of paraesthesiae and of anaesthetic areas, which are liable to damage by heat, abrasion or pressure. With LL, nodules appear on the skin, but neurological manifestations occur late in the disease. Large numbers of organisms are present in the nerves.

Diagnosis is reached by demonstration of characteristic histological changes (TL) or of mycobacteria in tissue (LL) in biopsy material. Treatment, the mainstay of which is dapsone and rifampicin, is designed to render the patient non-infective and to prevent further bacterial multiplication. *M. leprae* cannot be artificially cultured, but it will grow in the armadillo. A killed vaccine, which is given in combination with BCG to prevent leprosy, has been produced.

303

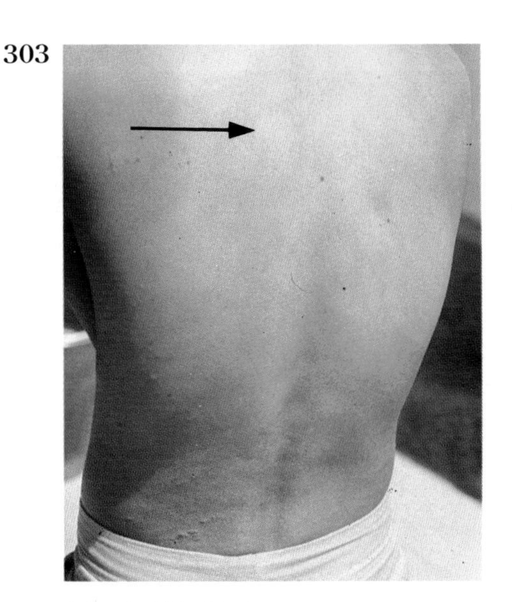

303 A child with lepromatous leprosy showing area of depigmentation.

304

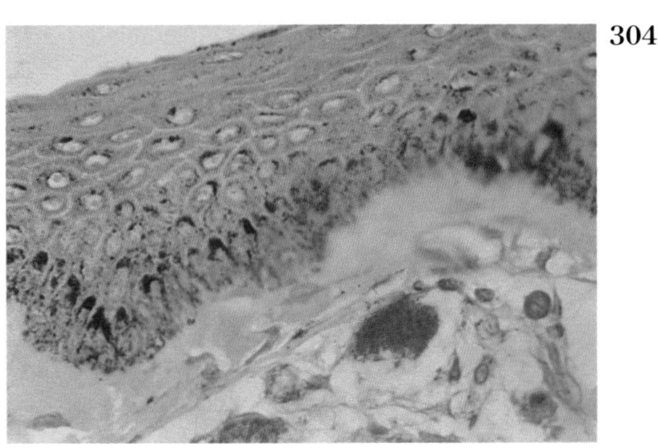

304 Ziehl–Neelsen stain of a section of skin, demonstrating alcohol-fast (pink) bacteria in the subcutaneous layers (× *400*).

Tetanus

Clostridium tetani is a gram-positive bacillus with a characteristic 'drum-stick' appearance (**305**). The bacterium is an obligate anaerobe but survives in the environment in the form of a spore which is highly resistant to drying, heating and disinfectants. It occurs naturally in the gastrointestinal tract of many animal species. For human infection to occur, two conditions are necessary: firstly, a wound that has a degree of necrosis must occur; and secondly, the wound must be contaminated with material containing *C. tetani* spores. If tissue necrosis is present, anaerobic conditions will be produced and the spores germinate into vegetative bacteria. The bacteria then release a toxin, tetanospasmin, which ascends peripheral nerves to the spinal cord, where it impairs inhibitory synapses. This causes muscle rigidity, spasm, and sympathetic overactivity.

305

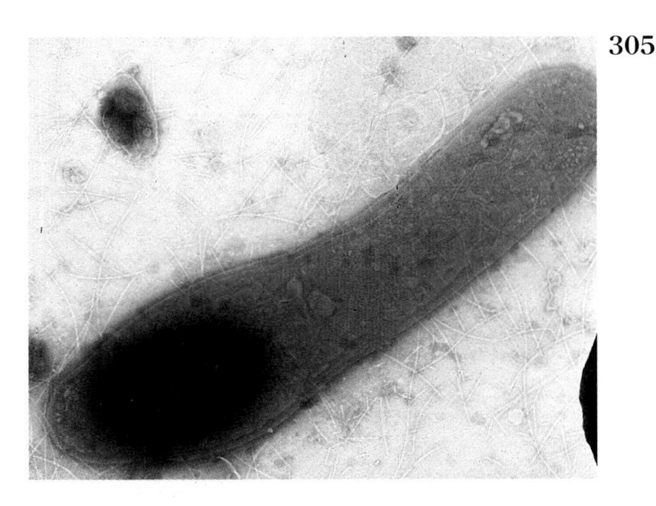

305 Negative-stain electron micrograph of *C. tetani* showing a terminal spore (× *12,000*).

The incubation period is usually 3-21 days; the further the initial injury is from the spinal cord, the longer the incubation period. The clinical presentation depends upon the nerves affected, but 50% of patients develop trismus or spasm of the masseter. As the disease progresses, spasm of other muscle groups occurs (**306 & 307**), affecting the jaws, neck, back and abdomen. The spasms, which are extremely painful, may be intense and prolonged, giving rise to opisthotonus.

Diagnosis is made on the basis of a history of an injury into which soil or faecal material (in particular) has been introduced, and the presence of trismus and other signs. Gram-stained film of the wound may occasionally reveal the bacterium, which may also be detected by culture.

Treatment involves neutralization of tetanospasmin with human antitoxin, debridement of the wound, careful and quiet nursing (stimuli such as noise or light will precipitate spasms) and an anticonvulsant regimen. The patients may need ventilatory support in severe cases. The mortality rate is 45–55%. Tetanus is entirely preventable. Tetanus toxoid given in the form of 3 injections 4 weeks apart, together with a booster 6 months later, produces protective antibody levels that persist for 5–10 years.

306

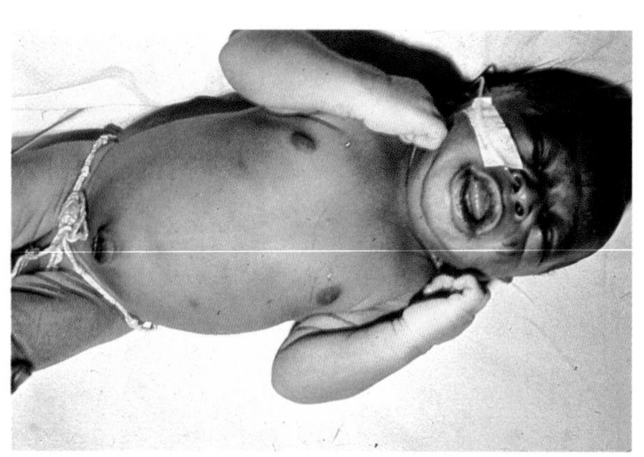

306 Neonatal tetanus showing severe spasm.

307

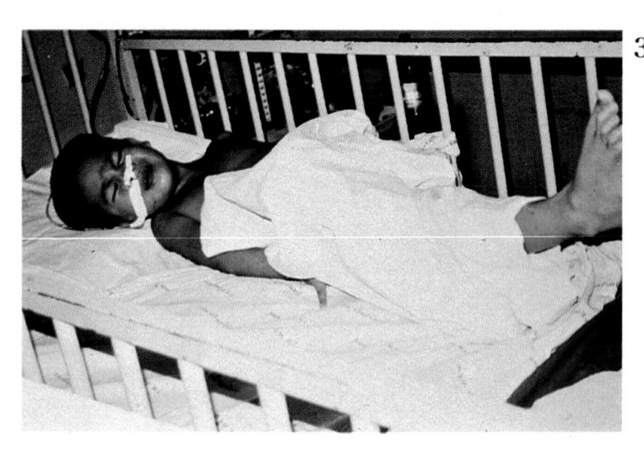

307 A child undergoing a severe painful tetanic spasm and trismus.

Botulism

Clostridium botulinum is a gram-positive anaerobic bacillus. Ingestion of the toxin, or growth of *C. botulinum* in the infant intestine, produces a descending flaccid paralysis. There are seven antigenically disparate types of toxin (A–G), but human disease is mainly due to toxins A,B,E,F and G. Toxin is produced by the heat-labile bacterium during growth at temperatures of between 3°C and 48°C. Spores in improperly processed acidic food can permit rapid toxin production. Outbreaks can be traced to canned fish, home preserves and even fruit yoghurt. *C. botulinum* spores are often ingested along with foods such as fruits, vegetables and honey, but it is only the infant intestine that is susceptible to colonization. The illness begins as a descending symmetrical motor paralysis that starts with the cranial motor nerves. It is extremely rare in the UK and Europe, and diagnosis depends upon clinical suspicion. Specific diagnosis requires detection of the organism or its toxin in food, the intestinal contents or in serum. The treatment is supportive, with antitoxin (horse) and, if the source of infection is a wound, penicillin G. The mortality in botulism is 20–25%. Scrupulous attention to detail in preserving foodstuffs and in cooking is needed for prevention. There is no vaccine.

7 Infections of the genitourinary tract

Urinary tract infection

During the neonatal period boys are more prone to urinary tract infections than girls, probably reflecting the blood-borne nature of infection. However, in infants and older children, girls are more liable to develop urinary tract infections, reflecting infections that ascend the shorter urethra. The incidence of both symptomatic and asymptomatic urinary tract infection in schoolgirls is about 2%.

Most commonly associated with urinary tract infections are gram-negative organisms of which *Escherichia coli* is the predominant organism, followed by *Klebsiella*, *Proteus* and, occasionally, coagulase-negative staphylococci (**Table 27**). Certain *E. coli* possessing K1 capsule and fimbriae (**308**) adhere to the epithelium of children with P blood group antigen and are more likely to cause infection.

Anatomical and functional abnormalities such as vesicoureteric reflux, obstruction, and urinary stasis from diverticula or from a neurogenic bladder, will predispose a child to infection. Vesicoureteric reflux (**309–311**) is one of the most common causes of recurrent urinary tract infection in children. Fortunately, the majority of cases correct themselves by the age of 5 years.

Diagnosis of a urinary tract infection is important and should be made on a clean urine sample (**312**). Pyuria ($>10\times10^6$/l) and a significant bacteriuria comprising a pure growth of $>10^8$/l should be seen from a clean catch sample of urine. In neonates and infants under 6 months, a suprapubic needle aspiration of urine may be necessary to obtain a pure specimen for immediate diagnosis.

When acute pyelonephritis is suspected, an ultrasound may show an echo-bright picture, and an enlarged inflamed kidney with small microabscess may be noted, as well as debris of cells and echo dense material in the bladder (**313**). An intravenous pyelogram (IVP) performed during an acute pyelonephritis may show an enlarged kidney, with squashing and crowding of calices within the renal pelvis (**314 & 315**).

Following treatment for an acute urinary tract infection, investigations should include an ultrasound, which will rule out most gross anatomical abnormalities and some causes of obstruction. A dimercaptosuccinic acid (DMSA) scan may demonstrate renal scarring as a consequence of the infection (**316**). Vesicoureteric reflux may be demonstrated by micturating cystography when the child is voiding urine.

Renal stones (**317 & 318**) are an uncommon predisposing cause of infection. However, there is a significant association between a *Proteus* spp. infection and renal stones.

Table 27. Organisms Commonly Associated with Urinary Tract Infections.

- *Escherichia coli*
- *Klebsiella aerogenes*
- Enterococci
- *Coagulase-negative staphylococci*
- *Proteus* spp.

308

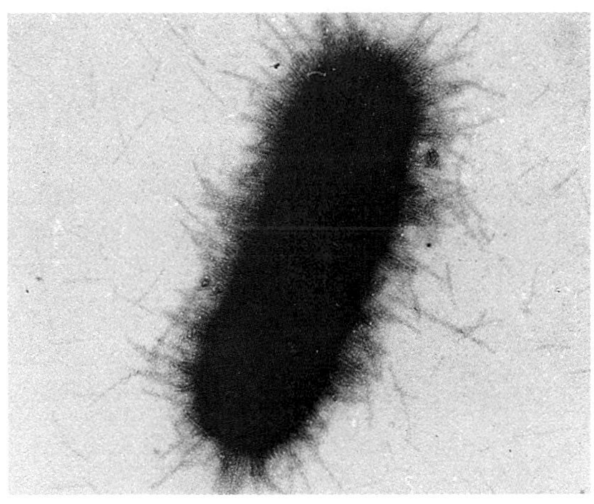

308 Negative-stain electron micrograph of *E. coli*. Fimbriae are clearly visible (× *7,000*).

309

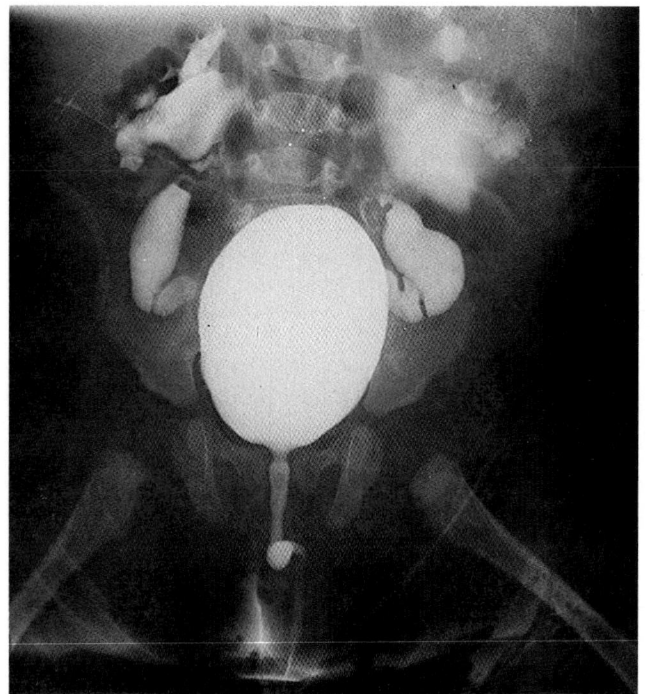

309 A retrograde cystourethrogram showing severe bilateral ureteric reflux and hydronephrosis, which predisposes to infection.

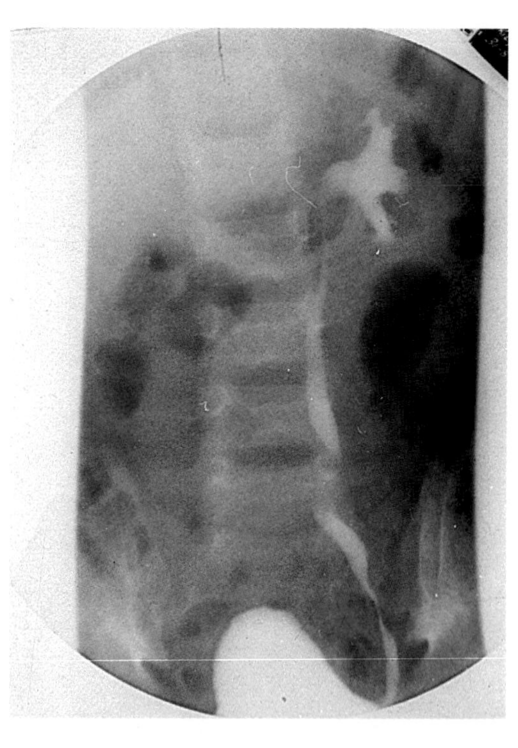

310 A retrograde cystourethrogram showing grade 4 reflux in the ureter of the left kidney.

311

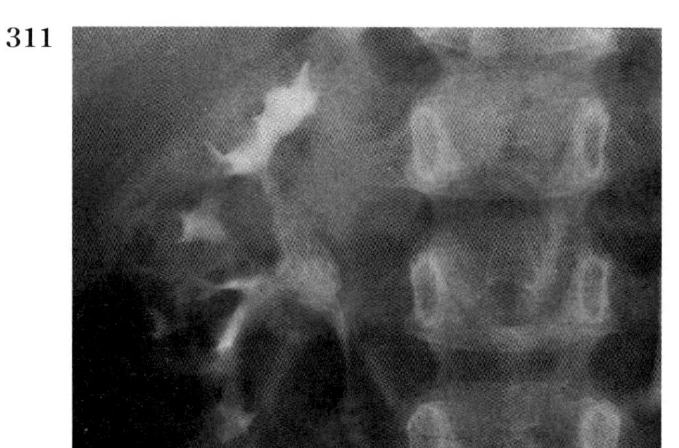

311 IVP of an acute pyelonephritis in the right kidney. Note how the renal pelvis is striated due to distension caused by reflux.

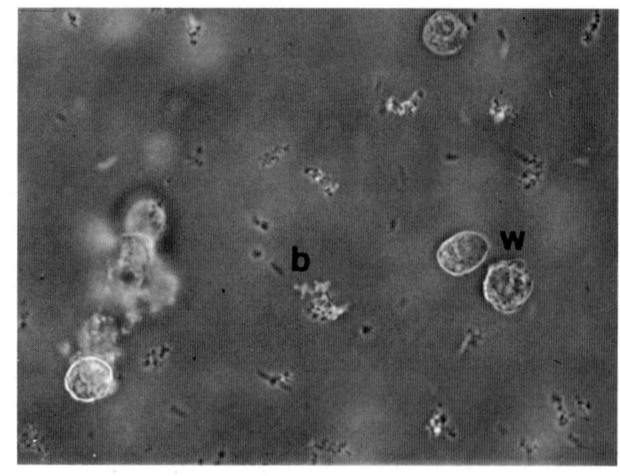

312 Wet film of urine from a mid-stream specimen of urine demonstrating white cells (w) and bacilli (b) (× *400*).

313

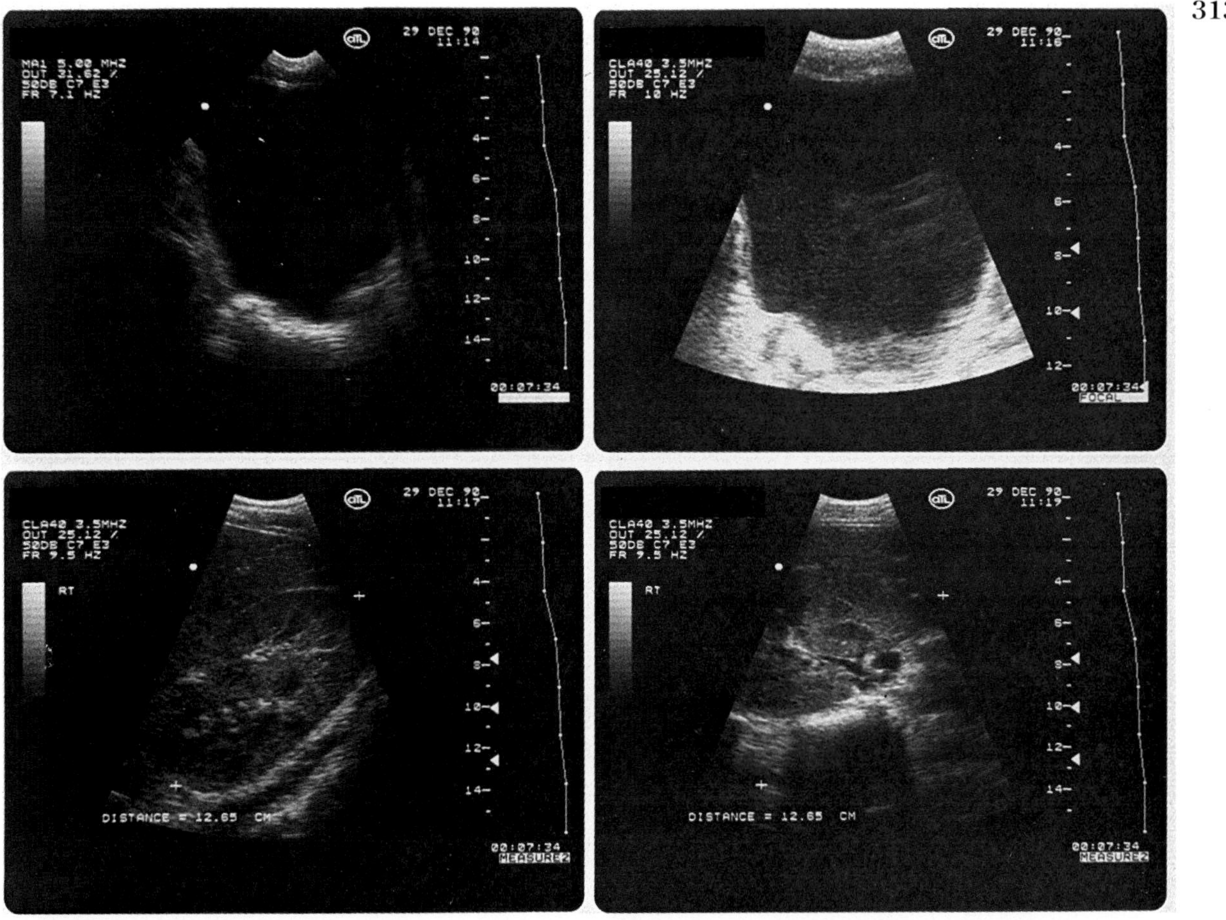

313 Ultrasound scan of a unilateral acute pyelonephritis. Note the scattered microabscesses in the echo-bright kidney.

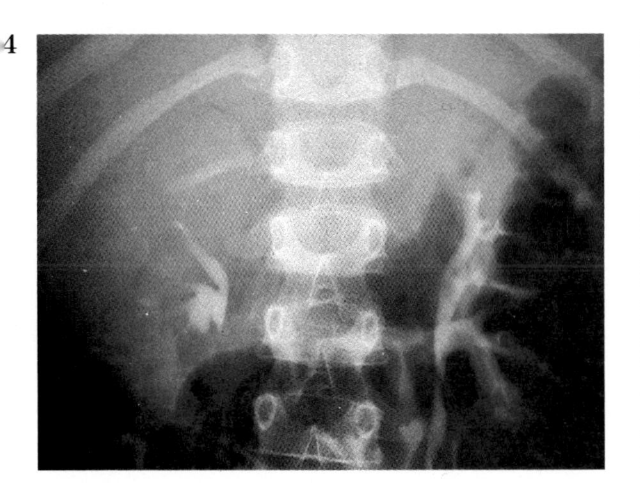

314 IVP showing features of acute pyelonephritis. The right renal calices are bunched together and the kidney is enlarged.

315

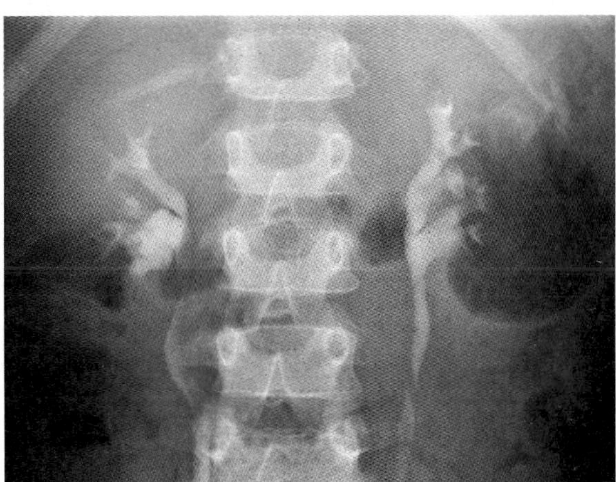

315 IVP of the patient in 314, four weeks later after treatment. A more normal caliceal pattern can be seen and the kidney has returned to a normal size.

316

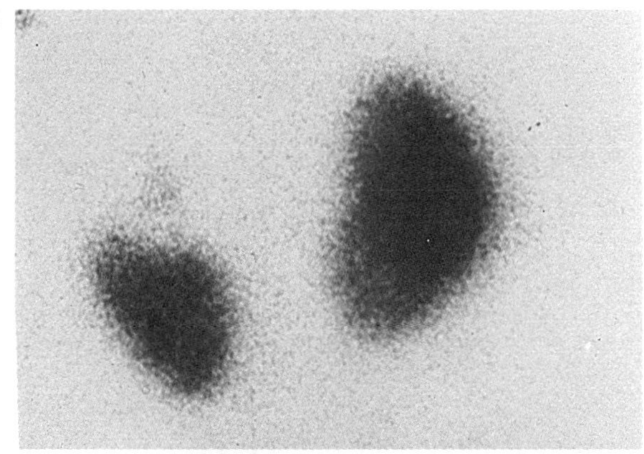

316 DMSA scan demonstrating poor radioisotopic uptake and renal scarring of the upper pole of the right kidney.

317

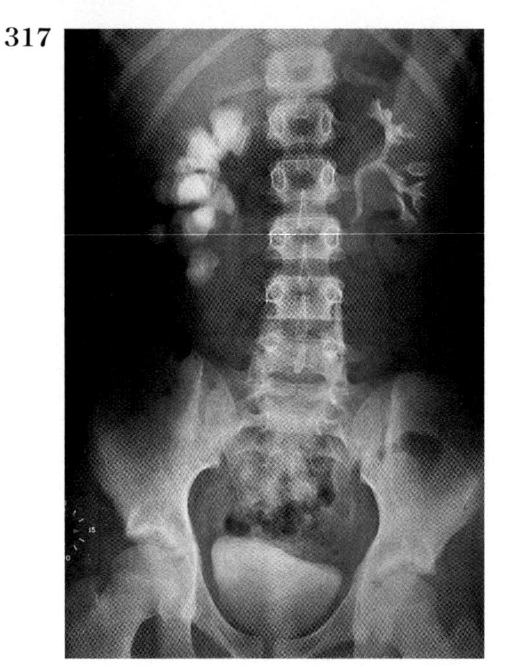

317 IVP demonstrating 'stag horn' calculus and clubbing in the pelvis of the right kidney.

318

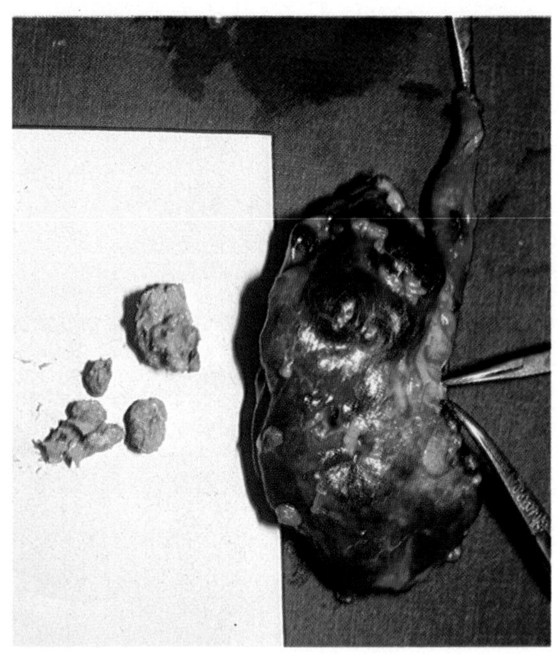

318 Stones removed from a scarred kidney after nephrectomy.

Chronic pyelonephritis

If left undetected and untreated, chronic infection of the kidneys will lead to contracted and scarred kidneys. An IVP may demonstrate reduced cortical thickness (**319**), and a DMSA scan (**320**) will reveal evidence of scarring, with loss of function demonstrable by poor radioisotopic uptake. If chronic infection remains untreated, chronic renal failure can develop (**321** & **322**). Hypertension and uraemia may necessitate nephrectomy, with the subsequent need for renal dialysis and eventual renal transplant.

Because of improved surveillance in developed countries, chronic pyelonephritis in children is now rare. However, in developing countries it is the single most common cause of chronic renal failure.

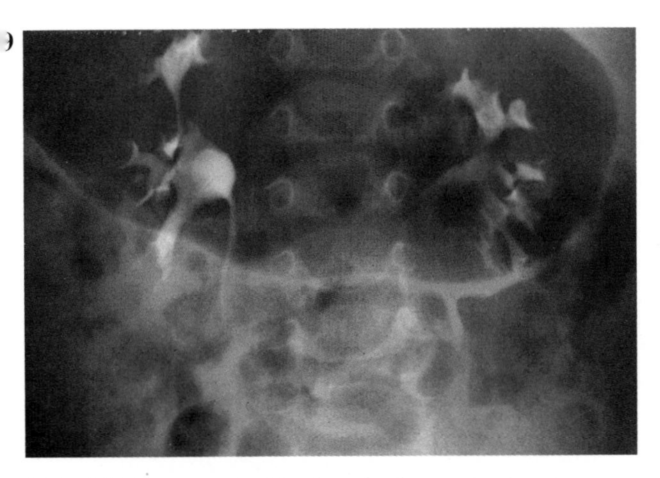

319 IVP demonstrating blunting of calices and reduced cortical thickness in the left kidney.

320

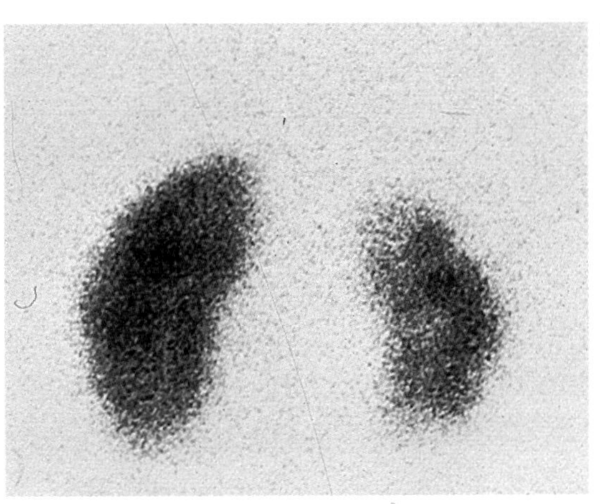

320 DMSA scan of the child in **319**, demonstrating a small left kidney with a reduced radioisotopic uptake (31%) in comparison to the right kidney (79%).

321

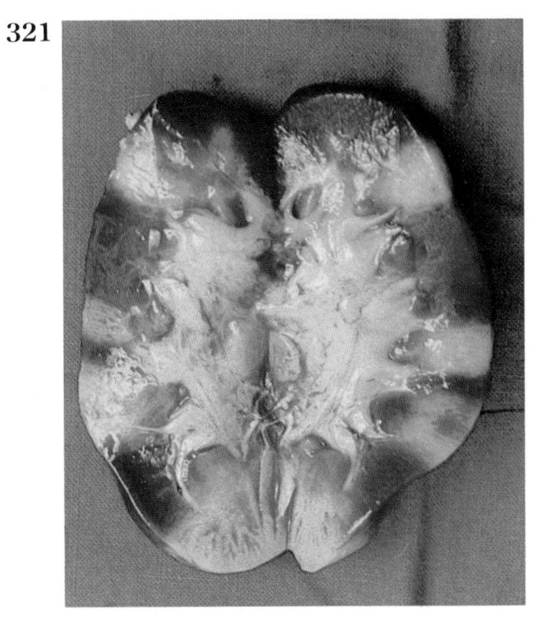

321 Longitudinal section of a right kidney, demonstrating characteristic reduced cortical thickness in chronic pyelonephritis and scarring. The section was made immediately after nephrectomy.

322

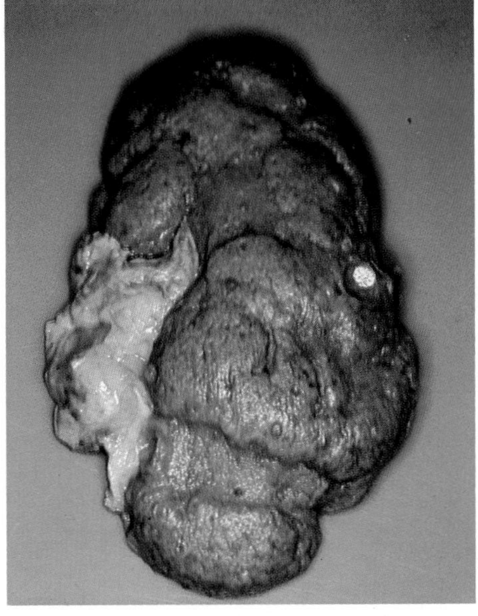

322 A left kidney with a cobbled surface due to scarring from repeated infections.

Renal tuberculosis

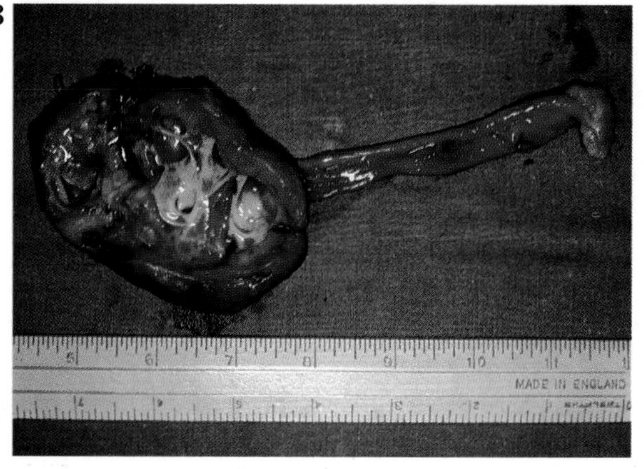

323 Renal tuberculosis showing caseation and destruction of parenchyma in a sectioned kidney.

Tuberculosis of the kidneys (**323**) is caused by blood-borne *Mycobacterium tuberculosis*. It occurs either as part of early bacteraemia or as part of miliary tuberculosis. It is rare in children and characteristically presents with painless haematuria. Diagnosis is made by taking early morning urine specimens. The fresh urine is examined and cultured for acid- and alcohol-fast bacilli. In order to prevent the emergence of drug resistance, antituberculous treatment with multiple drug therapy should continue for at least 9 months.

Renal abscesses

Renal abscesses may occur either as a complication of metastatic systemic infection or as a result of direct infection of the kidney. The presence of abscesses should be suspected if the acute symptoms for a urinary tract infection do not resolve with adequate antibiotic treatment. Ultrasound (**324**) and a radioisotopic DMSA scan (**325**) may suggest a diagnosis but the introduction of CT scanning (**326**) has allowed for very precise localization and diagnosis.

Treatment with a 2–3 week course of an antibiotic, which should include an antistaphylococcal agent, will often lead to resolution of the abscess, although surgical drainage may be necessary.

Clinically, suprarenal abscesses may present in the same way as a renal abscess. There is usually severe loin pain, and pus may track down into the inguinal region from the psoas muscle sheath (**327**).

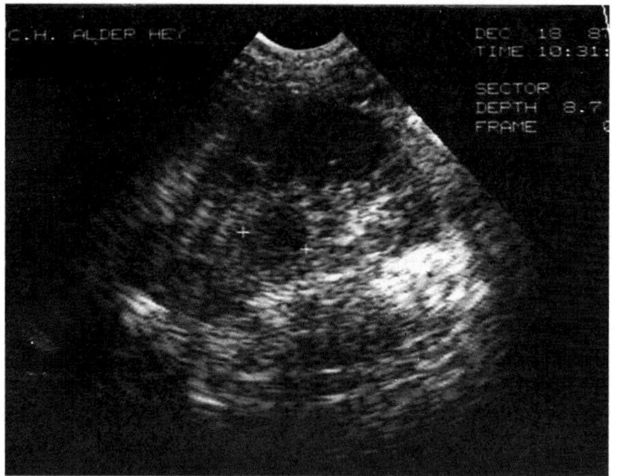

324 Ultrasound scan demonstrating a right renal abscess which is revealed as an echo-clear area between the two markers.

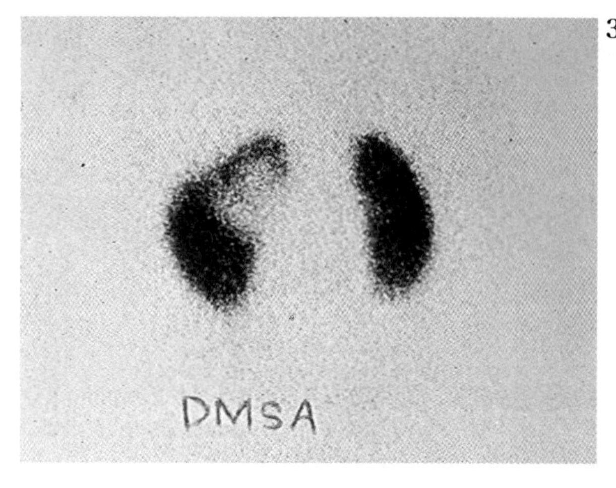

325 DMSA scan of the patient in **326**, reveals a filling defect and poor radioisotopic uptake in the right kidney.

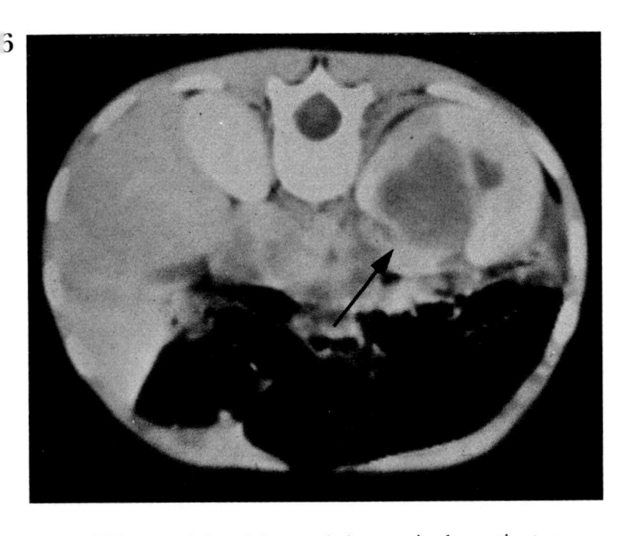

326 CT scan of the right renal abscess in the patient shown in **324** & **325**.

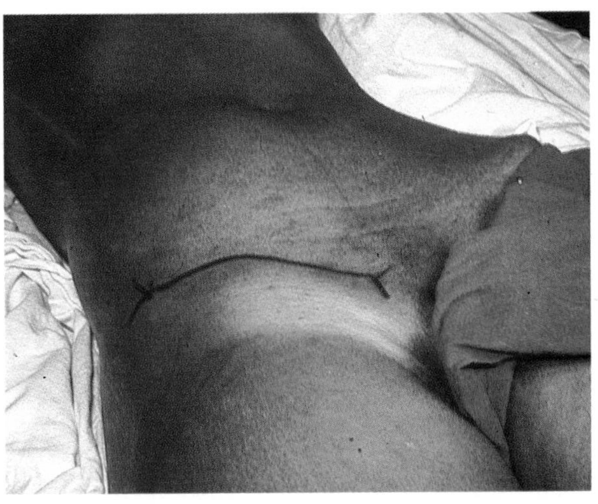

327 Right psoas abscess draining down the muscle sheath to the inguinal region.

Acute poststreptococcal glomerulonephritis

Acute poststreptococcal glomerulonephritis usually follows a recent infection of the throat or the skin by certain 'nephritogenic' strains of group A β-haemolytic streptococci (**328**). Haematuria (**329**), which may lead to oliguria and acute renal failure, is often a presenting symptom.

Some children develop oedema, with heart failure and pulmonary congestion. The blood pressure may rise, causing an acute encephalopathy. On light microscopy, most of the glomeruli appear enlarged, with diffuse mesangial cell proliferation and with an infiltrate of polymorphonuclear leukocytes (**330**). Electron microscopy reveals deposits of immunoglobulins and complement on the epithelial side of the glomerular basement membrane (**331**).

It is thought that poststreptococcal glomerulonephritis results from this deposition of immune complexes in the glomeruli. There may be evidence of a depressed serum complement (C3), and the anti-streptolysin O titre may be raised. However, acute poststreptococcal glomerulonephritis from skin infection does not produce a significant ASO titre. A better antibody marker is an elevated anti-DNAse titre. Rarely, acute glomerulonephritis may occur after infection with *Streptococcus pneumoniae* and *Streptococcus viridans*. Certain viruses may also cause acute glomerulonephritis, which is clinically indistinguishable from acute poststreptococcal glomerulonephritis.

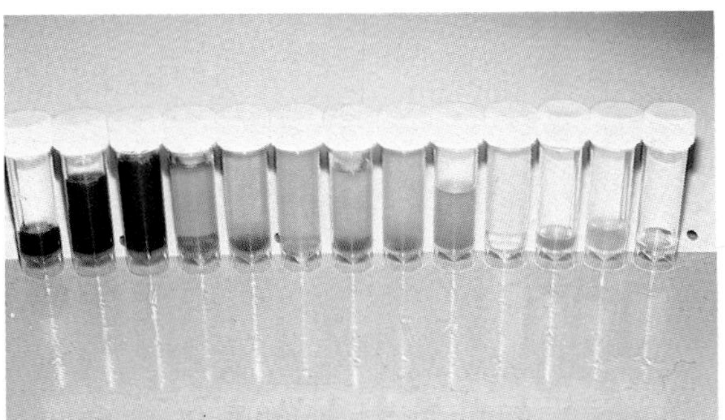

328 Acute glomerulonephritis demonstrating oedema of the ankles, and scabies burrows infected with *S. pyogenes*.

329 A series of sequential urine samples demonstrating the course of haematuria in acute glomerulonephritis.

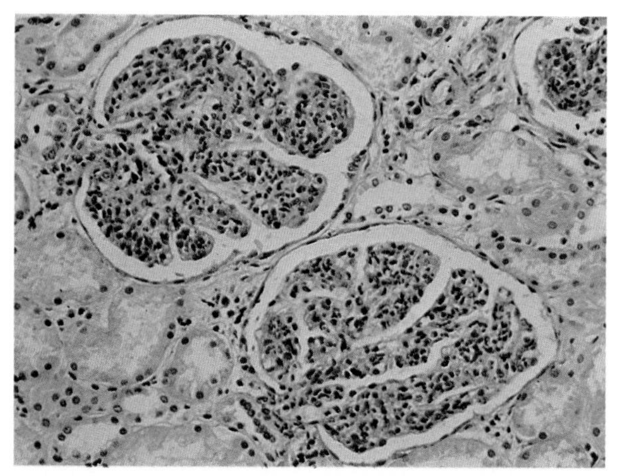

330 A renal biopsy specimen showing two glomeruli. There is increased cellularity with infiltration by neutrophils (× *200*).

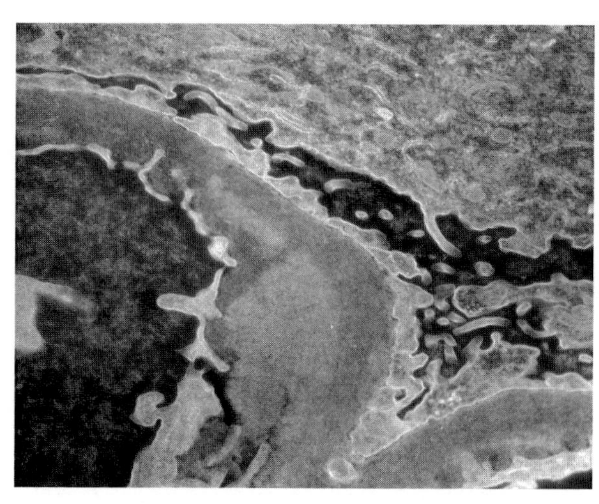

331 Electron micrograph of the basement membrane of a glomerulus. Immune complexes have been deposited as lumps (× *20,000*).

Haemolytic uraemic syndrome

Infections that arise at sites distant from the kidney may nevertheless affect the kidney, as is the case in haemolytic uraemic syndrome. This syndrome includes a haemolytic anaemia, thrombocytopenia and acute renal failure.

The haemolytic uraemic syndrome (**332**) is an important cause of acute renal failure in childhood. The condition has been associated with diarrhoea caused by a verocytotoxin (VT)-producing *E. coli* (VTEC) in temperate climates, and by *Shigella dysenteriae* Type I in hot climates. In the UK, a specific *E. coli* serotype, 0157:H7, which contains 2 verocytotoxins, VT1 and VT2, has been implicated in cases presenting with diarrhoea. The verocytotoxin of *E. coli* 0157:H7 may be detected from the stools of 63% of children with haemolytic uraemic syndrome if collected early in the illness.

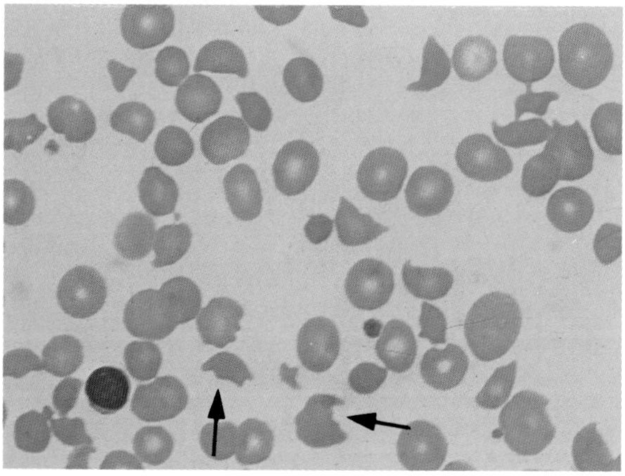

332 Blood film in haemolytic uraemic syndrome demonstrating fragmented red cells (× *500*).

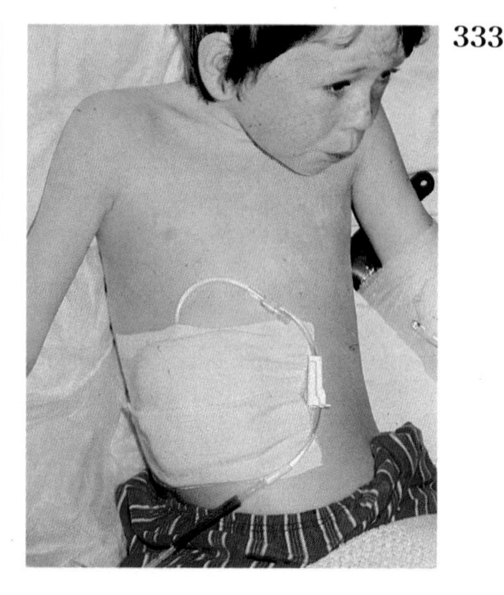

333 Peritoneal dialysis following acute renal failure due to the haemolytic uraemic syndrome.

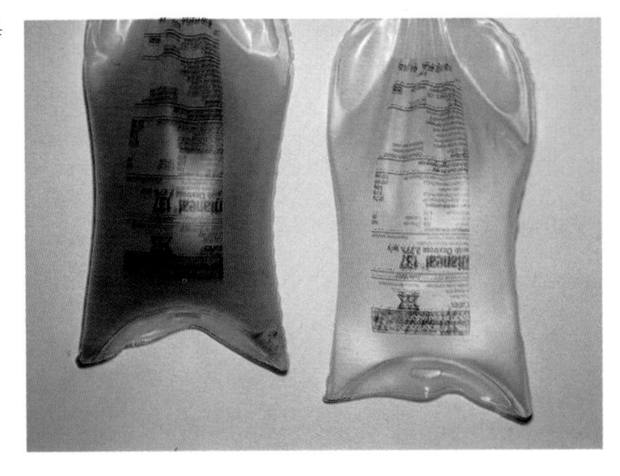

334 Infected dialysis fluid (in the left bag) from a patient with peritonitis acquired through faulty dialysis technique.

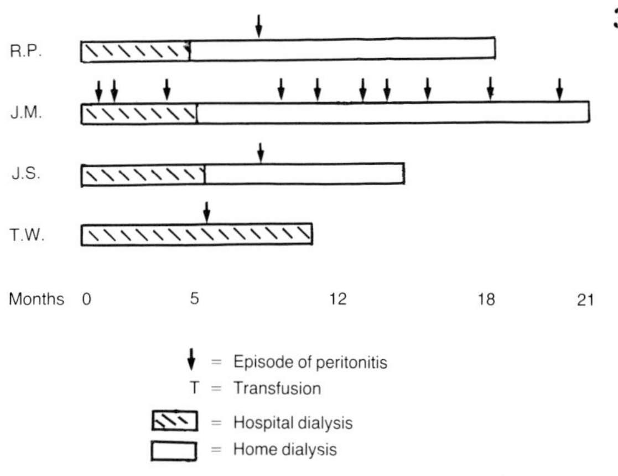

335 Fewer episodes of infection occur during peritoneal dialysis in hospital than at home.

The verocytotoxin causes a microangiopathy. A haemolytic anaemia then occurs and haemaglobinuria may contribute to the resulting acute renal failure. At the same time, symptoms caused by damage to the blood vessels may precipitate cerebral manifestations including convulsions and focal signs. Girls tends to predominate slightly among those who have diarrhoea as a presenting clinical feature of the syndrome. However, among those who present without diarrhoea, boys predominate and the prognosis appears to be poorer.

The acute renal failure may last from 2 to 4 weeks, and treatment of the haemolytic uraemic syndrome may require peritoneal dialysis (**333**). Care must be taken to prevent infection of the peritoneal cavity during dialysis. Home dialysis can be performed, but infection may occur if the family has not been adequately trained (**334** & **335**).

Balanitis

Balanitis is an acute infection of the glans penis and the prepuce (posthitis) (**336**). It may present clinically with dysuria, and the child may cry on micturation. Local antibiotic treatment may be all that is required, although in severe cases systemic antibiotics may occasionally be needed.

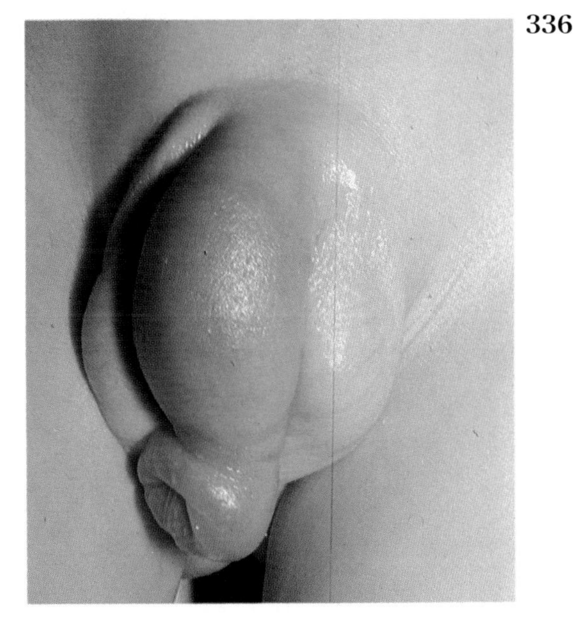

336 Acute balanitis.

Epididymitis and orchitis

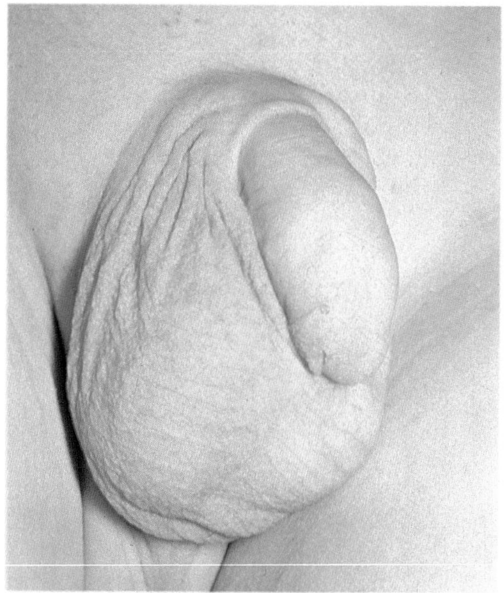

337 The swollen right testis of a boy with acute epididymo-orchitis.

Epididymitis and orchitis are rare infections in children. In most cases both testes are involved and if the swelling and pain are unilateral (**337**), torsion of the testes must be excluded. A broad-spectrum antibiotic such as cotrimoxazole should be given for 2 weeks.

Vulvovaginitis

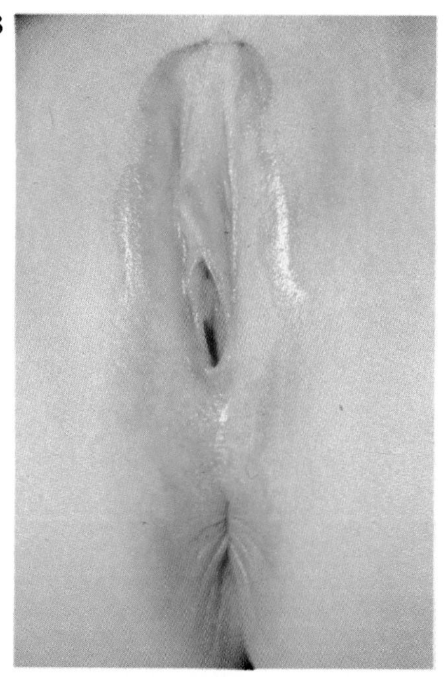

338 Inflammation of the vulva in a young girl with vulvovaginitis.

Non-specific vulvovaginitis is the most common cause of a vaginal discharge in prepubertal girls (**338**), often causing the parents more anxiety than the child. In many cases it is almost physiological, causing few symptoms other than staining of the knickers with a mucoid non-purulent discharge. The child may complain of irritation and dysuria.

The condition is sometimes caused by poor personal hygiene and all that may be necessary to achieve a cure is to advise parents on how to improve hygiene and to dress their child in loose cotton underclothes. Occasionally, threadworm (*Enterobius vermicularis*) infection may cause such intense perineal irritation that scratching can lead to inflammation and secondary infection.

Monilial vulvovaginitis may also occur in infants (**339**). It is uncommon in older children, but may arise in those who have been taking antibiotics for a prolonged period. Rarely, monilial vulvovaginitis may occur as a presenting symptom of diabetes mellitus. Treatment with topical nystatin cream or ointment will cure most cases.

Other organisms that may cause vulvovaginitis include *Haemophilus influenzae*, *Neisseria gonorrhoeae* and *Trichomonas vaginalis* (**340**). These should be treated with appropriate systemic antibiotics for 7–10 days.

In the young child a persistent foul-smelling vaginal discharge should alert a doctor to a possible self-inserted foreign body (**341 & 342**), which can cause chronic inflammation.

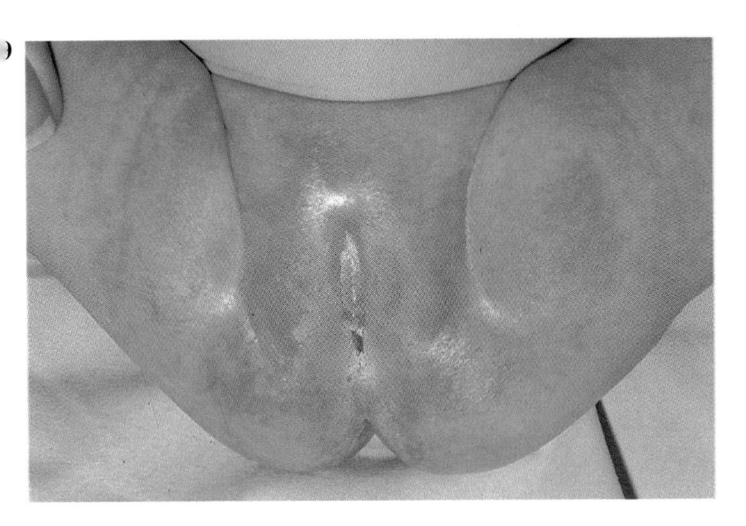

339 Vulvovaginitis from *C. albicans* infection.

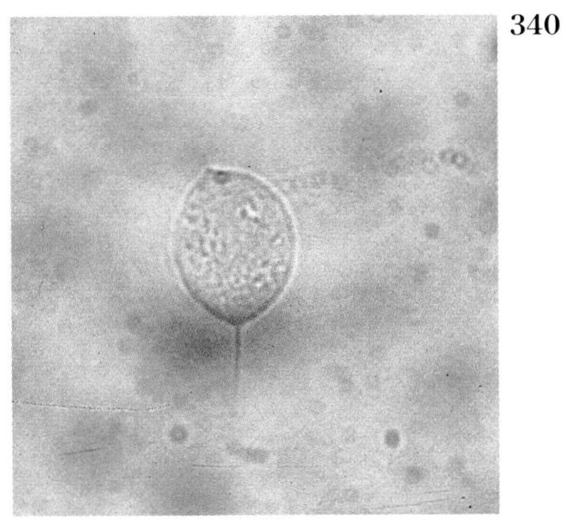

340 The protozoon *T. vaginalis*, which may be a cause of vaginal discharge in adolescent girls.

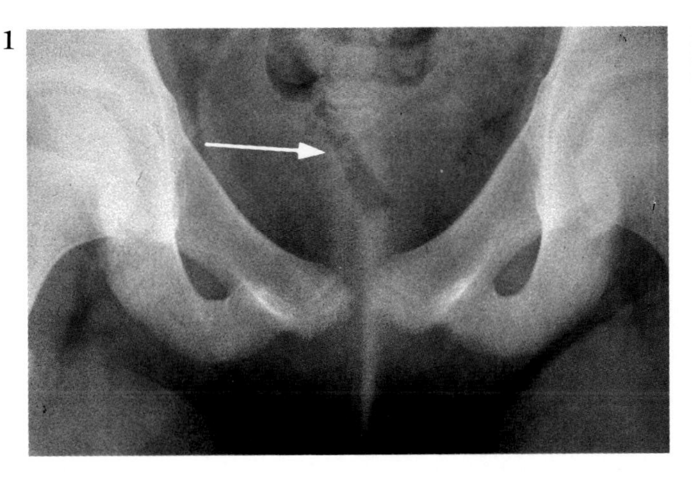

341 Plain X-ray of the pelvis, demonstrating a pen top inserted into the vagina. A secondary infection resulted.

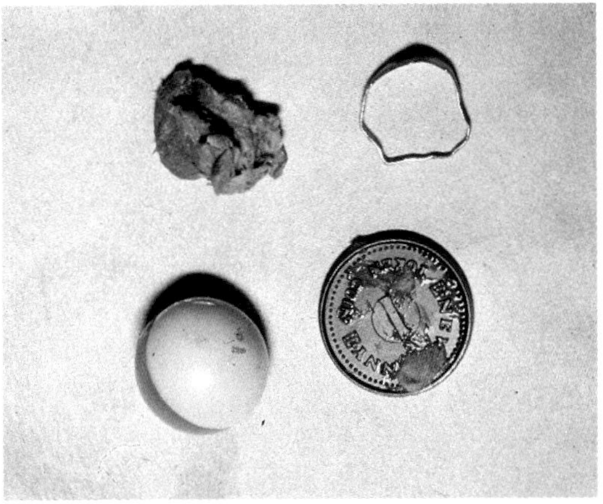

342 Foreign bodies taken from the vagina of a young girl with a vaginal discharge.

Vulval warts

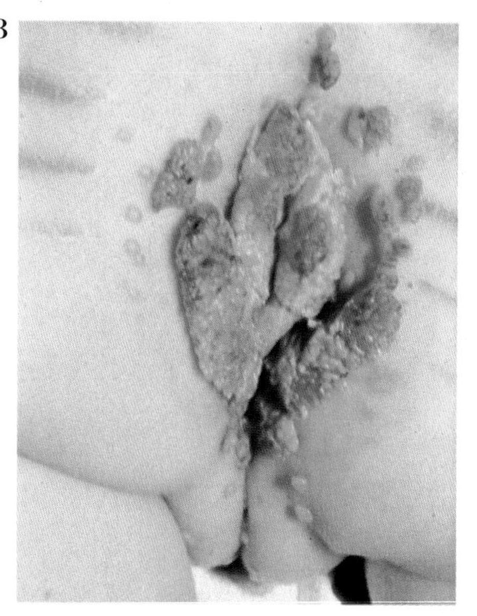

343 Vulval warts.

Vulval warts (**343**) may cause local irritation when conditions are moist and sweaty and there is friction in the perineal region. Treatment usually involves electrodesiccation. Podophyllin resin is not recommended since it can cause severe irritation if not applied with extreme care.

Genital herpes

Genital herpes (**344**) is usually caused by HHV2. In primary infections, painful bullous lesions that develop into shallow ulcers are common. Treatment with systemic and locally applied acylovir will shorten the course of the infection. Recurrence is common. Infection is more likely in pubertal girls, and in those who have suffered sexual abuse.

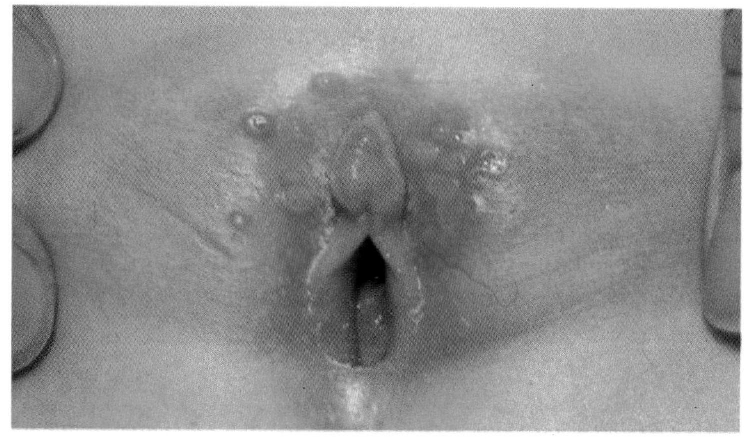

344 Genital herpes.

8 Exanthemata and enanthemata

Rashes often cause alarm to parents and pose a diagnostic dilemma to clinicians. Rashes can occur both on the skin (exanthemata) and on mucous membranes (enanthemata).

Measles

Measles is a highly infectious disease caused by a paramyxovirus (**345**) which has a helical RNA genome surrounded by a lipid envelope (120–250 nm diameter). There is only one antigenic type. The virus, which may be isolated from nasopharyngeal secretions, blood and urine, may remain viable outside the body for at least 36 hours. It primarily affects the reticulo-endothelial system and the endothelial cells of the blood vessels. Large, multinucleate, giant cells (Warthin–Finkeldey) may be found in secretions.

It is estimated that measles still causes over a million deaths annually in children under 5 years of age. It is spread by droplets and is very infectious. The incubation period lasts 10–14 days, and a prodromal period, usually 3–5 days' duration, is characterized by a low-grade fever with coryzal symptoms, a dry cough, and a non-purulent conjunctivitis which causes photophobia (**346** & **347**).

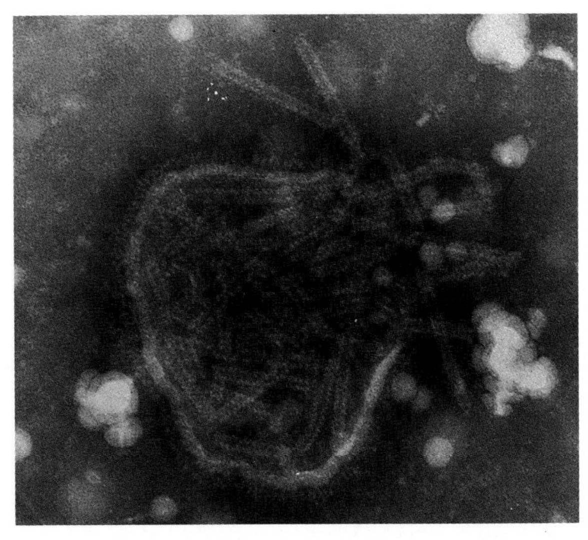

345 Negative-stain electron micrograph of measles virus which is a paramyxovirus (× *20,000*).

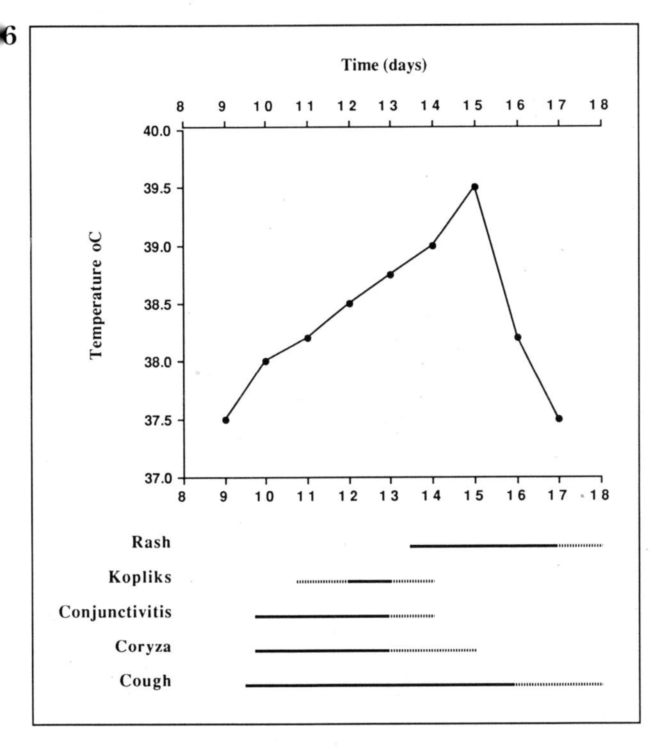

346 The clinical sequence of measles.

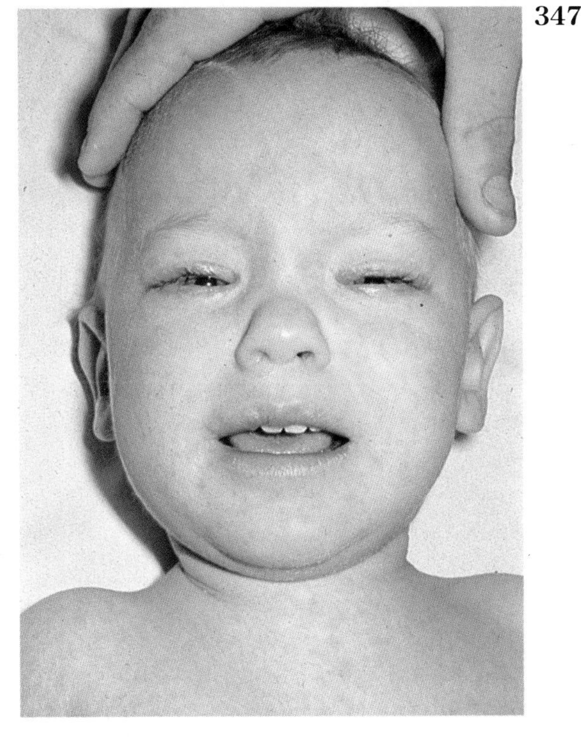

347 A child with measles showing the early clinical signs of conjunctivitis and the rash on the face.

An enanthem may be seen on the hard and soft palate. Koplik's spots (**348**), which are pathognomonic of measles, may be seen on the buccal mucosa and, occasionally, on the lower lip and palate. Koplik's spots consist of a serous exudate with a proliferation of endothelial cells. The spots usually disappear within 16 hours. As the characteristic morbilliform rash appears, the child's fever may rise above 38°C. The rash usually occurs at the hair line, spreading cephalocaudally over 48 hours (**349**). It is of a macular type (**350**), but a few petechiae may occur due to a transient thrombocytopenia (**351**). Areas covered by the rash of measles will subsequently desquamate fine scales of skin, and dark skin may demonstrate temporary hypopigmentation (**352**). The rash is immune-mediated and its appearance coincides with antibody production. The exanthem may not appear in T cell-deficient children. Rarely, haemorrhagic measles (**353**) may be a severe complication. In children who are deficient in vitamin A, superadded bacterial infection can occur. This may lead to permanent corneal scarring (**354**).

The most common complication of measles (**Table 28**) is pneumonia. Pneumonia may be caused by the virus itself. In some children a rapidly progressive giant-cell pneumonia of Hesch may progress to become fatal (**355**). A secondary bacterial invasive pneumonia can arise due to pneumococci, streptococci or staphylococci (**356**). However, such cases are more common in developing countries in malnourished children whose immunity is impaired. This impairment, together with the immunosupression from the measles virus itself, may lead to a reactivation of tuberculosis. In well-nourished children, gastrointestinal symptoms are

348

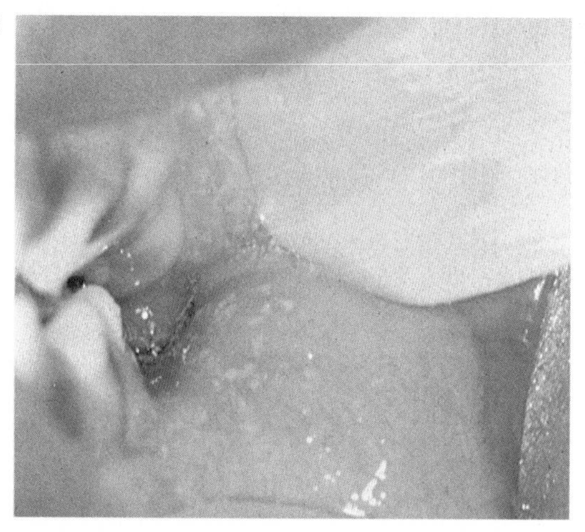

348 Koplik's spots in the buccal cavity.

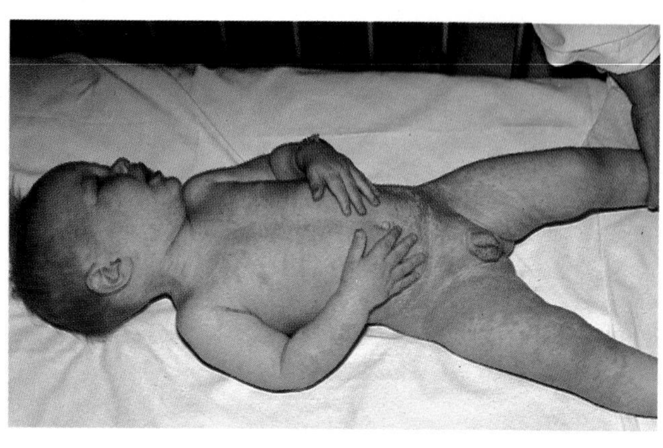

349 A child with measles demonstrating the morbilliform rash which spread cephalocaudally to the limbs.

350

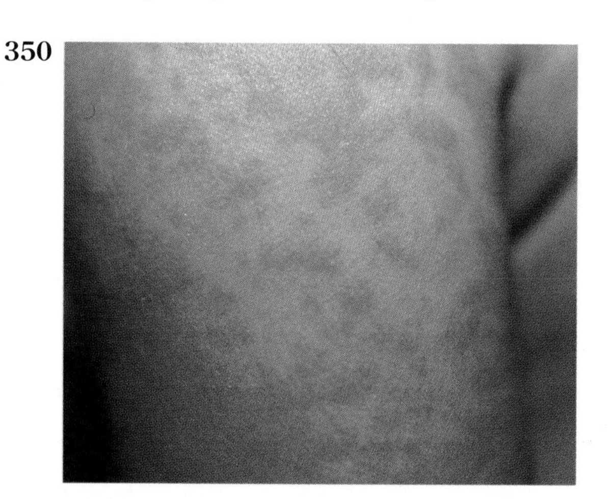

350 A close-up of the maculopapular measles rash.

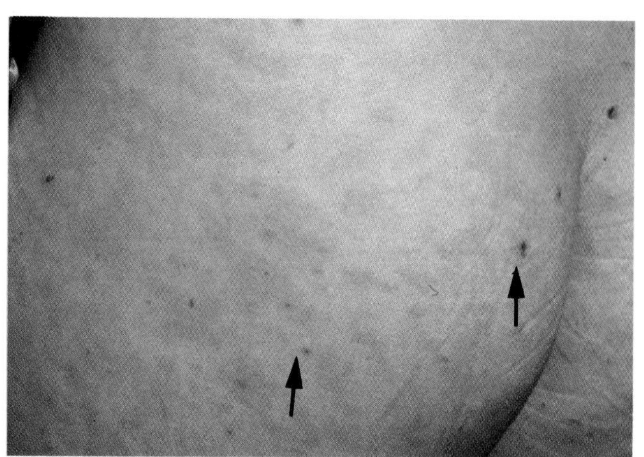

351 A measles rash demonstrating some scattered petechiae due to a transient thrombocytopenia.

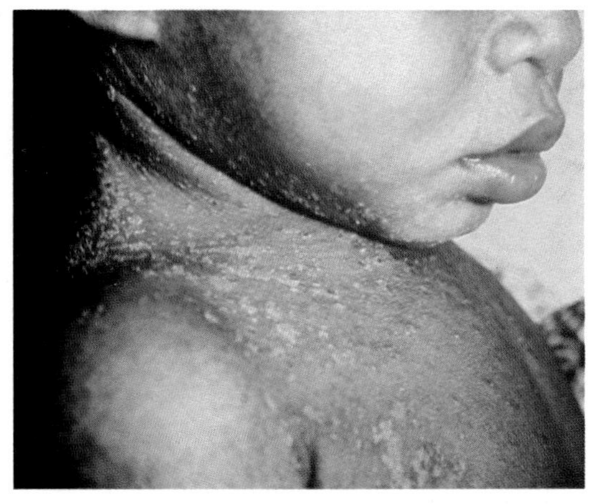

352 A measles rash demonstrating desquamation and hypopigmentation.

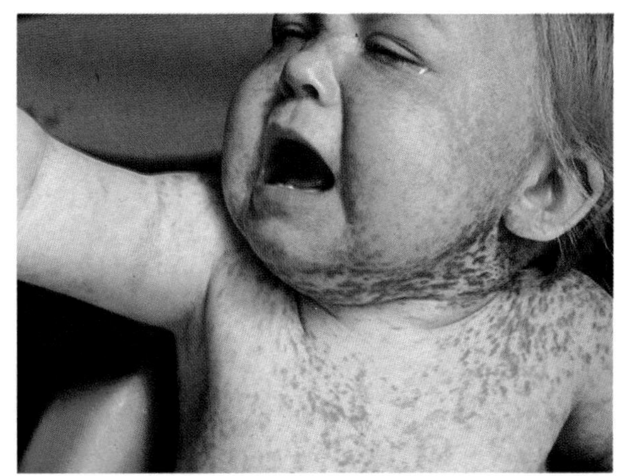

353 Haemorrhagic measles.

Table 28. Complications of Measles.

Upper respiratory tract	Croup Otitis media Laryngitis Sinusitis Mastoiditis
Lower respiratory tract	Viral pneumonitis Complicating bacterial pneumonia Giant-cell pneumonia Reactivation of tuberculosis
Central nervous system	Acute meningoencephalitis (1/1,000 cases) Subacute sclerosing panencephalitis (SSPE)
Haematological	Haemorrhagic measles Thrombocytopenia
Ophthalmic	Conjunctivitis and iritis Keratitis Corneal scarring } Associated with Blindness } vitamin A deficiency
Gastrointestinal	Diarrhoea, rare except in malnourished children in tropical climates
Cardiovascular	Myocarditis

relatively rare, but in children with malnutrition diarrhoea is a common feature and may precipitate kwashiorkor (**357**), an even more severe form of malnutrition.

Severe acute encephalitis (**358** & **359**) may occur in 1 in 10^3 children with measles. Examination of the CSF reveals a typical picture of aviral aseptic meningitis. There is a 15% mortality and a 10% morbidity associated with acute encephalitis. A late-occurring subacute panencephalitis can occur in approximately 1 in 10^5 cases. The child has usually encountered

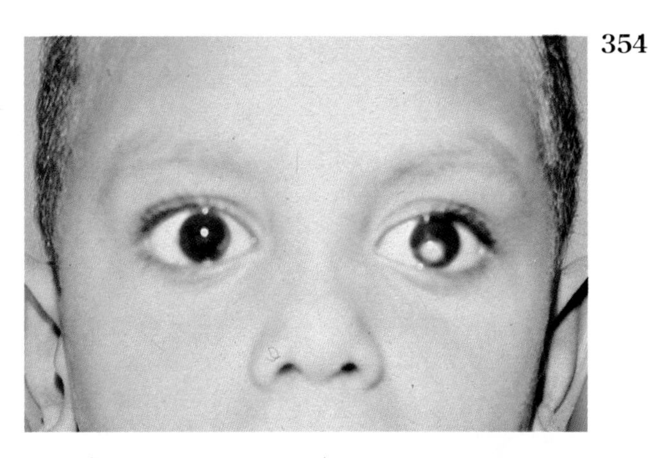

354 Corneal scarring following measles in a child who was deficient in vitamin A and developed severe measles keratitis.

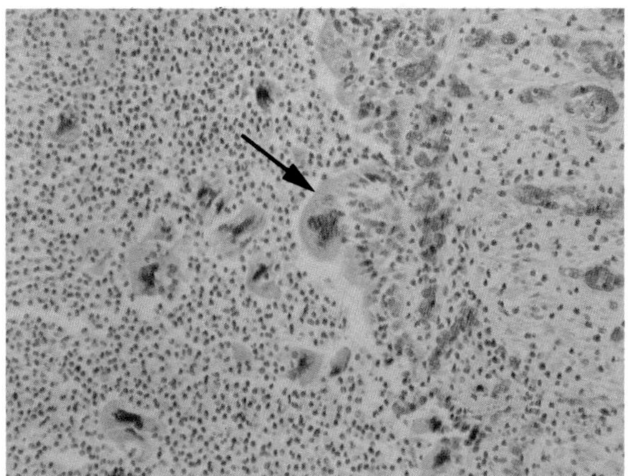

355 A section from a lung biopsy demonstrating multinucleate giant-cell pneumonia in measles (× *200*).

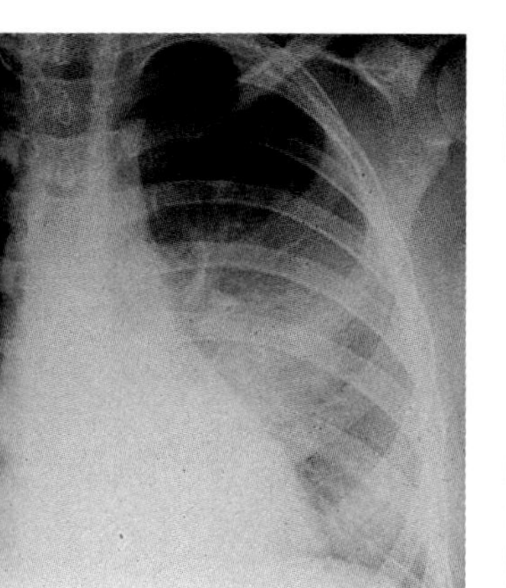

356 Chest X-ray showing secondary staphylococcal infection with abscess formation.

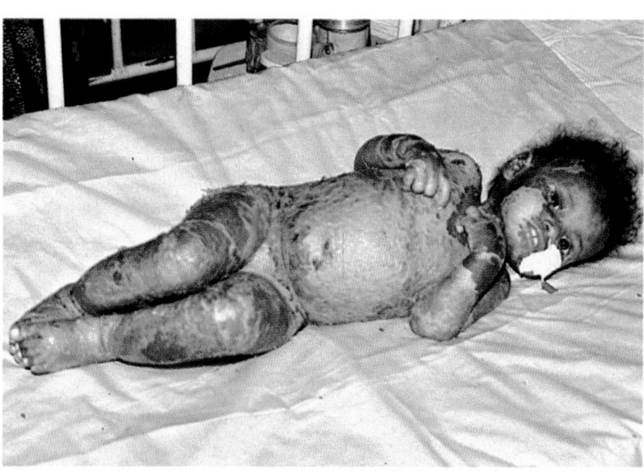

357 Kwashiorkor precipitated by measles.

measles in the first year of life, but does not develop the inevitably fatal encephalitis until the second decade.

The management of measles is symptomatic and involves treating the specific complications. Prevention is achieved with a live virus vaccine. In the UK, this is administered between the ages of 12 and 18 months as a triple vaccine combining measles, mumps and rubella cover, the MMR vaccine. In developing countries, vaccination may be recommended between 6 and 9 months because of the vulnerability of children once the maternal antibodies have disappeared. Vaccination of children as young as 4 months, using the Zagreb–Edmonston strain at a high dose, has been found to produce a significant antibody response, and provides good protection in the majority of children.

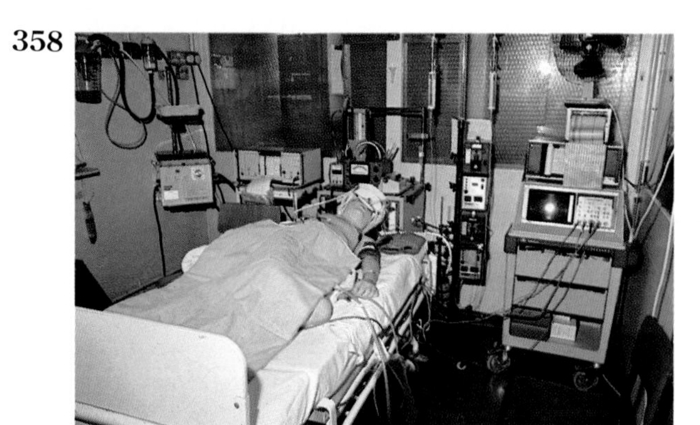

358 A nine-year-old boy on a ventilator owing to an encephalitis that presented two days after the rash appeared.

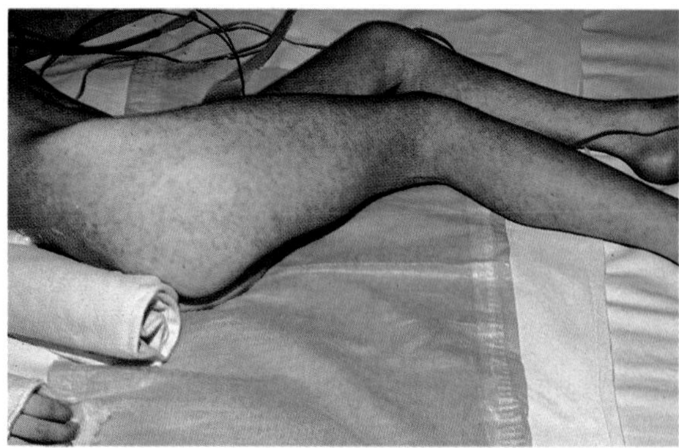

359 The same boy as in **358**, demonstrating the typical measles rash. Subsequently, he recovered fully.

Rubella (German measles)

Usually a mild infectious disease, rubella is caused by a togavirus. It is a single-stranded RNA virus with an icosahedral nucleocapsid which is 33 nm in diameter. During childhood as many as 50% of cases may be asymptomatic. The real danger of rubella virus lies in the threat to the developing fetus, because the virus can be transmitted transplacentally.

The incubation period lasts 14–20 days, and a brief prodromal period may be marked by mild fever. An enanthem then appears on the palate and a characteristic lymphadenopathy arises in the postauricular cervical (**360**) and postoccipital lymph nodes. The characteristic rash appears first on the neck and face, then travels in a cephalocaudal manner (**361**). It is often confluent on the face but tends to become more discrete over the upper limbs and trunk (**362**). The exanthem generally lasts 3–5 days but in some children it may be very ephemeral.

In adolescence a painful reactive arthritis may occur 5–7 days after the illness. The arthritis, which is more common in pubertal girls, usually affects the small joints of the hands (**363**). Usually appearing around the fifth day, it may last 2–3 weeks. Rarely, an acute encephalitis may occur (about 1 case per 6,000). During the acute phase of rubella a temporary thrombocytopenia may occur.

The virus can be detected in nasopharyngeal secretions from about 4 days before the onset of the rash until about 2 weeks later. Diagnosis is made by serology, using paired sera to detect a 4-fold rise in complement-fixing antibodies, or by detection of IgM antirubella antibody. During pregnancy it is important to distinguish rubella from parvovirus B19 infection, which may mimic rubella clinically but does not cause an embryopathy.

360

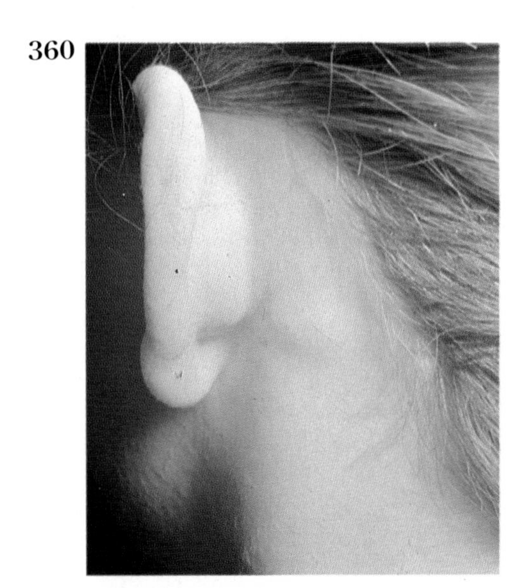

360 A child with rubella demonstrating postauricular lymph node enlargement.

361

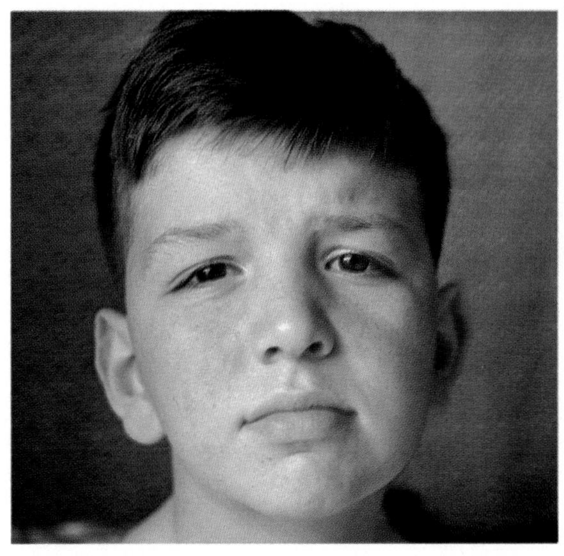

361 A child with rubella demonstrating the initially confluent rash on the face and neck.

362

362 A close-up of the rubella rash on the trunk. Small discrete areas of erythematous macules are visible.

363

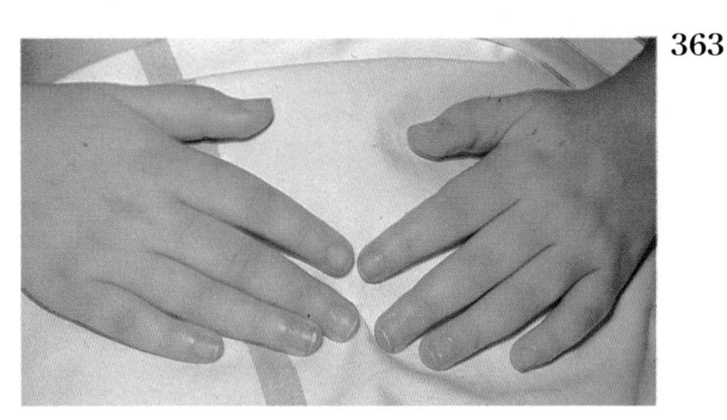

363 Postrubella arthritis in the metacarpal and interphalangeal joints.

Chickenpox (varicella–zoster)

364

364 Varicella virus from a chickenpox vesicle, demonstrating inflammatory cells (× *100*).

365

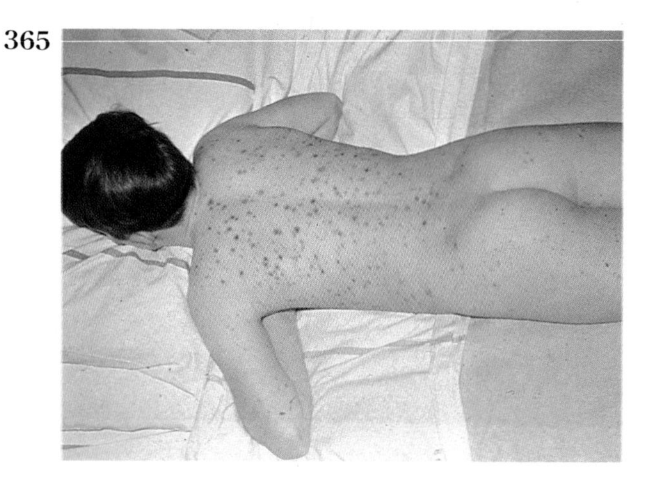

365 A child infected with varicella, demonstrating the typical centripetal distribution of the chickenpox rash.

366

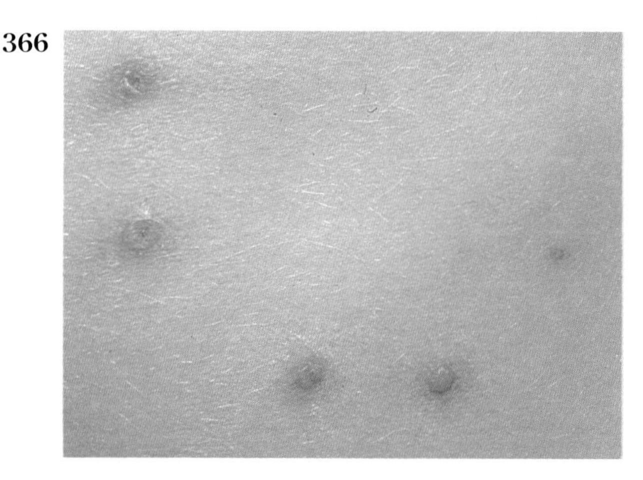

366 Varicella demonstrating all of the stages of evolution of the rash.

Varicella–zoster virus or human herpes virus 3 (HHV3) belongs to the herpes group of viruses, which have a double-stranded DNA genome within an icosahedral nucleocapsid surrounded by a lipid envelope that is 160 nm in diameter. The virus may be isolated from vesicular fluid (**364**) if it is aspirated at the first appearance of the lesions.

HHV3 causes two clinical diseases in man: chickenpox (varicella–zoster) and shingles (zoster). It is spread both by droplets and by contact with vesicles. Varicella is a highly infectious disease but it is usually a mild infection, except in immune-compromised children. The virus can cross the placenta, causing congenital chickenpox.

Chickenpox has a long incubation period of 14–20 days. The characteristic rash of lesions, which can be very itchy, may present first in the scalp. It then appears in crops over the whole body, being most concentrated over the trunk (**365**). In a process that takes only 12–18 hours, the typical lesions progress rapidly from macules to papules and vesicles, and then to pustules before finally crusting. New crops of spots appear successively over 2–3 days, so that lesions may be seen in all stages of evolution simultaneously (**366**). The typical vesicle has been likened to a teardrop because of its elliptical shape (**367**). It tends to crust from the centre, giving it an umbilicated appearance. Any mucous membrane can be involved including those of the tongue (**368**), vagina, rectum, pharynx, larynx and trachea, and the conjunctiva. Once crusting occurs, the child is no longer infectious. Provided that bacterial superinfection (**369**) does not occur, no residual scar is left.

Varicella is a severe disease in children who are immune-compromised for any reason. It may develop to become haemorrhagic and progressive, with a fatal outcome in about 7% of cases. One complication in children is viral pneumonia, which may later demonstrate calcification over both lung fields (**370**). Rare complications of chickenpox include arthritis, hepatitis, encephalitis, and an association with Reye's syndrome (**Table 29**).

Table 29. Complications of Chickenpox.

Bacterial infection
Pneumonia
Encephalitis
Reye's syndrome
Haemorrhagic chickenpox
Progressive disseminated disease in the immune-compromised

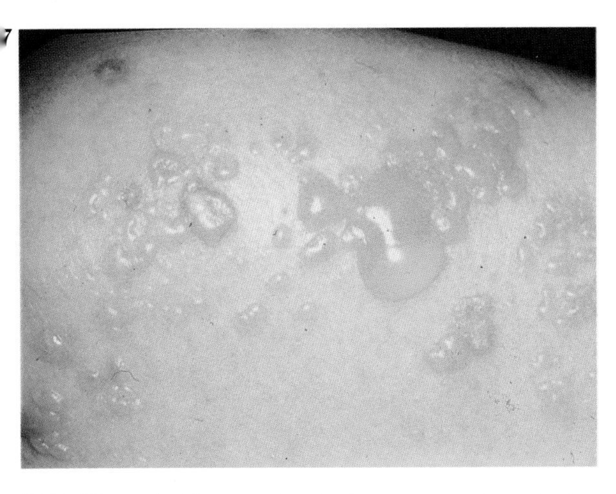

367 The typical 'teardrop' varicella papules and developing pustules with umbilication.

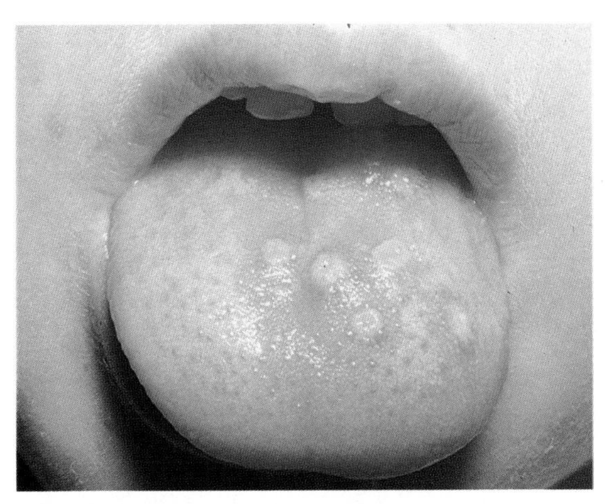

368 Varicella spots on the tongue.

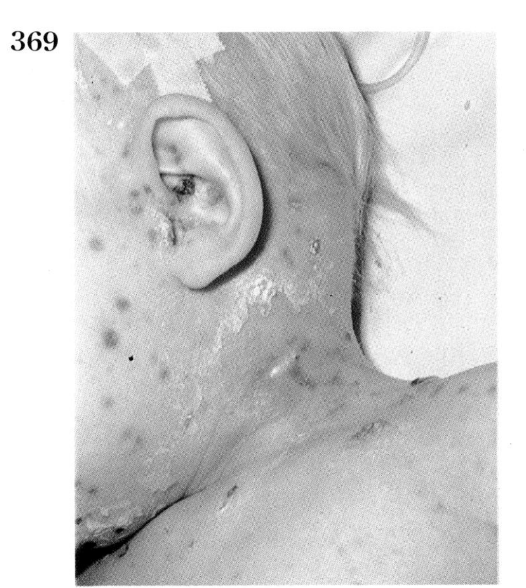

369 Varicella rash complicated by staphylococcal infection.

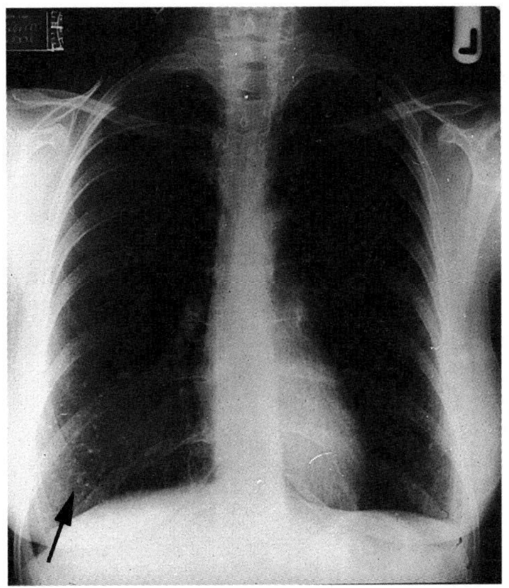

370 X-ray of varicella pneumonia showing small discrete areas of calcification, especially at the lung bases.

Herpes zoster (shingles)

Shingles, which is caused by reactivation of the VZV, can occur in normal children, but it is more likely to occur in children who are immune-suppressed for any reason. It may present in any dermatome when virus reactivates from latency in the corresponding dorsal root ganglion (**371**). Serious complications arise when the cranial nerves are involved, especially if the ophthalmic branch of the fifth nerve is affected, in which case damage to the eye may occur (**372**).

The shingles rash progresses through the same stages as those of varicella. There may be a few isolated lesions at sites distant from the main area of infection. The condition usually resolves over 2–3 weeks but a painful postherpetic neuralgia may persist for months afterwards.

A diagnosis can be rapidly made by electronmicroscopy and virus may be isolated from vesicular fluid. Fortunately in severe infection, treatment with acyclovir can be effective in shortening the course of the disease and it should certainly be used in the immune-compromised child.

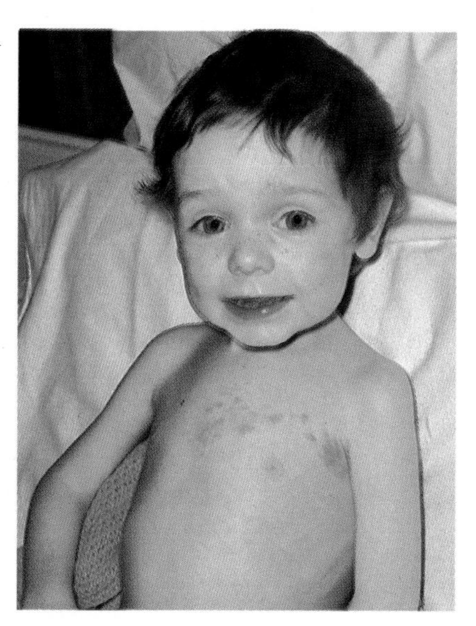

371 Herpes zoster (shingles) with a distribution of a left T7 thoracic dermatome.

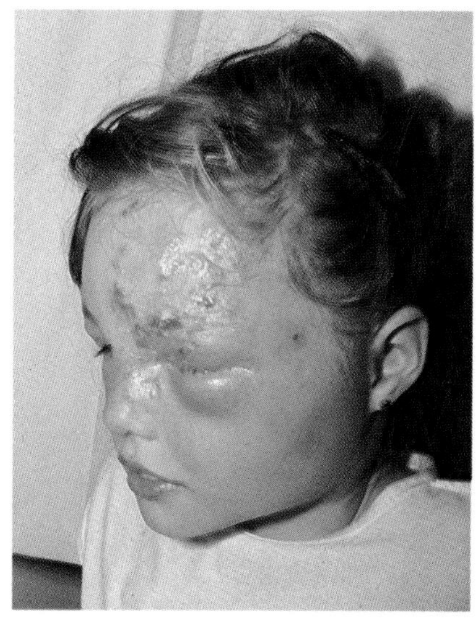

372 Herpes zoster affecting the ophthalmic division of left fifth cranial nerve.

Erythema infectiosum (fifth disease)

Erythema infectiosum is an exanthema of childhood caused by the human parvovirus B19. It has a single-stranded DNA genome and measures 22 nm in diameter. The incubation period is 7–10 days.

The rash is characterized by livid erythematous macular papular lesions which spread over the cheeks to give a 'slapped cheek' appearance (**373**). The edge of the rash is slightly raised but is not painful. The lesions fade from the face to migrate over the extensor surface of the limbs and onto the trunk. The distribution tends to be symmetrical. The progression of the disease usually takes 5–7 days, but occasionally recrudescences of the rash may occur over several weeks.

In older children and adolescents, parvovirus B19 may cause an arthritis which can take up to a month to resolve. A serious complication of the virus arises as a result of its predilection for development within erythroid bone marrow cells. An aplastic crisis, which is fortunately self-limiting, may occur in patients with haemolytic disease such as thalassaemia or sickle-cell anaemia. Parvovirus B19 can be transmitted to the fetus transplacentally and is a cause of non-transfusion hydrops fetalis. Although associated with miscarriage and stillbirth during the early pregnancy, no embryopathy has yet been defined.

373 Erythema infectiosum. The rash gives the child the characteristic 'slapped cheek' appearance.

Roseola infantum (exanthem subitum)

A common exanthema in infants and children, Roseola infantum is caused by the herpes virus that has been designated HHV6. Transmission is by droplets, usually from healthy asymptomatic adults who may shed the virus from the oropharynx. Infection, which is benign and self-limiting, is characterized by an abrupt onset of fever, and lasts for 2–4 days. As the fever subsides (**374**), a macular rash appears on the face and trunk (**375**), and there may be slight oedema of the eyelids.

Complications include acute febrile convulsions, and some children have been reported to develop a more severe illness which includes an acute encephalopathy, hepatitis, and diffuse lymphadenopathy with hepatosplenomegaly. Treatment is symptomatic. Diagnosis may be made by serology, demonstrating a 4-fold rise in antibodies on paired sera.

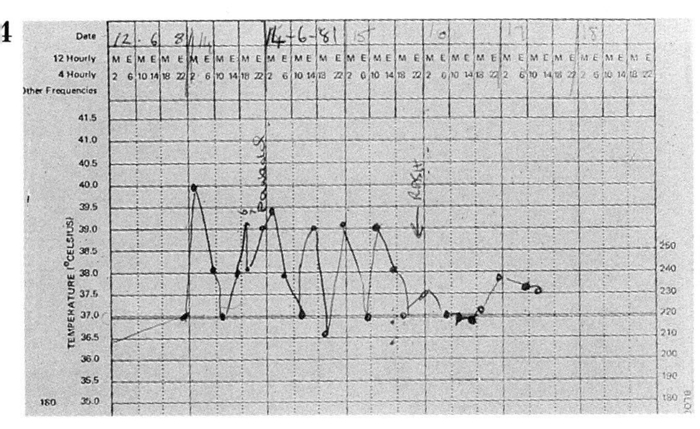

374 Temperature chart of a child with roseola infantum. There is a fall in temperature with the appearance of the rash.

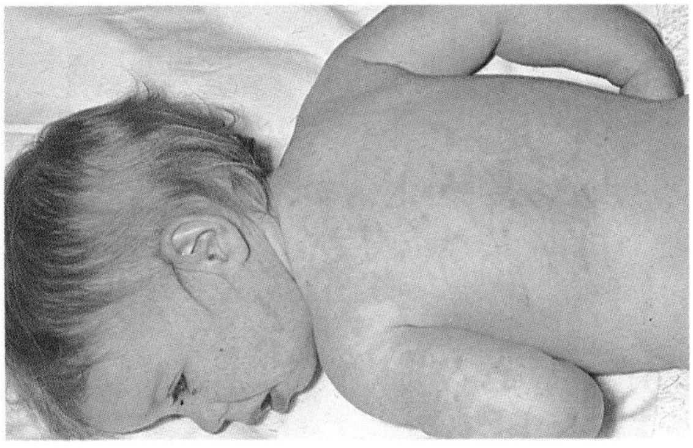

375 A child with roseola infantum. The delicate erythematous rash is clearly visible over the face and trunk.

Scarlet fever

Scarlet fever is caused by strains of group A β-haemolytic streptococci which elaborate an erythrogenic toxin. It may result from a streptococcal pharyngitis or, more rarely, from skin infections or infections of wounds or burns. There is usually a short (2–5 days) incubation period in which severe constitutional symptoms, such as fever, rigors, headache, vomiting and abdominal pain, may suddenly present. Usually, the pharynx becomes inflamed and is covered with a whitish membrane. This membrane may be present over the tongue, where the swollen papillae produce the characteristic appearance described as a

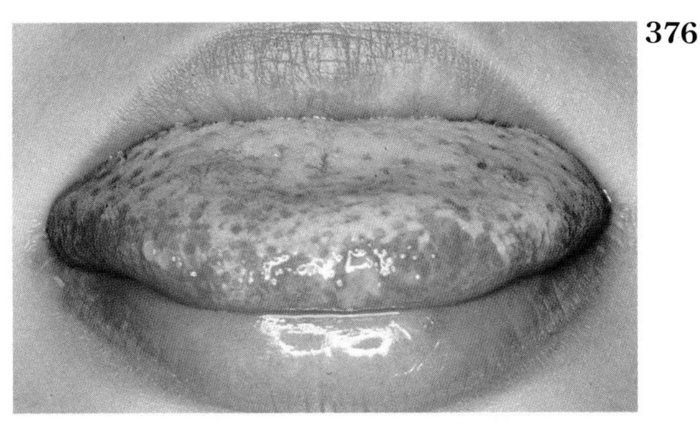

376 The characteristic white strawberry tongue of scarlet fever.

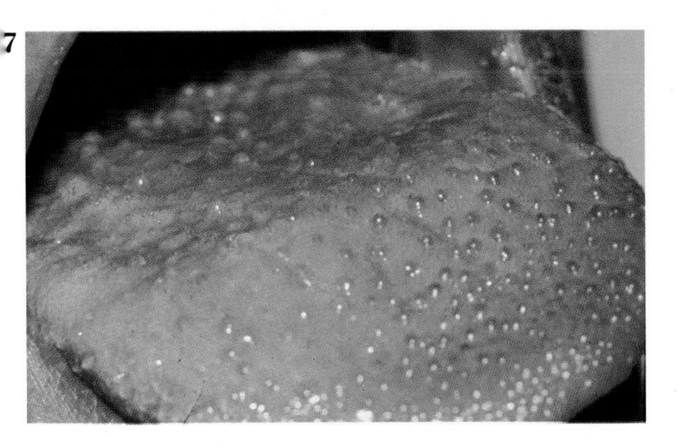

377 Hyperplasia of the papillae of the tongue in a child with scarlet fever.

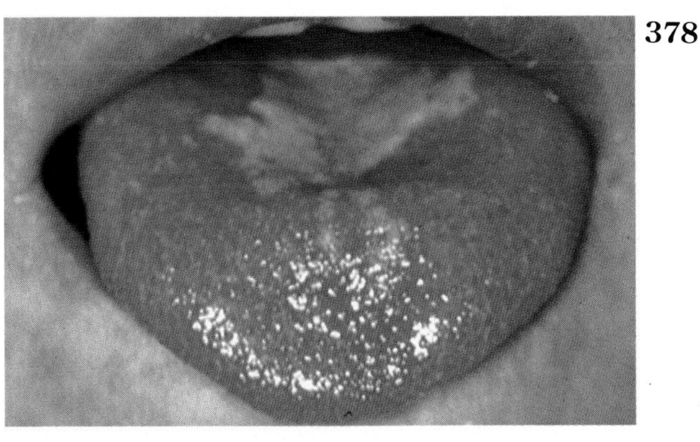

378 The characteristic red strawberry tongue after desquamation in scarlet fever.

'white strawberry tongue' (**376** & **377**). Within 48 hours the membrane desquamates, leaving the so-called 'red strawberry tongue' (**378**).

The exanthem usually starts on the face in the form of a diffuse erythematous flush which spares the circumoral region (**379**). It then spreads over the rest of the body as a fine punctate rash which feels like 'goose pimples'. The rash tends to blanche on pressure, but areas of hyperpigmentation occur in deep creases, particularly in the anticubital fossa. An important characteristic of scarlet fever is the desquamation that occurs on resolution of the rash. This usually starts on the face, evolves over the trunk and extremities (**380–382**). Large areas of desquamated skin may occur in some cases.

In the past, scarlet fever was a much feared, serious and potentially fatal infectious disease of children. However, since the introduction of penicillin it appears to have become a milder and less common disease.

379

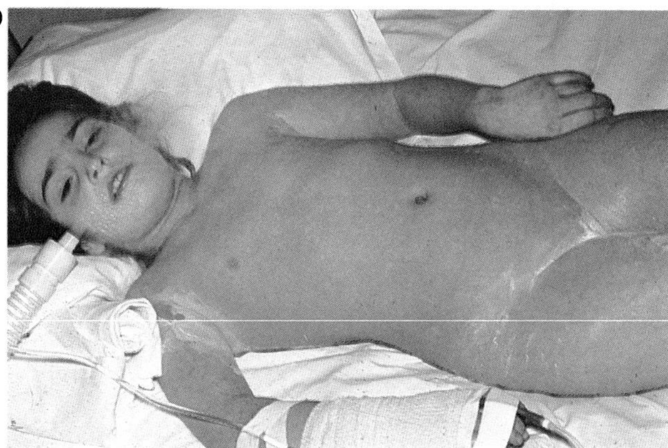

379 The scarlet fever rash is diffuse and there is circumoral pallor.

380

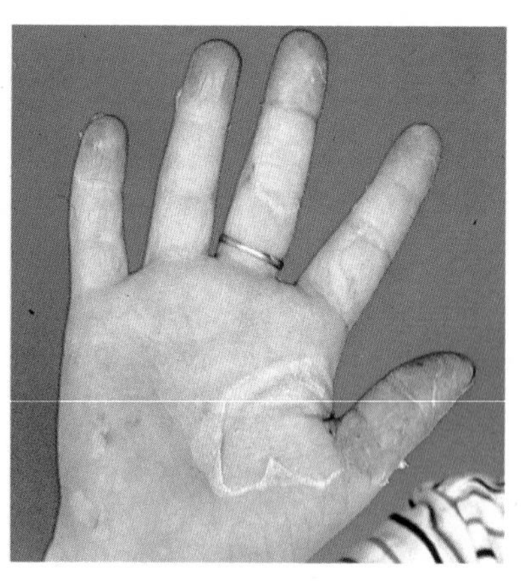

380 A child with scarlet fever demonstrating desquamation on the hands.

381

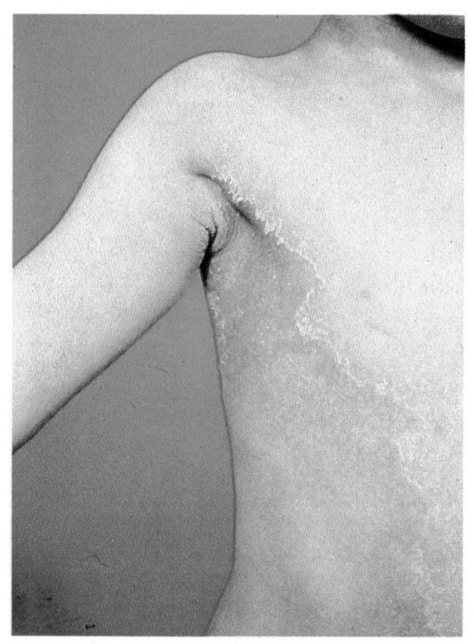

381 Scarlet fever showing desquamation spreading to the trunk.

382

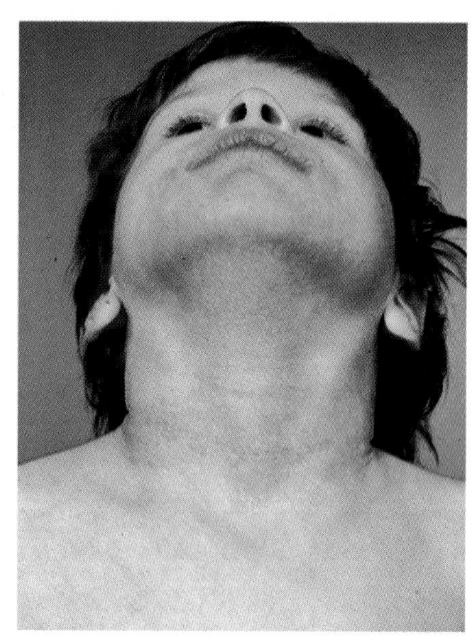

382 Scarlet fever with desquamation under the neck.

Infectious mononucleosis (glandular fever)

Infectious mononucleosis is caused by the Epstein–Barr virus (EBV or HHV5), which, like other herpesviruses, is a DNA virus. EBV is spread by droplet infection but close contact is needed for transmission. The virus has been associated with other clinical conditions such as Burkitt's lymphoma in Africa (**383**) and nasopharyngeal carcinoma in East Asia. Duncan's disease is a progressive and fatal form of EBV infection. It occurs in males who have an X-linked immune defect.

Infectious mononucleosis is so termed because of a characteristic increase in atypical peripheral blood monocytes. The virus infects B lymphocytes, but the atypical lymphocytes in the peripheral blood are T cells responding to infection (**384**). The incubation period is thought to last 10–17 days.

In infants and young children the infection is often mild or inapparent. In older children and adolescents the angiose type is a frequent presentation. There is a white exudate on the tonsils. (**385**). Diffuse lymphadenopathy is present especially in the cervical region. Oedema of the soft tissues may be present in association with lymphadenopathy (**386**). Hepatosplenomegaly is common. In 10–15% of cases a skin

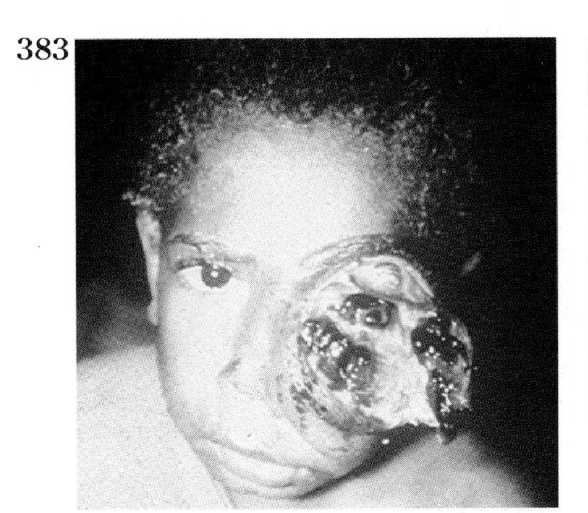

383 Burkitt's lymphoma is associated with EBV infection.

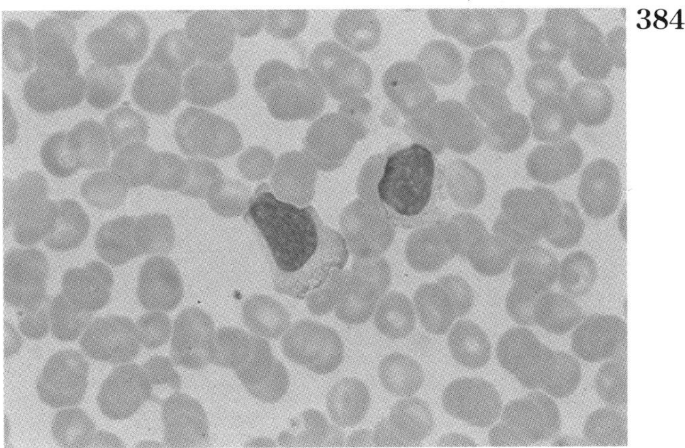

384 Infectious mononucleosis showing two atypical T lymphocytes with large dense nuclei (× *500*).

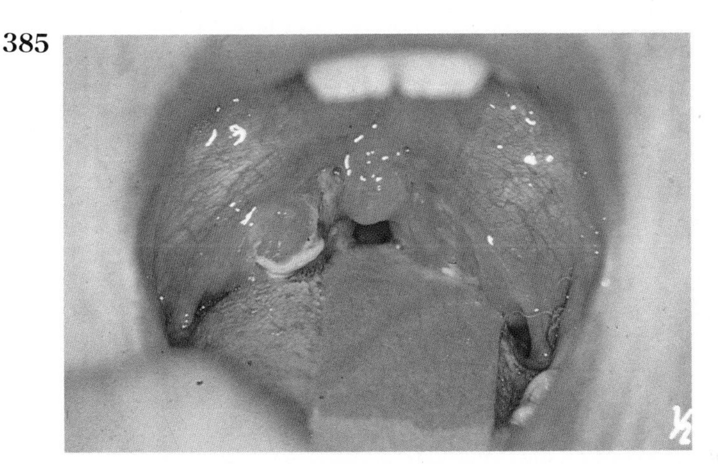

385 A white exudate on the tonsils of a child with infectious mononucleosis.

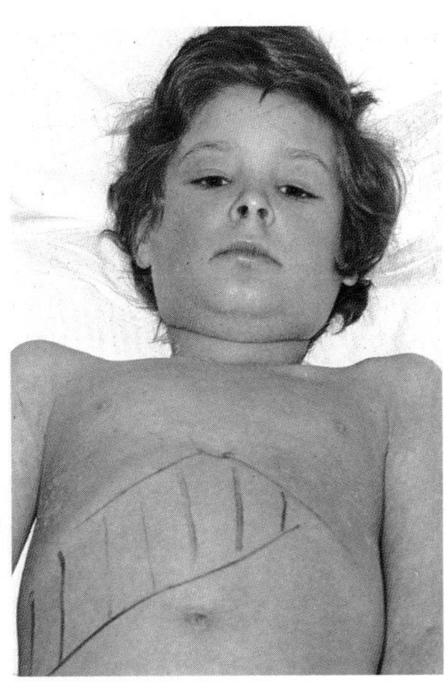

386 A child with infectious mononucleosis demonstrating cervical lymphadenopathy, oedema, hepatomegaly and a rash.

rash occurs. This often appears first on the face and then spreads over the whole body. It is erythematous with discrete areas over the trunk and limbs (**387**).

If a penicillin (especially ampicillin) is administered, a dramatic and widespread rash over the whole body may be precipitated. Complications are rare in children, but in adults and older children almost any system of the body may be involved and the clinical course may be prolonged (**Table 30**).

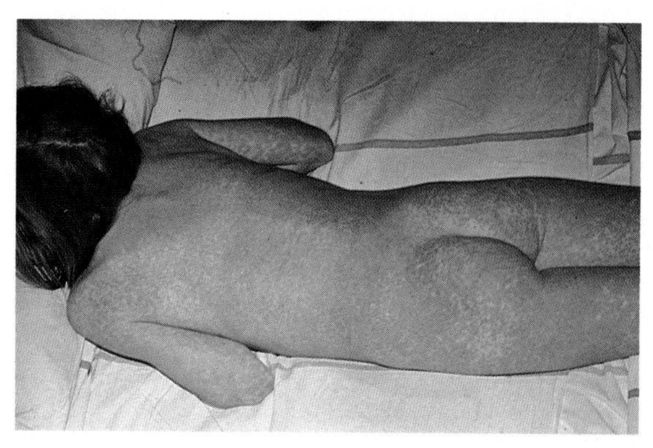

387 A typical discrete maculopapular rash on a child with infectious mononucleosis.

Table 30. Complications of Infectious Mononucleosis.

Hepatitis with hepatosplenomegaly
Pharyngitis with cervical lymphadenopathy
Reactive arthritis
Guillaine–Barré postinfective polyneuritis
Encephalitis
Meningitis
Pneumonitis
Carditis

Mumps (epidemic parotitis)

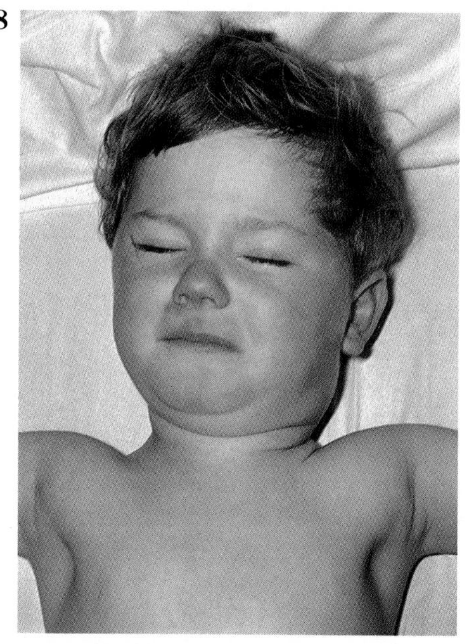

388 A child with mumps. The parotid gland is enlarged, hiding the angle of the jaw.

Mumps is a common and usually mild infectious disease of childhood. It is caused by an RNA paramyxovirus and is spread by droplet infection. In 30–40% of cases the disease may be asymptomatic. Mumps has an incubation period of 14–24 days and in some children there is a short prodromal period of 24–48 hours when some myalgia, pain in the parotid glands and, occasionally, a headache may be experienced. Fever is usually low grade and below 38°C. The first clinical signs are usually of pain and swelling in one or both of the parotid glands. Parotid swelling usually affects one side before the other, giving the face an asymmetrical appearance (**388**). Any of the salivary glands may be involved, but the parotid glands are the most commonly affected, followed by the submaxillary and submental glands. Redness and swelling of the orifices of the Stensen's and Wharton's ducts may also occur.

The one serious complication of mumps is meningoencephalitis which occurs in approximately 3.5 cases per 10^3. Males appear to be affected more frequently than females. It is clinically indistinguishable from other types of meningoencephalitis, and the CSF reflects the typical picture of aseptic meningitis.

Occasionally, sensorineural deafness, which is usually unilateral and may be temporary or permanent, is a complication. Other complications such as orchitis, oophoritis, or pancreatitis are rare in children, but they may present in postpubescent adolescents and young adults (**Table 31**).

Table 31. Complications of Mumps.

Meningoencephalitis	Nephritis
Deafness	Thyroiditis
Orchitis	Myocarditis
Oophoritis	Arthritis
Epididymitis	Thrombocytopenia
Pancreatitis	

Coxsackie A and B virus and ECHOvirus exanthemata

Although Coxsackie viruses and ECHOviruses are classified as enteroviruses, they cause a variety of conditions that are not necessarily associated with gastrointestinal symptoms (**Table 32**). A whole range of rashes may occur including scarlatiniform, morbilliform, petechial and vesicular types. Those that have a characteristic appearance are described. Enteroviruses are a genus comprising over 70 types. Part of the Picornaviridae family, they have a single-stranded RNA genome and a virion that is 27 nm in diameter.

Hand, foot and mouth disease is caused by Coxsackie A virus (types 4, 5, 7, 9 and 16). Vesicles appear in crops on the palms of the hands (**389**), the soles of the feet (**390**), and in the mouth. The illness is usually relatively insignificant and self-limiting.

ECHOvirus may also cause an exanthematous illness (**391**). ECHOvirus types 4, 9 and 16 have been particularly associated with a vesicular rash, which may be petechial. The lesions may be widely spread over the body including the face.

389

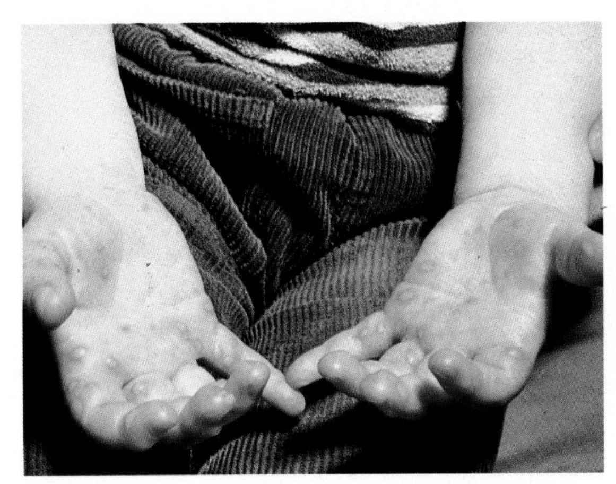

389 Discrete papules on the hands of a child with Coxsackie A infection. (Hand, foot and mouth disease.)

Table 32. Illness Associated with Coxsackie and ECHOvirus infection.

Enterovirus	*Serotype*	*Disease*
Coxsackie A	A5, 10 and 16	Hand, foot and mouth
	A2–6, 8 and 10	Herpangina
Coxsackie B	B3, 5 and others	Epidemic myalgia (Bornhölm disease)
	B3, 4	Neonatal disease
	B3, 4 and others	Myocarditis
ECHOvirus	4, 9 and 16	Aseptic meningoencephalitis

390

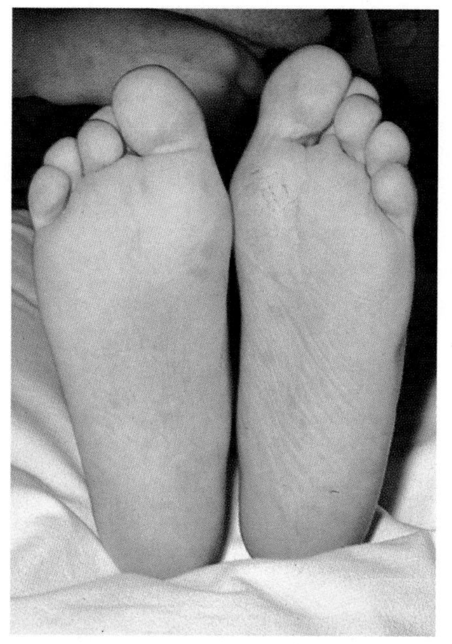

391

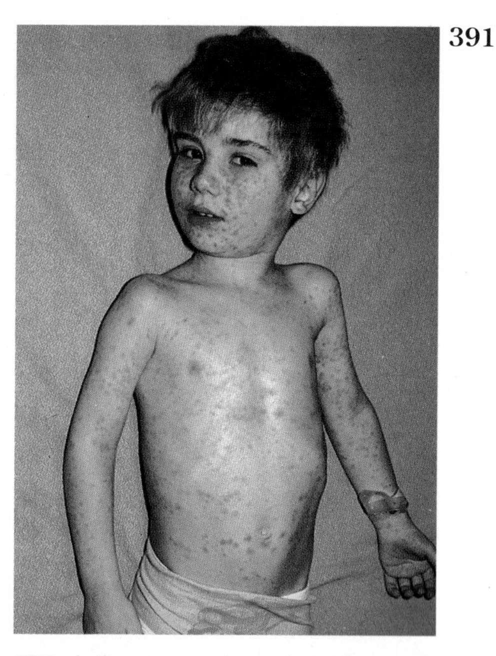

390 Discrete papules on the feet of a child with Coxsackie A infection. (Hand, foot and mouth disease.)

391 A discrete maculopapular rash caused by ECHOvirus.

Adenovirus exanthemata

Adenoviruses, which are double-stranded DNA viruses, have also been associated with a variety of rashes including scarlatiniform, rubelliform and morbilliform types (**392** & **393**).

392

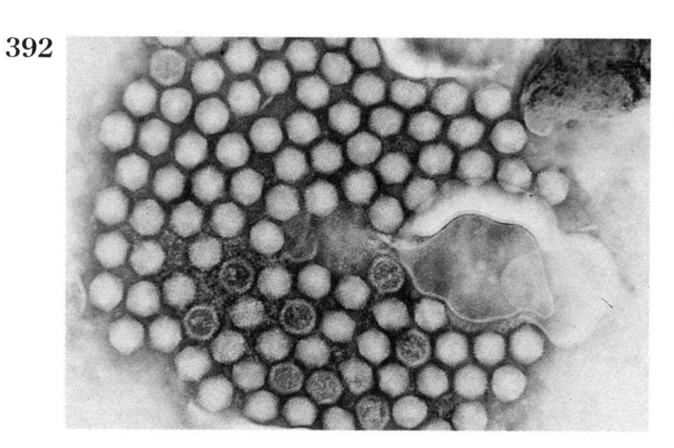

392 Negative-stain electron micrograph of an adenovirus, which may be associated with a variety of rashes (× *26,000*).

393

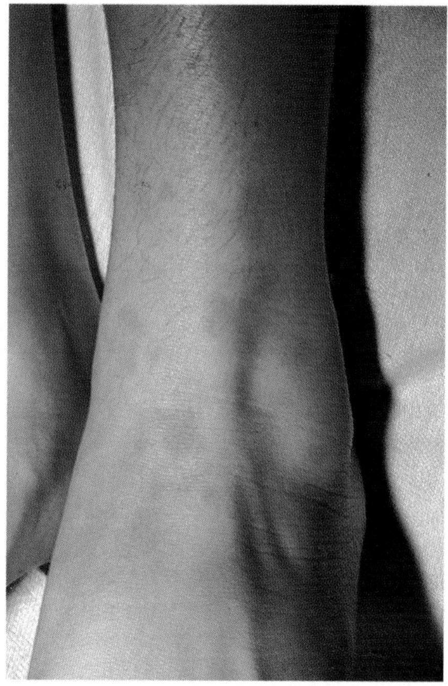

393 An adenovirus-associated rash.

Erythema multiforme

As the name suggests, erythema multiforme has a wide variety of clinical presentations. At one extreme, there may be a rash limited to certain areas of the skin (Hebra's disease). At the other, a severe systemic illness associated with inflammation of all mucocutaneous junctions may occur (Stevens–Johnson syndrome). Erythema multiforme has been associated with many infectious diseases as well as with other trigger factors (**Table 33**). The exact pathophysiological mechanism that causes the condition is unknown.

In the mild disease the rash is usually asymmetric and characteristic target (iris or bull's-eye) lesions are seen (**394**). In the more severe Stevens–Johnson syndrome the child may be ill with a fever, malaise, arthralgia and upper respiratory symptoms. All mucocutaneous junctions may be affected, including those of the nose, eyes and mouth (**395**), as well as those at the anal, vaginal and urethral orifices (**396**).

394

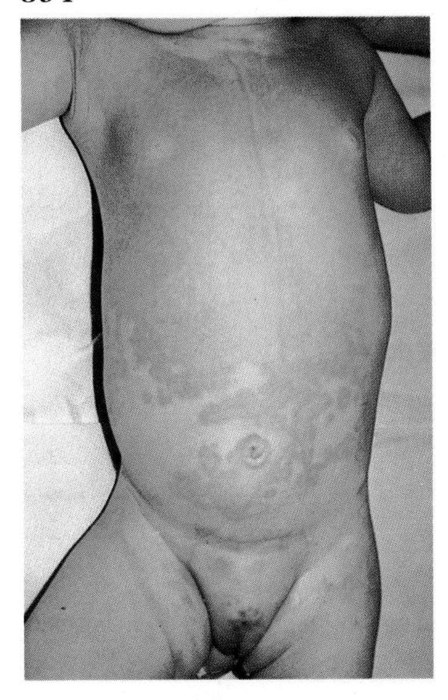

394 A polymorphic rash with typical 'target' lesions in a child with erythema multiforme.

395

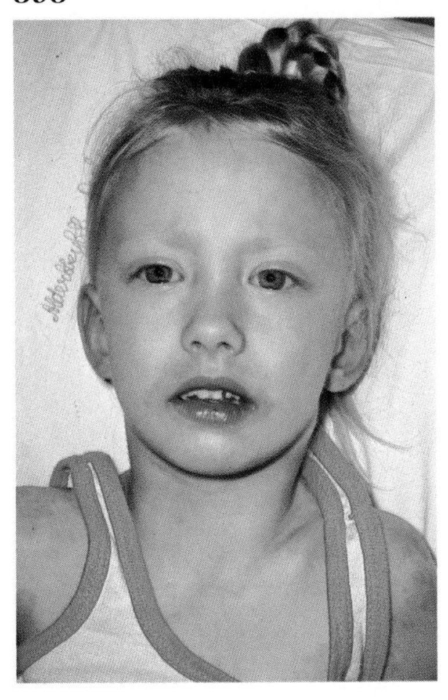

395 Mucocutaneous involvement of the mouth and conjunctivae in Stevens–Johnson syndrome.

396

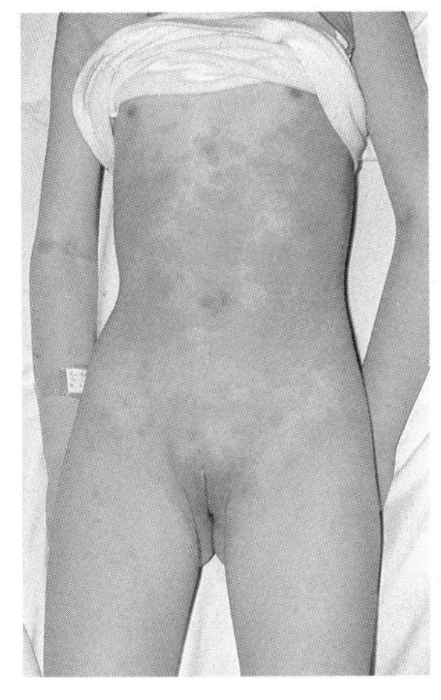

396 Involvement of the vagina and other mucocutaneous junctions in Stevens–Johnson syndrome.

Table 33. Conditions and Trigger Factors Associated with Erythema Multiforme.

Infections	*Drugs*	*Vaccines*	*Others*
Mycoplasma pneumoniae	Antibiotics	Antitoxins	Connective-tissue disease
Bacterial pneumonia	Anticonvulsants	BCG	Malignancies
Meningitis	Aspirin	Polio	Contact dermatitis
Cholera	Codeine		
Typhoid	Quinine		
Measles	Others		
Mumps			
Herpes simplex			
Psittacosis and other chlamydial infections			
Glanders			
Malaria			

Erythema nodosum

Erythema nodosum is thought to be a dermal manifestation of a hypersensitivity reaction to various viral, bacterial and fungal infections (**Table 34**), as well as to some drugs. It is characterized by tender erythematous nodules which usually arise on the extensor and anterior surfaces of the lower (**397**) and upper limbs and, occasionally, on the head and face. The lesions are due to a vasculitis with an infiltration of inflammatory cells. The nodules usually disappear within 2 or 3 weeks without leaving any scarring.

397

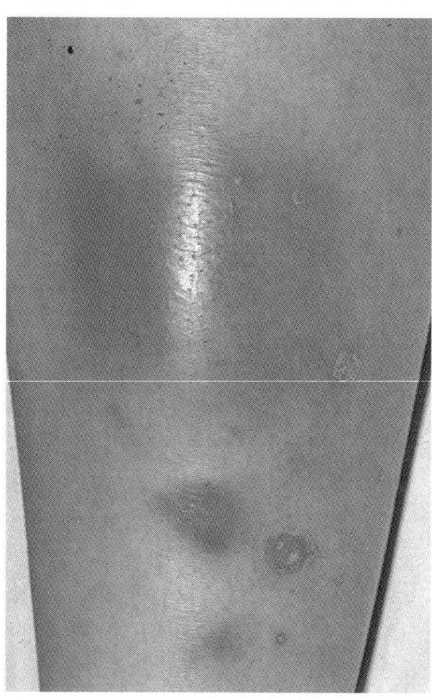

397 Erythema nodosum on the shin. This condition is associated with several infections including TB and streptococcal infections.

Table 34. Infections Associated with Erythema Nodosum.

Tuberculosis	Syphilis
Streptococcal infection	Gonorrhoea
Leprosy	Histoplasmosis
Mycoplasma pneumoniae	Coccidiomycosis
Whooping cough	Trichophytosis
Lymphogranuloma inguinale	Sarcoidosis
Measles	

9 Infections of the skin, soft tissue and bone

Skin and soft tissue

Viral infections

Cutaneous manifestations of viral infections may arise either by direct inoculation into the skin, or as a result of a viraemia. In general, direct inoculation produces localized lesions, whereas viraemia produces more widespread rashes. The generalized rashes may be due either to the replication of virus in the skin (e.g. chickenpox), or to an immune reaction to viral antigens in the skin (e.g. measles). Localized infections are caused by herpesviruses, poxviruses and papillomaviruses.

Herpes simplex virus

Herpes simplex or HHV1 is a neurotropic α-herpesvirus which produces a primary infection in the mouth. The infection, which is generally acquired from siblings or parents, is usually inapparent to mild, but it may also produce gingivostomatitis (**398**). Virus tracks back along the trigeminal nerve to the trigeminal ganglion, where it remains latent. In some individuals the latent virus reactivates, passes back along the nerve and produces a typical vesicular 'cold sore' at the vermillion border of the lips (**399**). This secondary infection or recrudescence can occur with monotonous regularity. Factors leading to recrudescence include fever, colds and sunburn.

The primary infection need not occur only in the mouth. Herpetic whitlows (**400**) may develop, especially if the child is a finger or thumb sucker at the time of the primary oral infection. In such circumstances, virus tracks back along sensory nerves to become latent in the cervical ganglia. Reactivations do occur into the skin, be they recurrences of whitlows (**401**) or recrudescences in the other areas of skin (**402**). The resulting vesicle contains large numbers of infective virus particles (about 10^7/ml). If viral inoculation into an inflamed skin occurs, it may lead to a more widespread infection. For example, inoculation into an area of napkin dermatitis can produce a florid infection (**403**) and inoculation into eczematous skin can give rise to a widespread and life-threatening infection, eczema herpeticum (**404**). Infections do not usually require treatment, but some, such as eczema herpeticum, will require intravenous acyclovir.

398

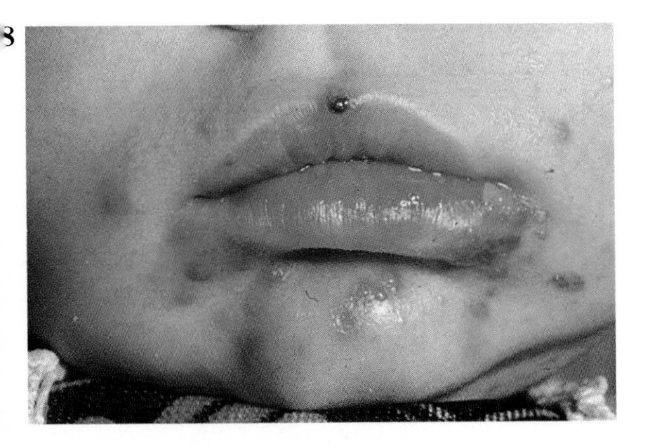

398 Primary herpes gingivostomatitis.

399

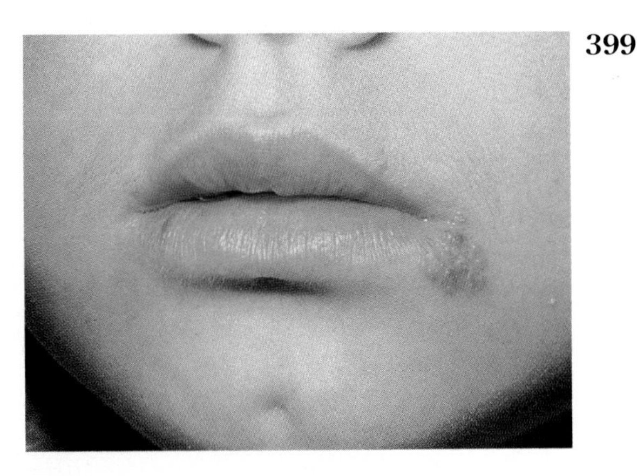

399 A cold sore or secondary Herpes labialis infection.

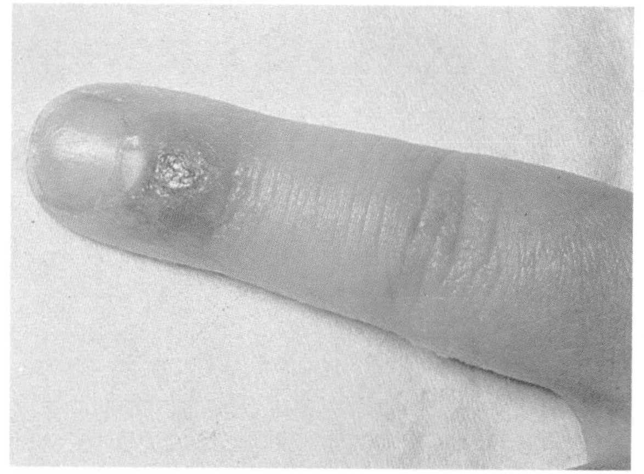

400 A primary herpetic whitlow.

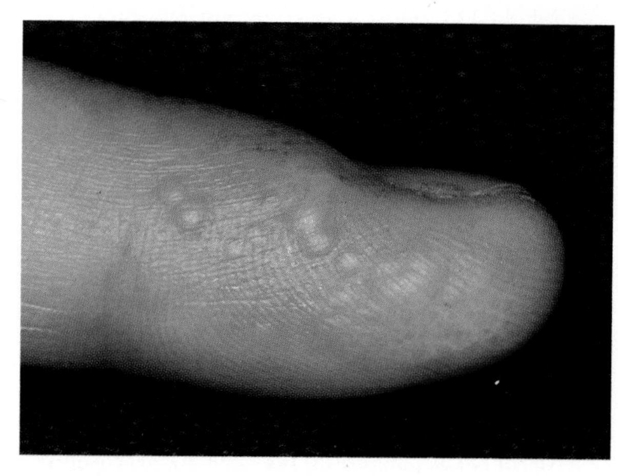

401 Recurrent or secondary Herpes simplex infection on the finger.

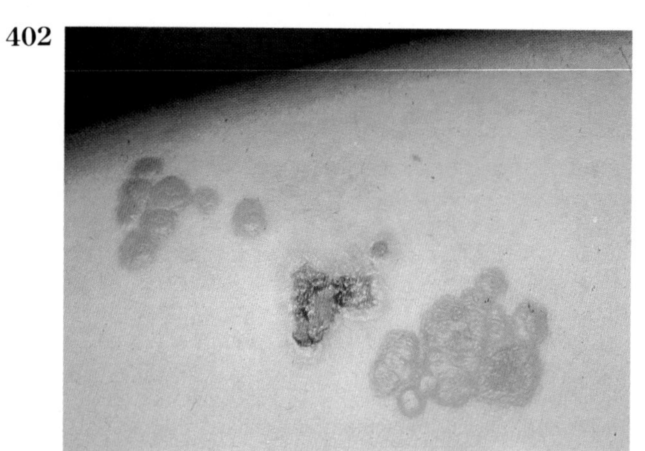

402 Recurrent Herpes simplex infection on the shoulder.

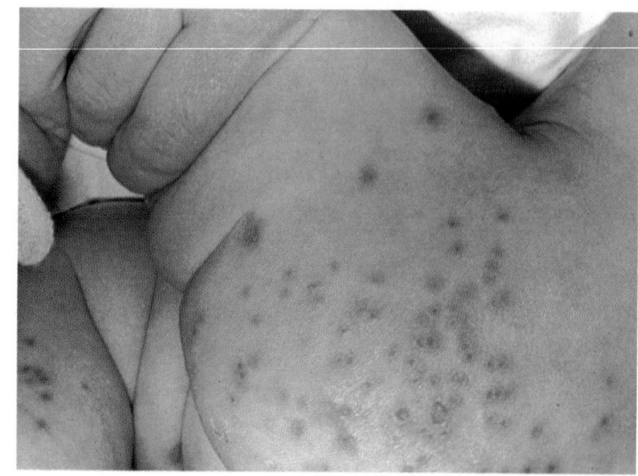

403 Herpes simplex infection of the nappy area.

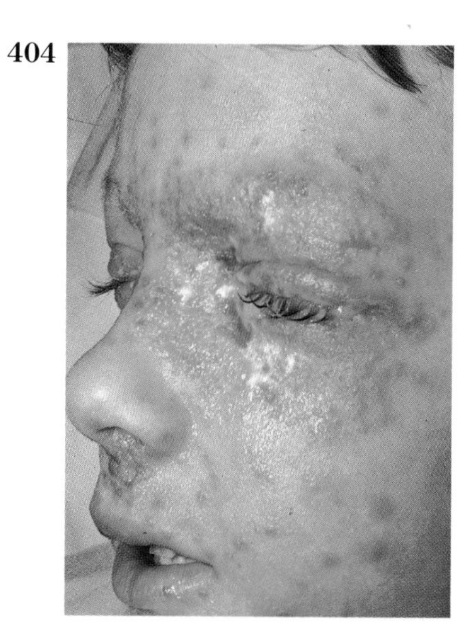

404 Eczema herpeticum or Kaposi's varicelliform eruption.

Varicella–zoster virus

Varicella–zoster virus or HHV3 may reactivate in childhood to produce shingles (**405**). This is not an indication for investigation of possible immunodeficiency. It is part of the normal spectrum of recrudescence.

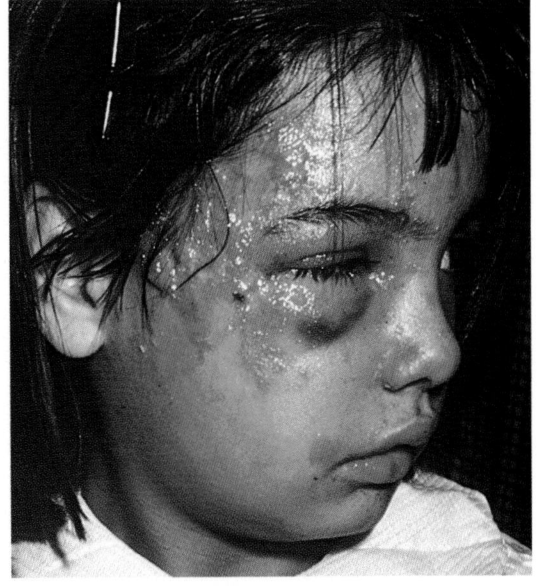

405 Shingles involving the ophthalmic division of the trigeminal nerve.

Human papillomaviruses

Human papillomaviruses (HPV) are small unenveloped DNA viruses (**406**) that produce cutaneous and mucosal warts. HPV1 and HPV2 are the most common types. Lesions may be papular (plane warts) (**407**) or nodular (**408**), and can occur on any part of the skin including the perianal region (**409**) or the feet (**410**), where they are commonly called verrucas. Depending upon the site of the wart, treatment usually involves cryotherapy, trichloracetic acid, currettage or podophyllin.

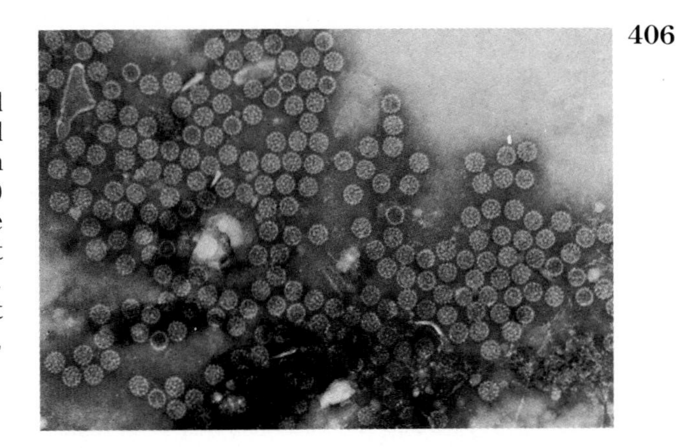

406 Negative-stain electron micrograph of human papillomavirus (× *20,000*).

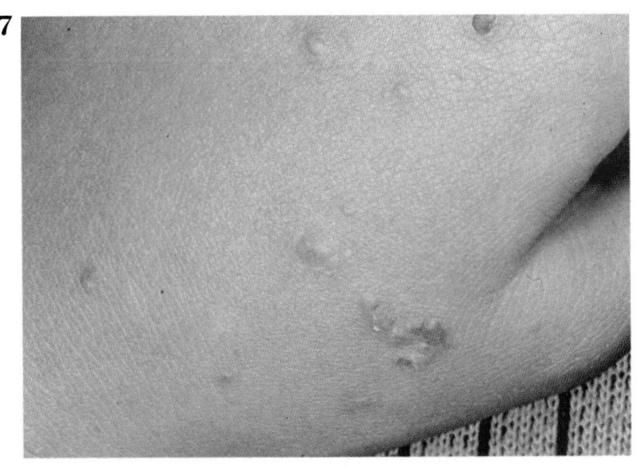

407 Plane warts.

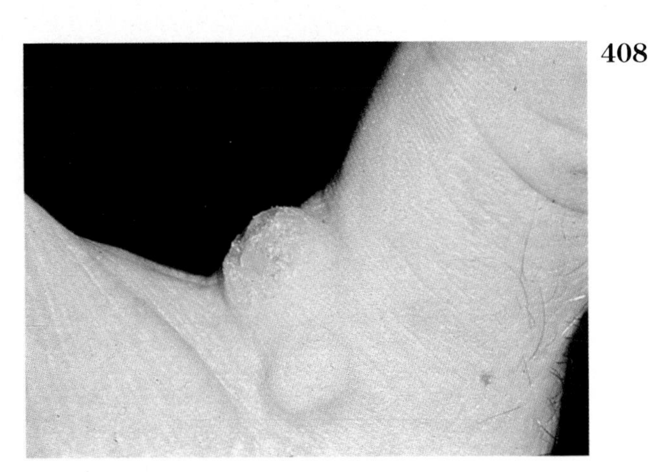

408 A nodular wart.

409

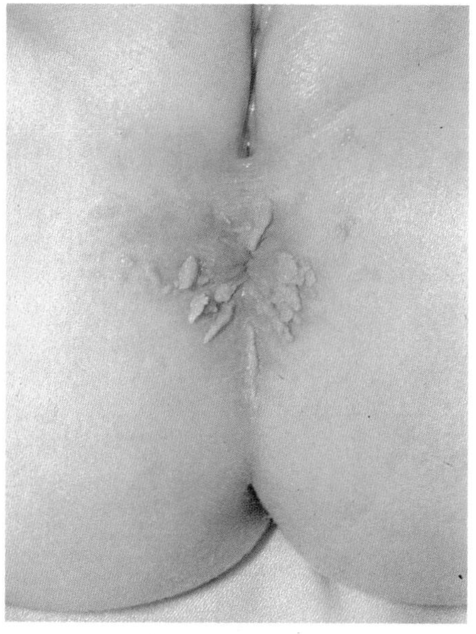

410

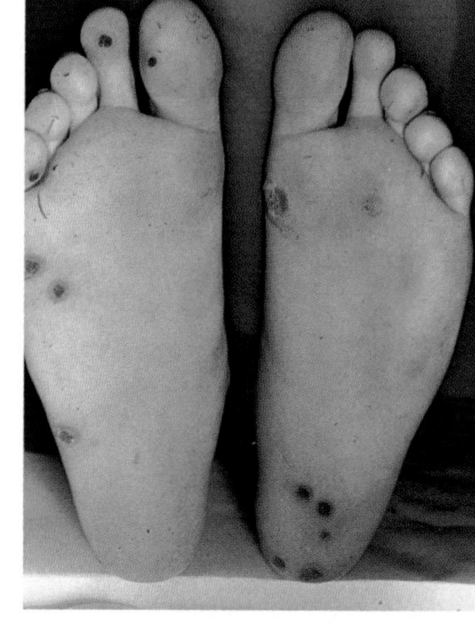

409 Perineal warts in a sexually abused child.

410 Plantar warts or verrucas.

Poxviruses

Molluscum contagiosum is a benign self-limiting disease that is caused by an, as yet, uncultivable and unclassified poxvirus. On electronmicroscopy, a large (300nm in diameter) virus described as looking like a ball of string (**411**), is seen. It has a worldwide distribution and affects children and young adults most commonly. Clinically, lesions present as single or multiple dome-shaped smooth papules (**412**). The infection is spread by close contact, with an incubation period of 2–7 weeks, and persists for months. Treatment, if required, involves curettage of each lesion.

The parapoxvirus infection orf or contagious ecthyma (**413**) is a zoonosis acquired from sheep. It usually produces a solitary lesion on the hand (**414**) within 3–6 days of handling infective granulomas on the mouth of a sheep or lamb. The lesion begins as an erythematous papule which enlarges to a granulomatous ulcer, persisting for up to 6 weeks.

411

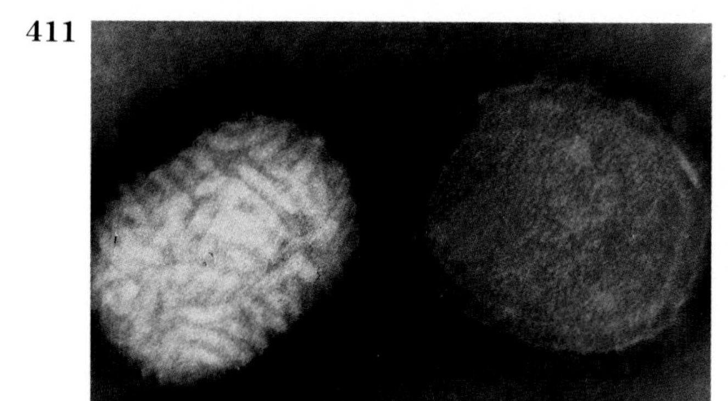

4

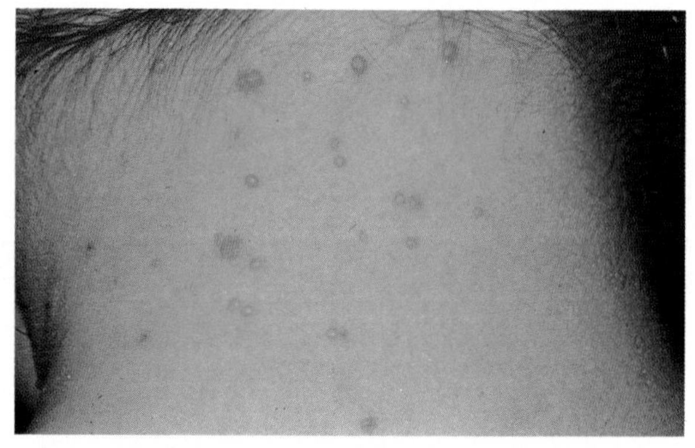

411 Negative-stain electron micrograph of molluscum contagiosum virus (× *50,000*).

412 The characteristic fleshy lesions of molluscum contagiosum.

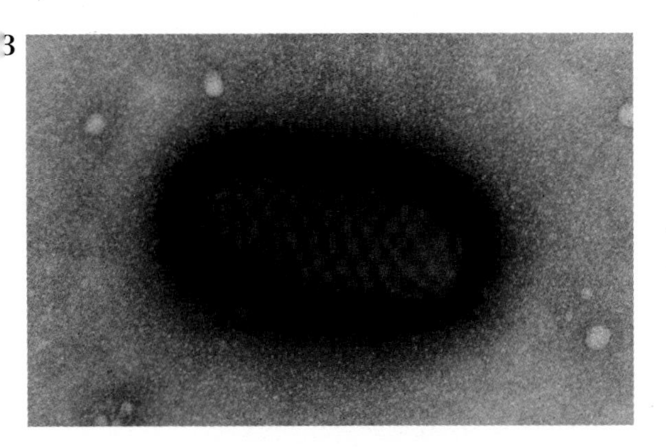

413 Negative-stain electron micrograph of orf virus (× *10,000*).

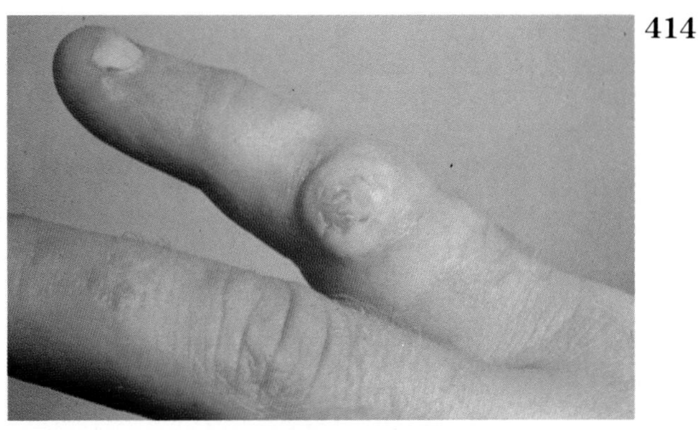

414 A characteristic orf lesion on a finger.

Bacterial infections

The bacterial pathogen most often associated with cutaneous infection is *Staphylococcus aureus*. Infection of hair follicles or of sebaceous glands may lead to the formation of carbuncles (**415**) or furuncles, which in the immune-compromised may develop into deep abscesses (**416**). Infection with *S. aureus* of phage group II may lead to the development of impetigo, which is often bullous (**417**) and heals with the characteristic golden crusting (**418**). *S. aureus* may also colonize and infect eczematous skin (**419**).

Impetigo may also be caused by *Streptococcus pyogenes* (**420**), with or without *S. aureus*, and it should be remembered that streptococcal skin infections may

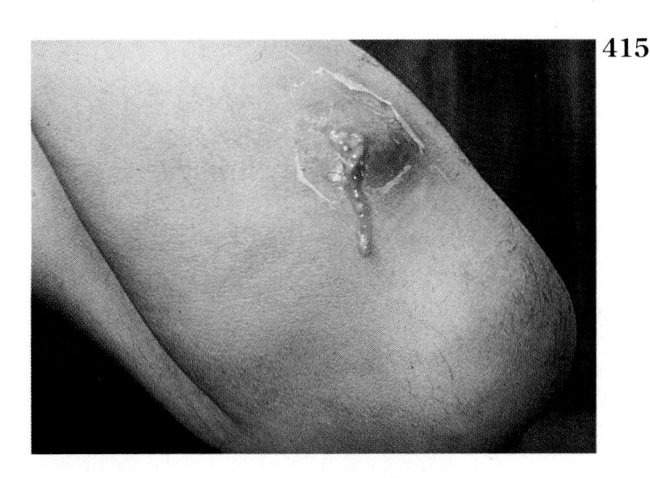

415 A carbuncle discharging pus (which contained *S. aureus*).

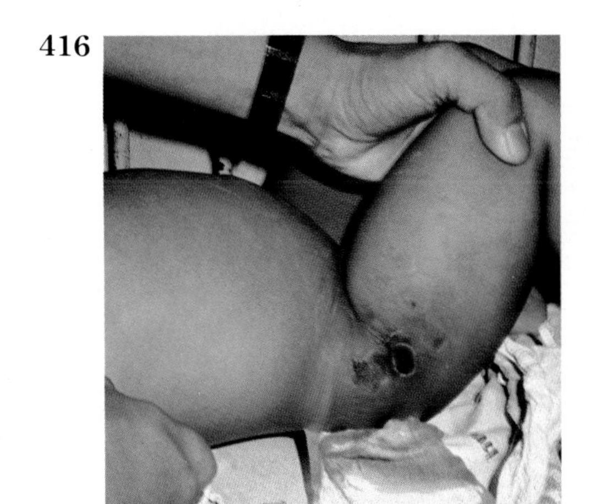

416 A deep abscess due to *S. aureus* in an immune-compromised child.

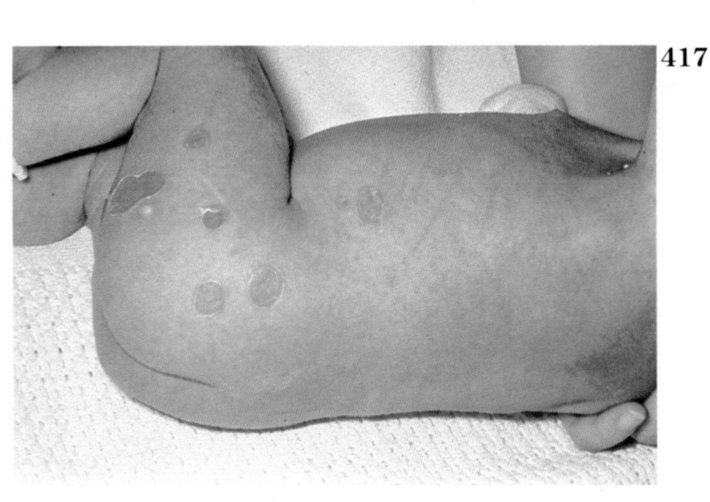

417 Bullous impetigo due to *S. aureus* of phage group II.

lead to the development of glomerulonephritis. Because *S. pyogenes* generates hyaluronidase it is also able to produce more spreading infections, such as erysipelas (**421**). It is also important to note that in children under 7 or 8 years of age, *H. influenzae* (b) can produce cellulitis of the face (**422**) or of the extremities. Insect bites may also become infected with *S. aureus* or *S. pyogenes*, giving rise to large purulent lesions (**423**).

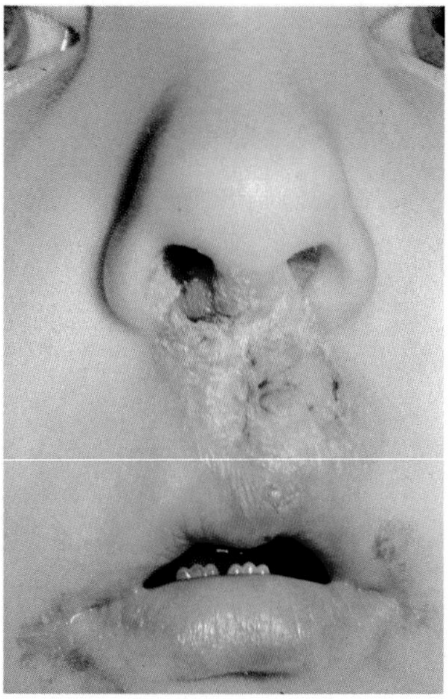

418 The typical golden crust of impetigo.

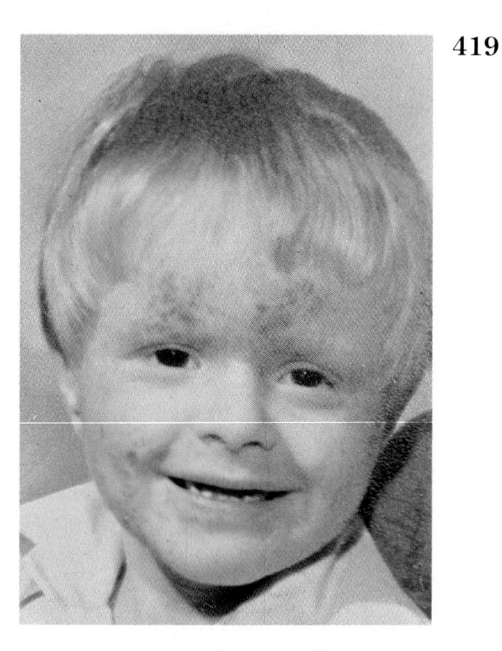

419 Eczematous skin infected with *S. aureus*.

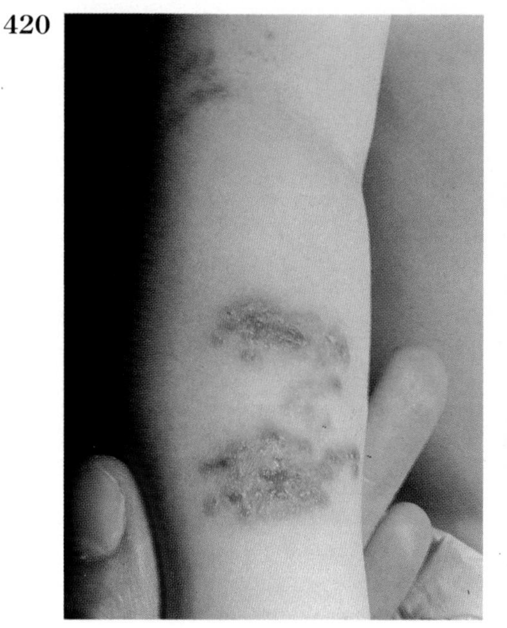

420 Impetigo due to *S. pyogenes*.

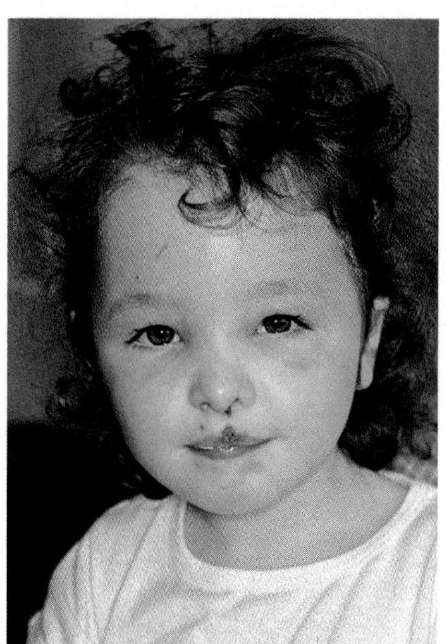

421 Erysipelas on the forehead.

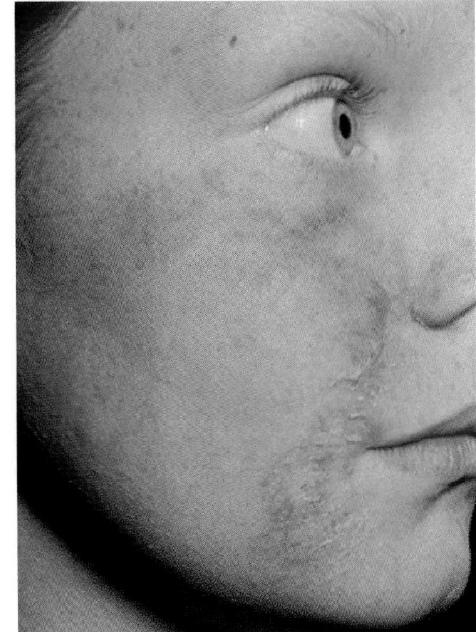

422 Facial cellulitis due to *H. influenzae*.

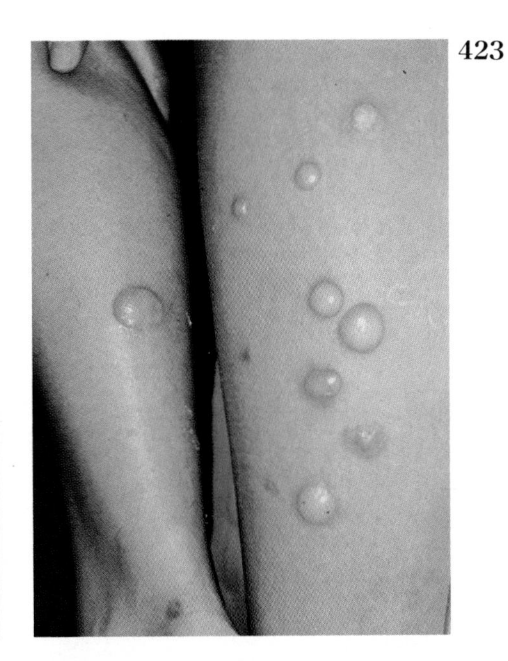

423 Insect bites infected with *S. aureus*.

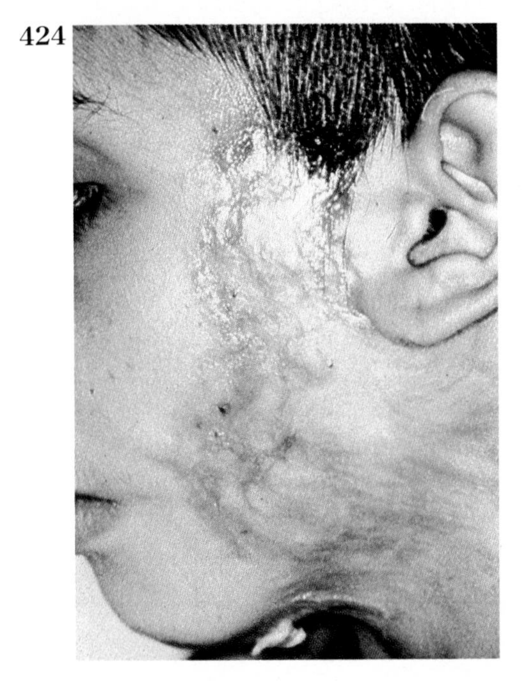

424 Lupus vulgaris (a skin infection) due to *M. tuberculosis*.

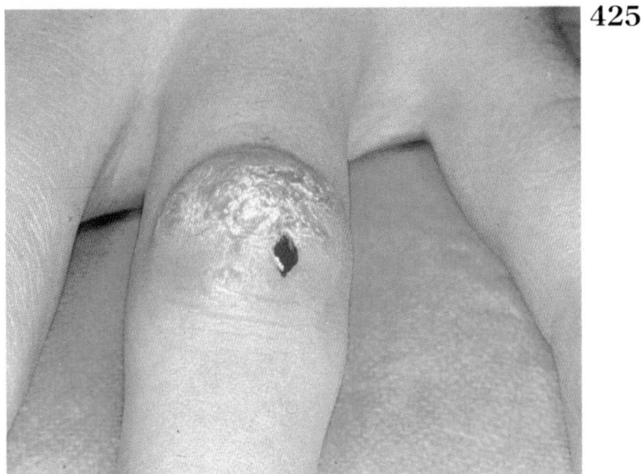

425 Skin infection due to *M. marinum* (swimming-pool granuloma.)

Mycobacteria such as *M. tuberculosis* and *M. marinum* may infect the skin to produce indolent lesions. *M. tuberculosis* produces lupus vulgaris (**424**), but is often associated with other manifestations of tuberculosis. In contrast, *M. marinum* produces localized granulomatous (**425**) or ulcerative lesions where the organism has been inoculated into grazes, often sustained by children while climbing out of swimming pools.

Cervical adenitis may follow a *S. pyogenes* tonsillitis (**426**). In such cases the lymph node tissue may be totally replaced by pus containing neutrophils and chains of gram-positive cocci (**427**). In countries with a low prevalence of tuberculosis, mycobacteria may also cause cervical adenitis (**428**). In such cases the infection is usually due to *M. avium/intracellulare*, but elsewhere *M. bovis* or *M. tuberculosis* is more likely to be responsible. Surgical excision is often the only way to achieve a specific diagnosis, and in the case of *M. avium/intracellulare*, excision is often curative. However, it may lead to the development of a chronically discharging sinus (**429**). Antituberculous therapy is indicated for tuberculous adenitis, but *M. avium/intracellulare* is often resistant. In such instances, erythromycin therapy may prove beneficial.

Although not directly an infective condition, napkin dermatitis (**430**) results from the breakdown of urea in urine by urease liberated by either *Proteus* spp. or *Ureaplasma urealyticum*. Urea is hydrolysed to pro-

426

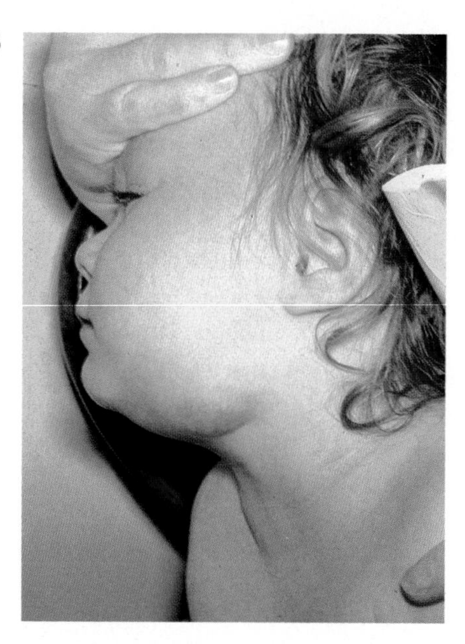

427

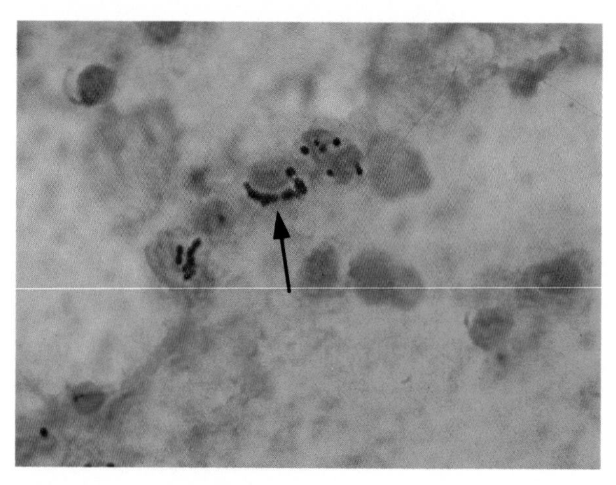

426 Cervical adenitis following a streptococcal tonsillitis.

427 Gram-stained pus from a cervical abscess, with pus cells and a chain of gram-positive cocci (× *1,000*).

428

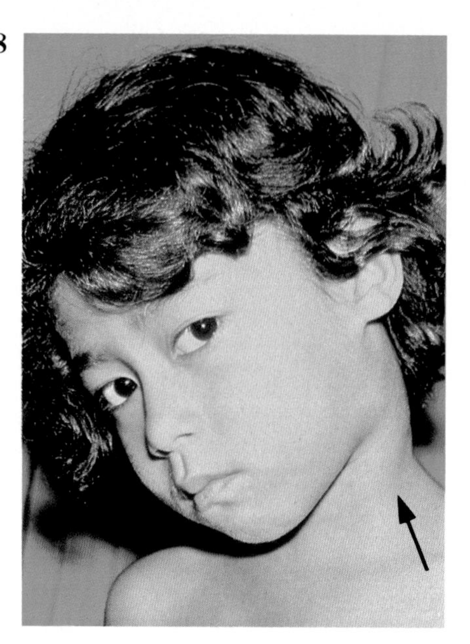

428 Tuberculous adenitis.

429

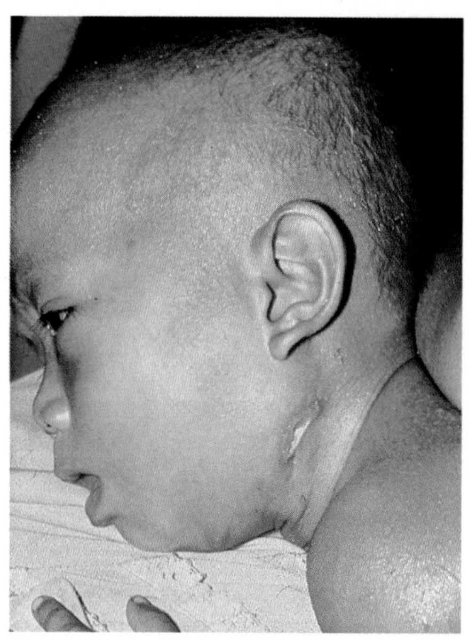

429 A discharging sinus following tuberculous adenitis.

duce ammonia, which is then held close to the skin by the nappy, giving rise to a red and inflamed area that is susceptible to infection by Herpes simplex (**403**) or *Candida albicans* (**431**).

430

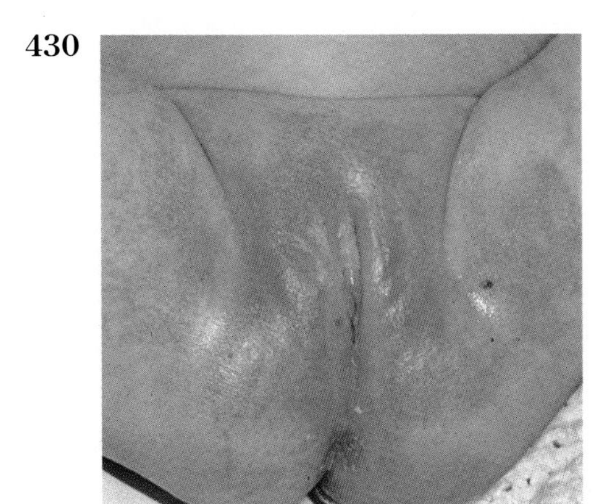

430 Florid inflammation in napkin dermatitis.

431

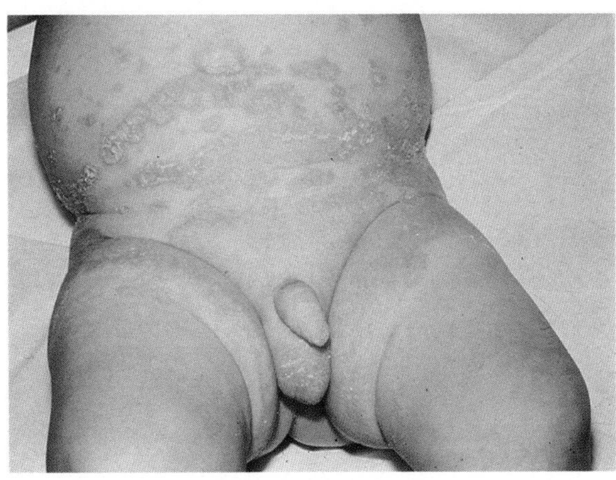

431 *C. albicans* infection of the nappy area.

Fungal infections

In addition to infecting inflamed napkin areas, *Candida albicans* can also produce intertrigo in skin folds (**432**) and may also cause paronychia (**433**).

Dermatophytes are a group of fungi that have evolved mechanisms to enable them to survive and grow in keratinized epithelium. They are divided into three groups: geophilic, zoophilic and anthropophilic (**Table 35**). Geophilic dermatophytes are found in soil and dust, and only two species infect man. Several zoophilic dermatophytes can infect man, and they generally tend to produce much more florid infections than the others. Epidemics of infection can occur with both zoophilic and anthropophilic dermatophytes. The term 'tinea', which is Middle English for moth, is used to prefix these infections, as the lesions are said to be like moth-holes in clothes. Dermatophytes infect keratinized layers in the skin (tinea corporis, tinea faciale, tinea cruris, tinea manuum or tinea pedis), hair (tinea capitis, tinea barbae) or nails (tinea unguium).

Table 35. Classification of Dermatophyes.

Geophilic		
Microsporum gypseum		
M. fulvum		
Zoophilic		
M. canis	*Tricophyton equinum*	
M. nanum	*T. verrucosum*	
M. distortum	*T. mentagrophytes*	
	T. quinckeanum	
Anthropophilic		
M. audouinii	*T. tonsurans*	*Epidermophyton floccosum*
M. ferrugineum	*T. violaceum*	
	T. soudanense	
	T. schoenleinii	
	T. megninii	
	T. yaoundii	
	T. rubrum	

432

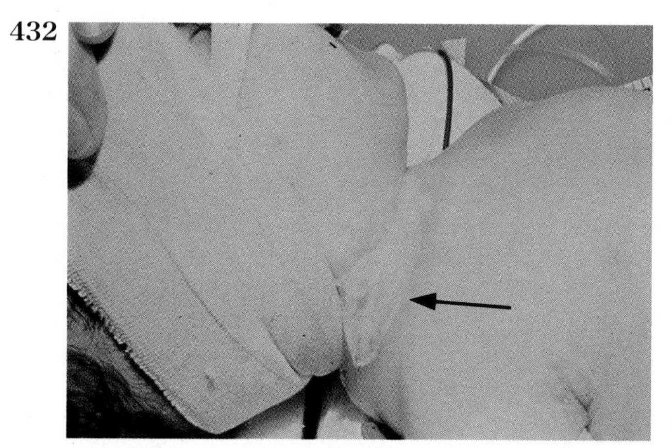

432 Intertrigo due to *C. albicans*.

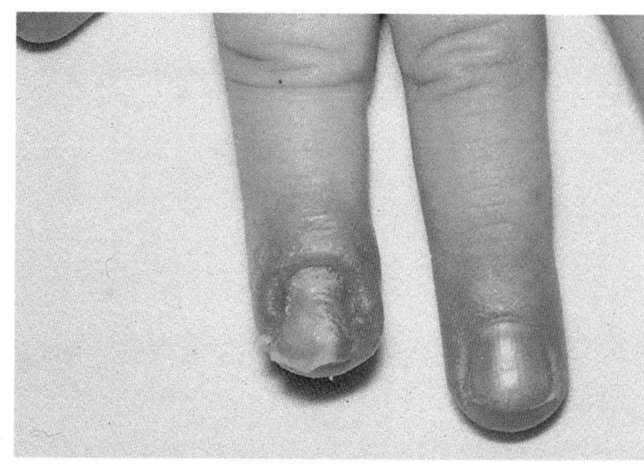

433 Paronychia due to *C. albicans*.

434

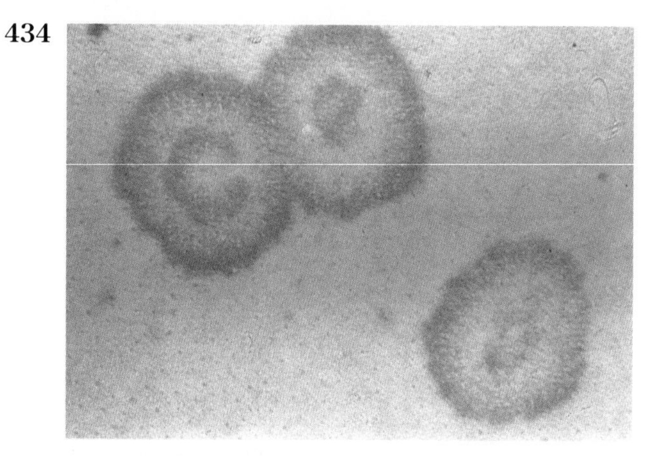

434 Ringworm due to *M. audouinii*.

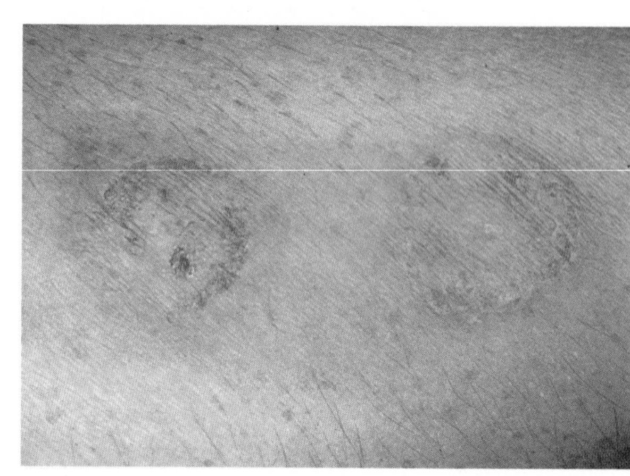

435 Florid inflammatory ringworm due to *M. canis*.

436

436 Tinea capitis.

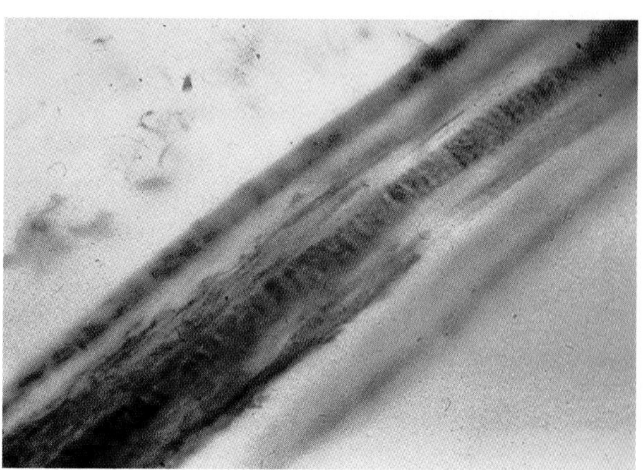

437 A close-up of hair demonstrating endothrix.

On the skin the lesions are also known as ringworm (**434**) because the radially spreading dermatophytes induce a raised area of inflammation that gives the appearance of a worm just beneath the skin surface. Zoophilic species tend to produce much more inflammation (**435**). Infection of hair follicles produces tinea

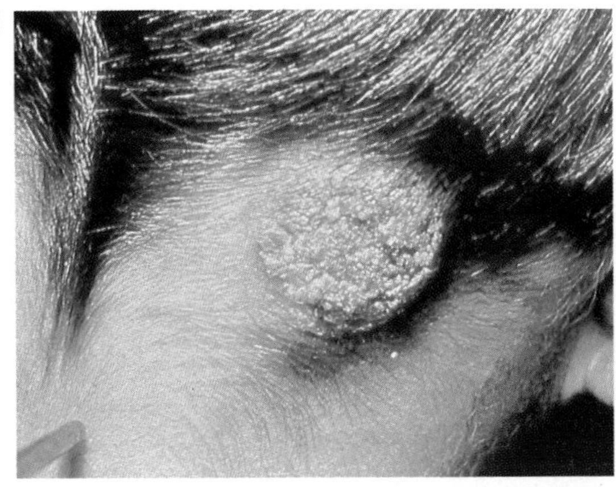

438 A kerion.

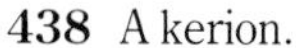

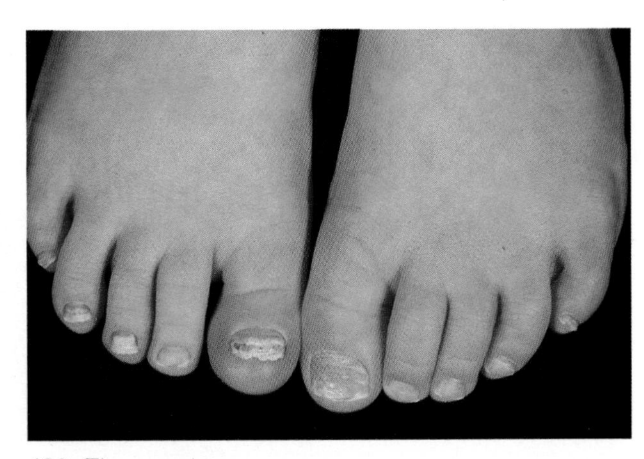

439 Tinea unguium.

capitis, which is the most common manifestation in children (**436**). Dermatophytes grow at the same rate as the hair, invading new keratin as it is formed (**437**). This produces scaling of the scalp and partial alopecia with cases of broken hairs. With zoophilic dermatophytes in particular, a boggy inflammatory ulcerative swelling known as kerion (**438**) may develop. Tinea unguium in children most frequently involves the toenails. Brownish discoloration of the nails, hyperkeratosis and separation of the nail from the nail bed occurs (**439**).

Diagnosis is reached by taking scrapings of skin, hair or nail, adding potassium hydroxide (KOH), and examining the samples under the microscope. Hyphea and arthrospores will be visible. Speciation requires cultivation (at 25°C) of the dermatophyte on Sabouraud's agar (**440**).

Treatment is with griseofulvin, which is concentrated in the stratum corneum. In order to reach the fungal hyphae, prolonged treatment is needed. Some imidazoles, for example ketoconazole, may be effective.

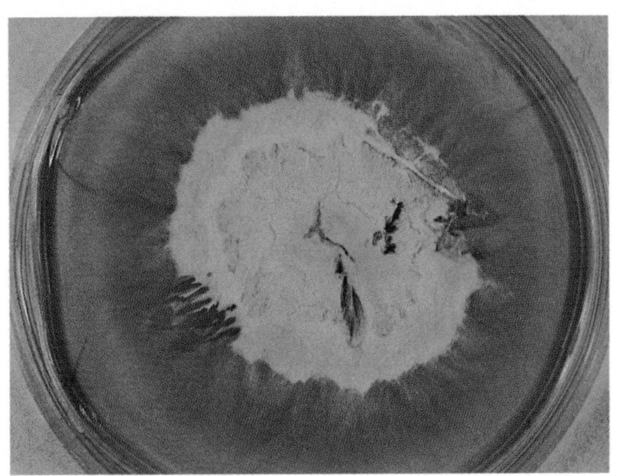

440 *M. canis* growing on Sabouraud's agar.

Infestations with arthropods

Sarcoptes scabei

Sarcoptes scabei infestation is spread by close contact and has a high prevalence in conditions of poor hygiene. The gravid female (**441**) burrows into the horny layer of the skin (**442**) and lays her eggs. After 3–4 days the eggs hatch to produce larvae, which leave the burrow to mature over a 2-week period. The cycle then recommences. The male is seldom seen since it does not survive copulation. The bur-

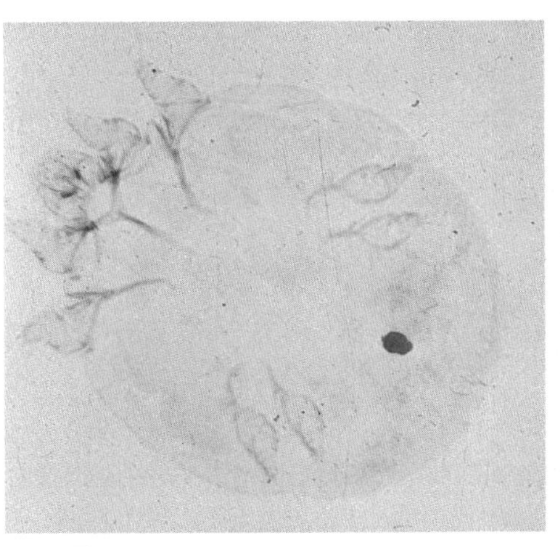

441 The scabies mite (*Sarcoptes scabei*).

rowing produces intense and severe itching, and lesions are found predominantly on the wrists, palms, anterior axillary folds (**443**), lower abdomen and buttocks. Secondary infection of the lesions with *S. aureus* or *S. pyogenes* can be a major problem.

Treatment is with lindane lotion or permethrin cream. The whole family (or community) may need treatment.

442

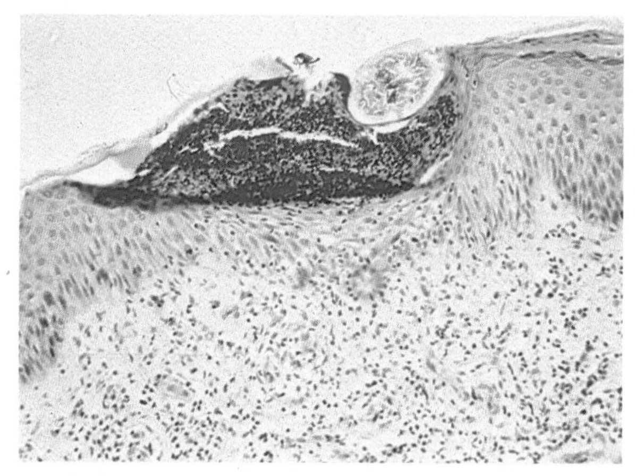

442 A section of skin showing the scabies mite in its burrow.

443

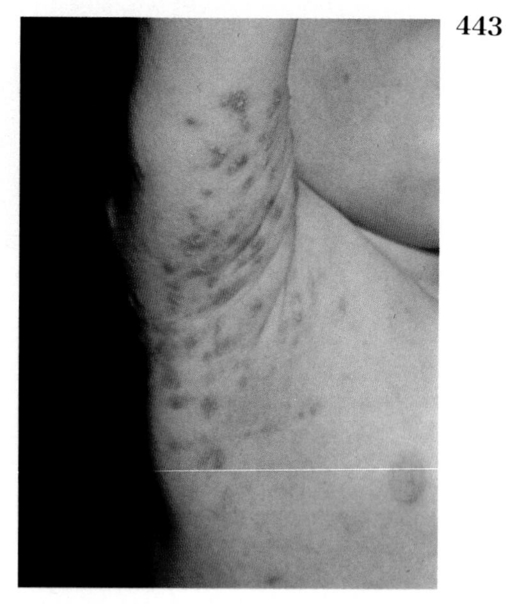

443 Intense scabies infestation.

Pediculus capitis

Pediculus capitis is the head louse. Infestation produces profound itching. The adult louse (**444**), which lives on blood sucked through the skin, may be seen meandering through the scalp and eyebrow hairs. The female lays eggs (200–500), commonly known as nits, which are glued on to hairs (**445**). The larvae hatch 6–10 days later, maturing within 1–2 weeks. Treatment is with carbaryl or malathion shampoo.

444

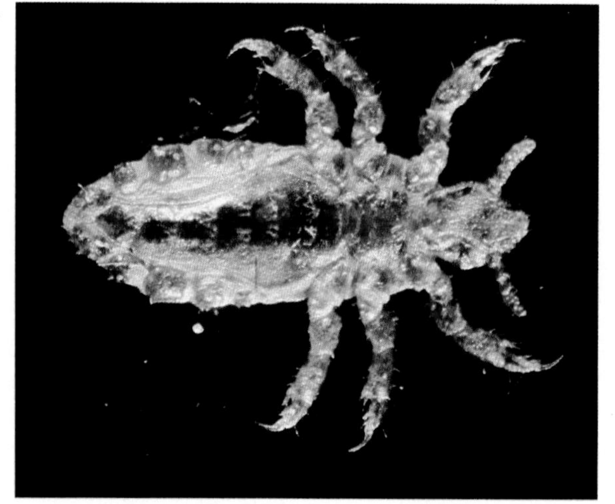

444 An adult headlouse (*Pediculus capitis*).

4

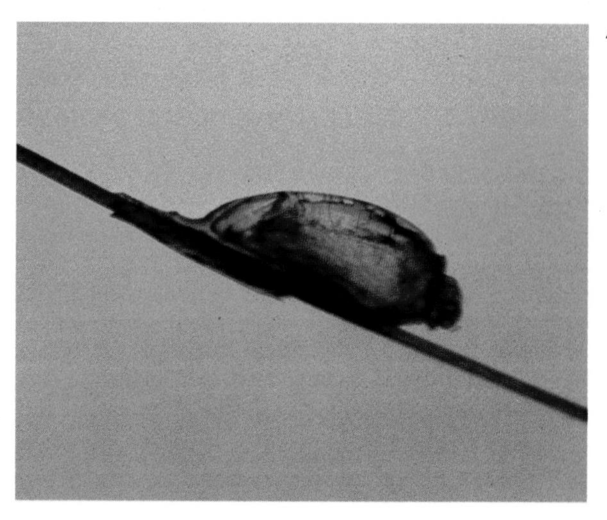

445 A headlouse egg (nit) stuck to a hair.

Ocular infections

Ocular infections are quite common in children, and are most often self-limiting. Infection may be of the eyelids (blepharitis), the glands of Zeiss (sty), the Meibomian glands (hordeolum), the lacrimal system (dacryocystadenitis), the conjunctivae, the cornea (keratitis), the whole eye (endophthalmitis) or the surrounding tissue (orbital cellulitis).

The main aetiological agents affecting the eyelid and lacrimal system are *S. aureus*, *S. pyogenes*, *S. pneumoniae* and *H. influenzae*. The pathogens associated with conjunctivitis are shown in **Table 36**. Viruses are the most common agents, often being associated with outbreaks of conjunctivitis. They tend to produce lymphoid hyperplasia (follicles), hyperaemia and a watery discharge, that is a follicular conjunctivitis (**446**). The most common bacterial cause of conjunctivitis is *H. influenzae*. Beginning with watering and irritation of the eye, conjunctival infection develops with a mucopurulent exudate. In rare cases, infection may spread to cause orbital cellulitis (**447**), which requires urgent treatment with intravenous antibiotics as extension into the CNS is common.

Herpes simplex can pose particular problems, as it is capable of causing conjunctivitis and blepharitis (**448**) as a primary infection. Recurrence may also produce conjunctivitis in some, but in others, for reasons that are unclear, keratitis followed by the development of dendritic ulcers (**449**) occurs.

Finally, papillomaviruses may produce papillomata on the eyelids or even on the conjunctivae (**450**).

Table 36. Aetiology of Conjunctivitis.

Viruses	Adenovirus (8, 19) – Epidemic keratoconjunctivitis
	Adenovirus (3, 7) – Pharyngoconjunctival fever
	Enterovirus (70) – Haemorrhagic conjunctivitis
	Coxsackievirus (A24) – Haemorrhagic conjunctivitis
	Herpes simplex virus
	Varicella–zoster virus
	Newcastle disease virus
Bacteria	*H. influenzae*
	S. pneumoniae
	S. aureus
	N. gonorrhoeae
	N. meningitidis
	Moraxella spp.
	S. pyogenes
	B. catarrhalis
	P. aeruginosa
	Chlamydia trachomatis

446

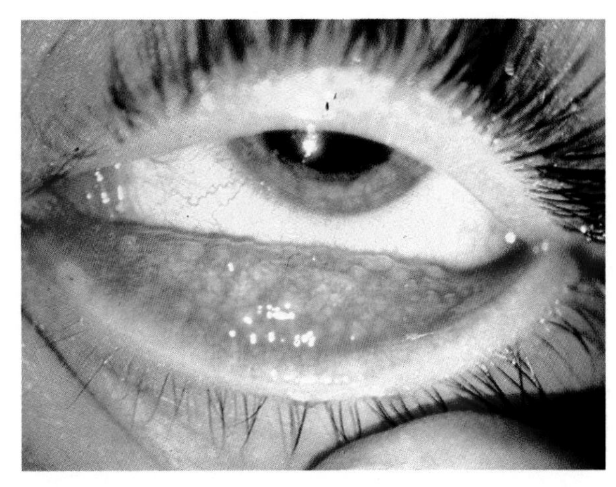

446 Follicular Herpes simplex conjunctivitis.

447

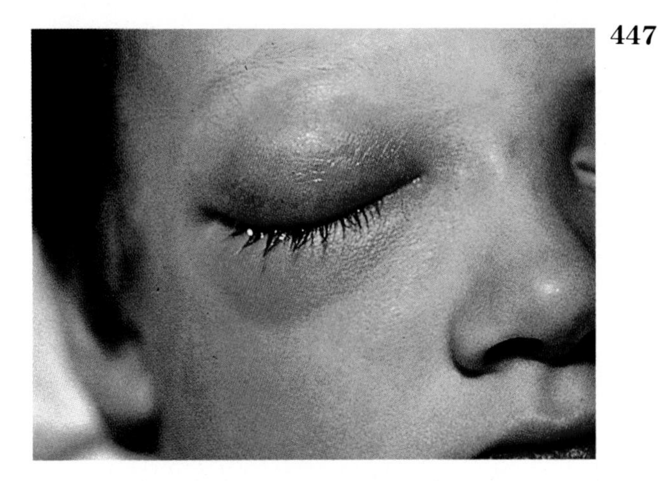

447 Orbital cellulitis due to *H. influenzae*.

448

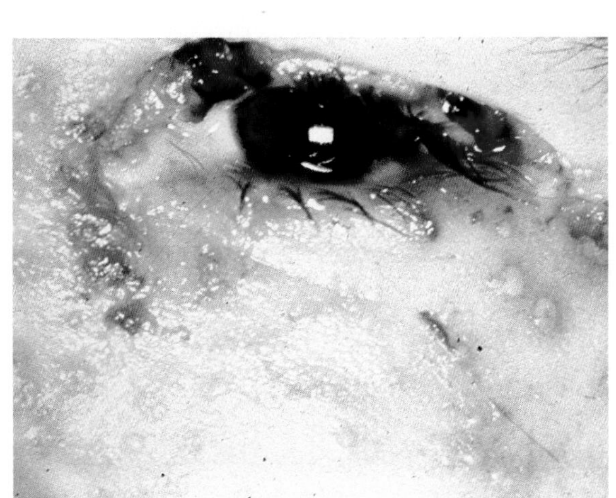

448 Herpes simplex blepharitis.

449

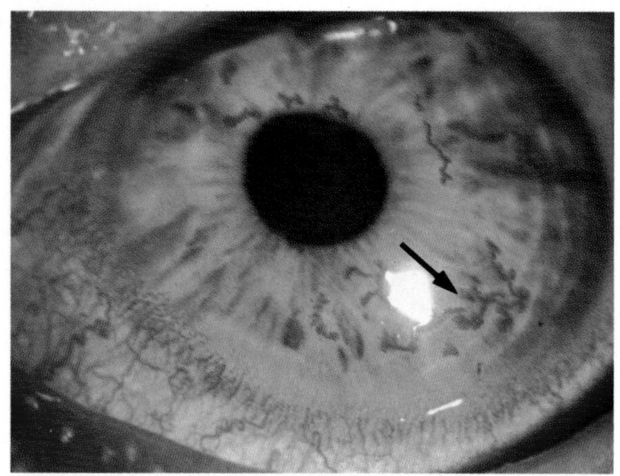

449 Multiple dendritic ulcers on the cornea.

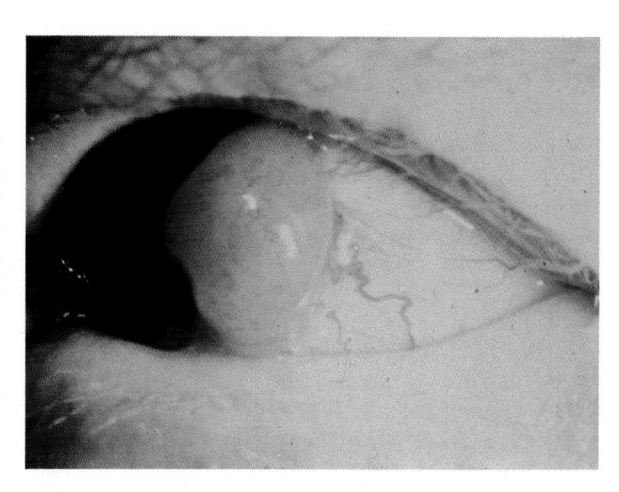

450 A conjunctival papilloma.

Infection of bone and joints

Approximately 1 in 5,000 children under 13 years of age are diagnosed as having osteomyelitis. Infection is almost three times more common in males. The majority (90–95%) of infections are due to *S. aureus* (**451**). *H. influenzae* and *S. pyogenes* account for most of the remainder, although *Salmonella* spp. may cause osteomyelitis, especially in patients with sickle-cell disease.

451

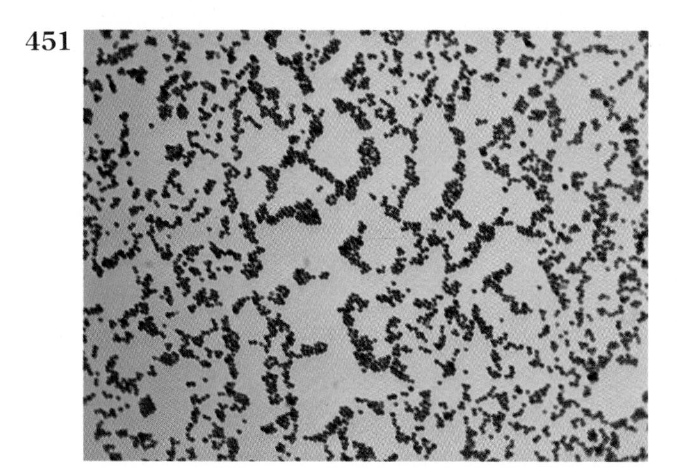

451 Gram-stained film of *S. aureus* (× *1,000*).

Infection, which is usually haematogenous and, in general, involves the long bones (at the metaphyses adjacent to the epiphyseal growth plates), normally presents as pain in the affected limb, with tenderness on palpation. If there is bacteraemia, the patient will be febrile. Diagnosis depends upon clinical acumen and laboratory and radiological investigation. There is often a neutrophilia, together with a rise in acute-phase proteins. Blood culture may also be positive (up to 60% of cases). X-ray changes in surrounding tissue may be visible 3 days after onset, but these can easily be missed. The classical changes of bone destruction and periosteal new bone (**452**) take from 10–21 days to develop. Bone scans using technetium–99m polyphosphate are a valuable adjunct to diagnosis, except in neonates. **453** shows a technetium–99m scan of the case shown in **452**. Occasionally pus may be obtained from bones that have been drilled to relieve pressure (**454**). If the patient is already receiving antibiotics, cultural techniques must be modified to try to inactivate the antibiotics.

Treatment should be parenteral initially, with administration of antibiotics that cover the major pathogens and that penetrate into bone, for example cloxacillin or cephalosporins. There is a significant relapse rate if treatment is maintained for less than 3 weeks; the usual duration of therapy is 4–6 weeks.

Skeletal tuberculosis (bone or joint) is likely to develop in 1–5% of children whose initial infection is left untreated, becoming clinically apparent 1–3 years later. The bones most often affected are those of the spine, knee and hips. Tuberculous spondylitis most frequently affects the thoracic spine (**455**), with extensive wedging of the vertebral body leading to kyphosis or Pott's disease (**456**). Treatment requires both chemotherapy and orthopaedic support.

Osteomyelitis may also arise from penetrating wounds or compound fractures, the microbiology and treatment of which can be very complex. Compound fractures will cause muscle necrosis and, if *Clostridium pefringens* is inoculated into the wound, gas gangrene (**457**) may result. Consequently all patients with compound fractures should be given prophylactic penicillin unless thay have a proven hypersensitivity.

Chronic osteomyelitis may follow surgical procedures, major trauma or inadequately treated acute osteomyelitis. Patients present with a painful non-functioning limb, a chronically draining sinus, and severe radiological changes (**458**). The infection may be polymicrobial including *S. aureus*, *H. influenzae*, *Pseudomonas aeruginosa*, coliforms and even anaerobes. Treatment requires surgical intervention and appropriate antimicrobial chemotherapy, but the outlook is not good.

Acute arthritis may result either from invasion of a joint by bacteria or as an immunological phenomenon (reactive arthritis). Patients present with fever, a painful, swollen, reddened joint (**459**) and a reluctance to use the limb. The knee and hip joints are most frequently affected. Septic arthritis may arise from extension of osteomyelitis, or by itself. Pathogens associated with septic arthritis are *S. aureus*, *H. influenzae* and, less frequently, enterobacteria including *Salmonella* spp. Treatment involves drainage and appropriate antimicrobial chemotherapy. Reactive arthropathy may arise in certain individuals (HLA (human leukocyte antigen) B27-positive) following infection in other sites by *Shigella*, *Salmonella*, *Yersinia*, *Campylobacter*, *Chlamydia* or *N. meningitidis*. Disease usually resolves spontaneously within 10 days. Severe cases may need intra-articular corticosteroids.

452

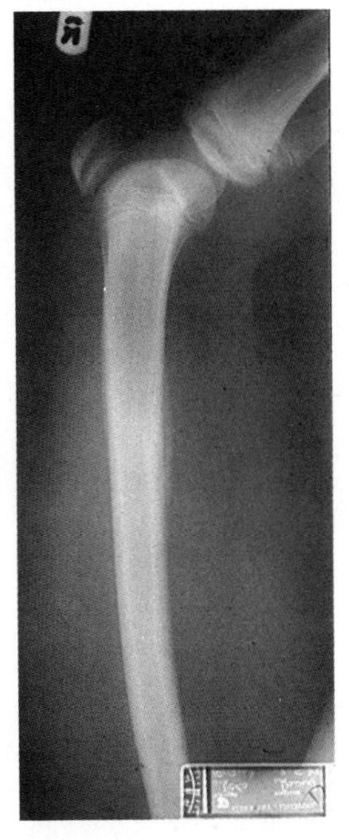

452 X-ray demonstrating osteomyelitis of the tibia.

453

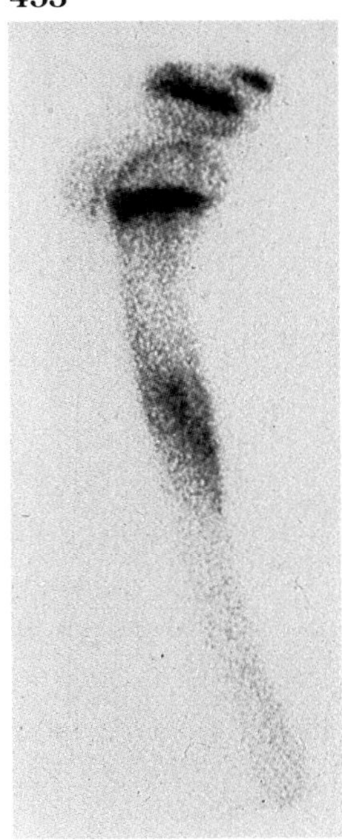

453 Technetium–99m scan of the same limb.

454

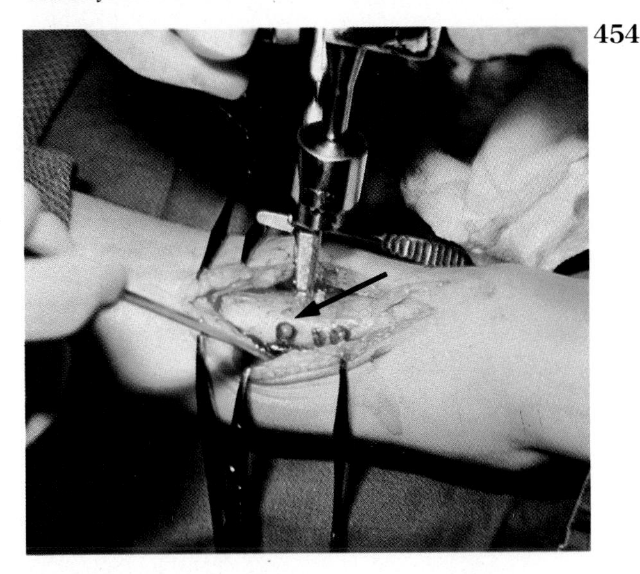

454 Drilling to drain pus in a case of osteomyelitis.

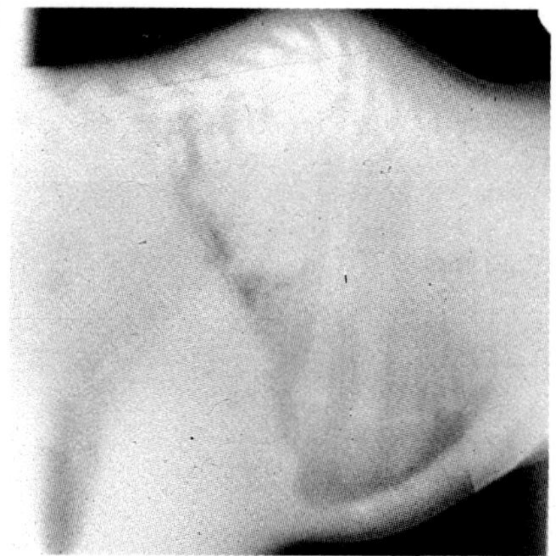

455 Lateral chest X-ray demonstrating kyphosis due to spinal tuberculosis.

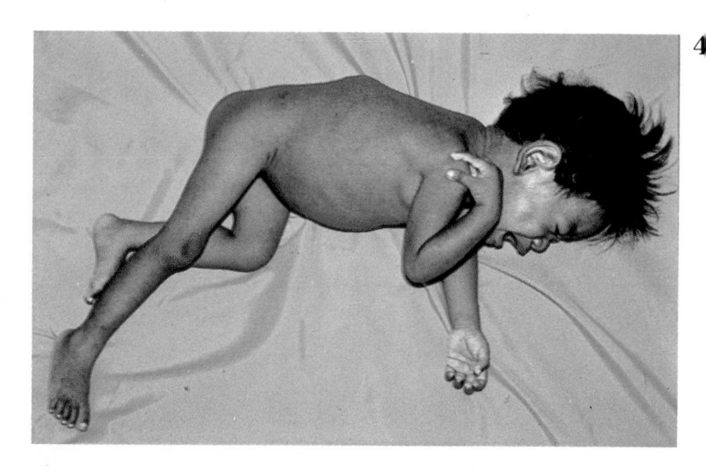

456 Spinal tuberculosis or Pott's disease.

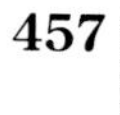

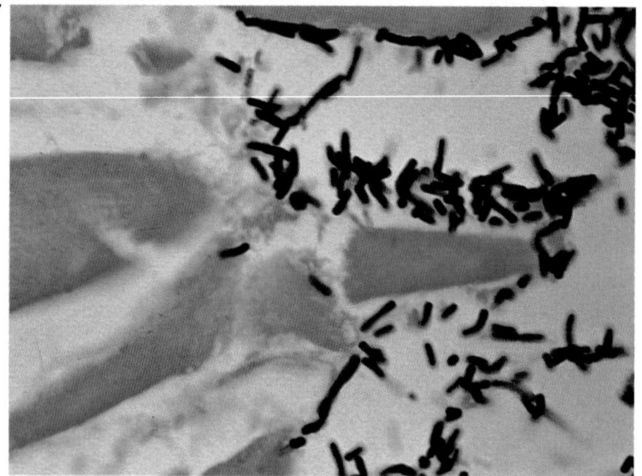

457 A section of muscle from a case of gas gangrene due to *C. perfringens* (× *1,000*).

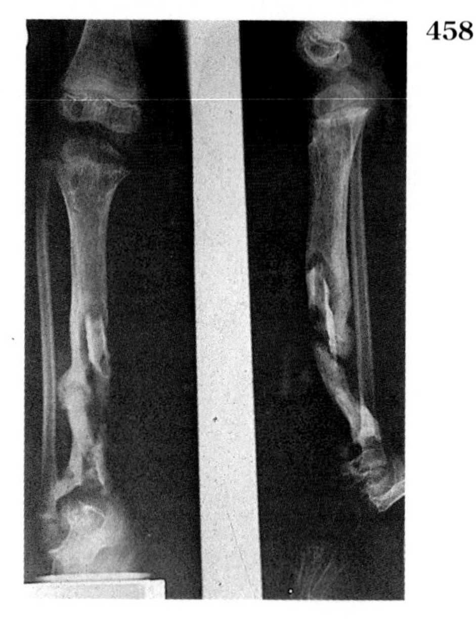

458 X-ray demonstrating chronic osteomyelitis of the tibia.

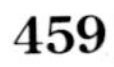

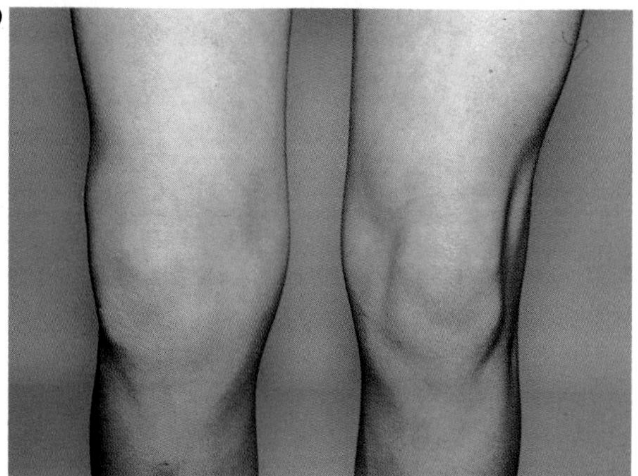

459 A case of septic arthritis.

10 Fever of unknown origin

The original definition of fever of unknown origin (FUO), also known as pyrexia of unknown origin (PUO), was of an illness persisting for 3 or more weeks, with temperatures of 38.4°C or higher on several occasions. Although such a description is of value when investigating fever in adults, it is less useful for children. A more practicable definition for children has been proposed by several authors, and FUO in children is currently defined as the occurrence of a fever lasting more than a week in a child of whom a careful and thorough history and examination, together with preliminary laboratory investigations, have failed to reveal the probable aetiology. The inclusion of the duration factor (i.e. more than 1 week) and results of laboratory investigations will exclude cases of occult bacteraemia (often pneumococcal) and children in the prodromal stage of various infectious diseases.

Under normal circumstances the human body temperature is maintained within 1–1.5°C of 37°C, temperature regulation being mediated by centres in the anterior and posterior hypothalamus. Early studies demonstrated that bacterial endotoxin (from the outer membrane of gram-negative bacteria) was a potent cause of fever, and the endotoxin was termed exogenous pyrogen. However, it became apparent that this was not the sole mediator of fever since, for example, viruses and gram-positive bacteria were also able to produce fever. A pyrogenic factor released from neutrophils was described, the liberation of which could be stimulated by, amongst other factors, endotoxin. This factor was termed endogenous pyrogen and the molecule was subsequently purified and its gene was cloned and called interleukin-1 (IL-1). IL-1 is produced not only by neutrophils but also by other haemopoietic cells and by many epithelial and endothelial cells. In addition to its pyrogenic activity, it also promotes thymocyte proliferation, is a growth factor for T-helper and B-lymphocytes and induces synthesis of acute-phase proteins and other cytokines (e.g. IL-6). Other hormones, such as adrenaline, prostaglandins and progesterone, are also able to produce fever.

Production of fever is an important defence mechanism. Since most pathogenic micro-organisms are adapted for optimal growth at normal body temperature, a raised temperature inhibits their growth. In addition, many immune functions, such as phagocytosis, are enhanced at slightly higher temperatures. In FUO there is a prolonged febrile response to an infectious agent, or inappropriate secretion of IL-1 or other pyrogenic hormones, or inappropriate stimulation of hypothalamic thermoregulatory centres.

The causes of FUO are shown in **Table 37**. In most surveys infection accounts for 29–52% of cases.

Table 37. Causes of Fever of Unknown Origin.

Infections	*Other causes*
Abscesses: liver, pelvic, subphrenic, perinephric	Sarcoid
Bacterial endocarditis	Collagen diseases: Still's disease, polyarteritis nodosa (PAN), systemic lupus erythematosus (SLE)
Brucellosis	Malignancies: neuroblastoma, Hodgkin's lymphoma, hypernephroma
Cholangitis	Drugs: atropine, amphotericin B, antibiotics, isoniazid, diphenyl hydantoin, etc.
Glandular fever: EBV, CMV, *Toxoplasma gondii*	Diabetes insipidus
Hepatitis viruses A, B and C	Familial Mediterranean fever
Histoplasmosis	Fabry's disease
Malaria	Familial dysautonomia
Mastoiditis, sinusitis	Granulomatous colitis
Osteomyelitis	Infantile cortical hyperostosis
Psittacosis	Pancreatitis
Pyelonephritis	Thyrotoxicosis
Q fever	
Rickettsia spp.	
Spirochaetes: *Leptospira* spp., *Borrelia recurrentis*	
Trypanosomiasis	
Tuberculosis	
Tularaemia	
Typhoid, paratyphoid and occasional salmonelloses	
Visceral larva migrans	

Abscesses

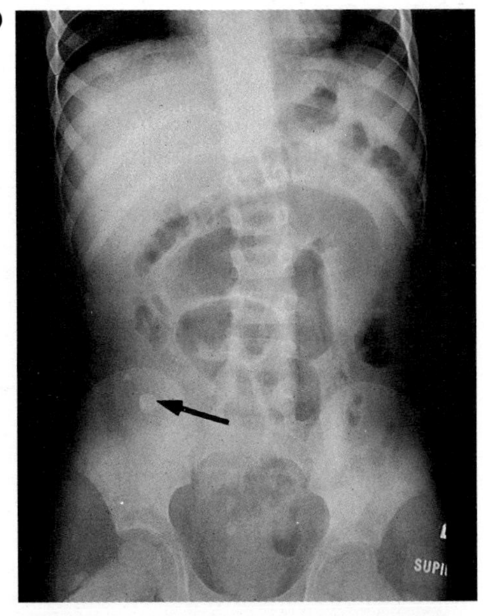

Intrabdominal abscesses may arise following intestinal surgery or perforation. The bacteria most often isolated are *Staphylococcus aureus*, *Streptococcus milleri*, *Escherichia coli*, together with various anaerobes such as *B. fragilis*. The site of the abscess generally depends upon the site of intestinal perforation, thus a ruptured appendix may give rise to an appendiceal abscess (**460**) or pelvic abscess (**461**). Blood culture may provide a diagnostic clue, as will the neutrophil count, which is generally very high. However, specific diagnosis depends upon ultrasound, CT scans and gallium scans. Treatment must involve drainage (**462**), as well as administration of antibiotics that cover the most likely pathogens.

460 Abdominal X-ray of a child with an appendiceal abscess. A faecolith caused gangrene and perforation of the appendix.

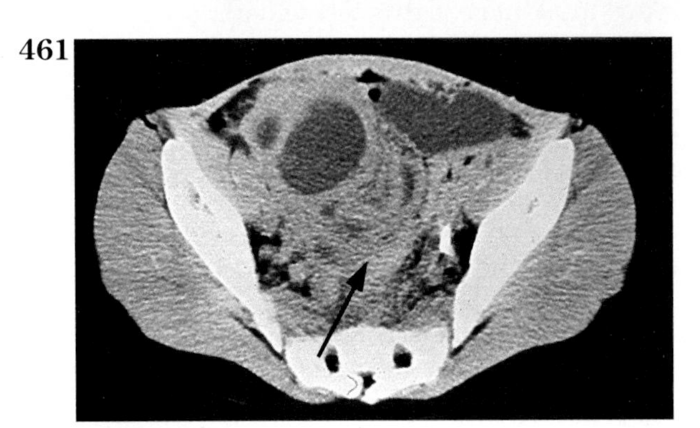

461 CT scan of a large pelvic abscess.

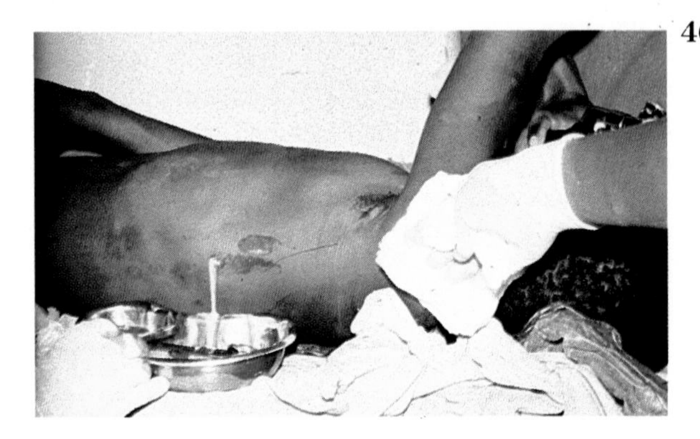

462 Draining an abdominal abscess under less than optimal conditions.

Brucellosis

Brucellosis has a worldwide distribution but it has been eradicated from some temperate countries. Infection with *Brucella* spp. is transmitted to man principally from goats (*B. melitensis*), cattle (*B. abortus*, *B. suis*), sheep (*B. melitensis*) and pigs (*B. suis*, *B. abortus*). Usually, transmission is either by drinking infected milk or by contact with infected animals. In the latter case, infection is usually from aerosols that are either inoculated into the conjunctivae or inhaled. Bacteria are conveyed to the local lymph nodes, where they are either destroyed or they multiply to establish a bacteraemia. They are then removed by macrophages of the reticuloendothelial system, which are unable to kill them, and granulomas develop. The incubation period can vary from as little as a week to as long as 6 months but it commonly lasts 1–3 weeks.

Acute brucellosis may commence with sudden chills and rigors, together with a high, swinging temperature (38–39°C). The patient becomes toxic and ill with anorexia, malaise and fatigue. There may be splenic enlargement (**463**) and the liver may be tender but there are few other clinical signs. Diagnosis is made on the basis of blood culture and the peripheral blood count, which often shows a leucopenia with a decrease in neutrophil numbers. In many cases the illness subsides within 2 weeks. However, it may recur, leading to subacute brucellosis or undulant fever. This may present with recurrent persistent fever, together with malaise, fatigue and back pain. Apart from splenomegaly, there may be few other signs. Complications may arise in bones and joints (spondylitis in particular), the CNS (chronic meningitis), the cardiovascular system (endocarditis), and the liver and spleen (granulomas and abscesses).

Diagnosis, most importantly, depends upon suspicion of brucellosis. Blood cultures may be positive, and pus from abscesses (and even bone marrow aspirates) should be cultured. Detection of IgM anti-brucella and brucella agglutinating antibodies are useful techniques. Treatment requires antimicrobials that can penetrate macrophages, for example, cotrimoxazole and chloramphenicol. The prognosis is generally good and mortality rates are low (1–3%).

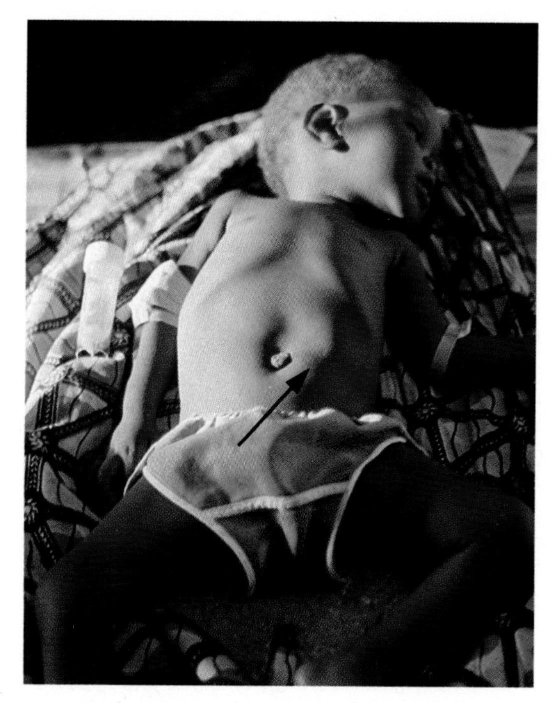

463 Splenomegaly in a child with brucellosis.

Glandular fever

Glandular fever or infectious mononculeosis has been covered earlier (p. 66). It may be due to infection with EBV, CMV, or *Toxoplasma gondii*. It must be remembered that it is not just with EBV infection that antibiotics such as ampicillin may produce a severe rash (**464**).

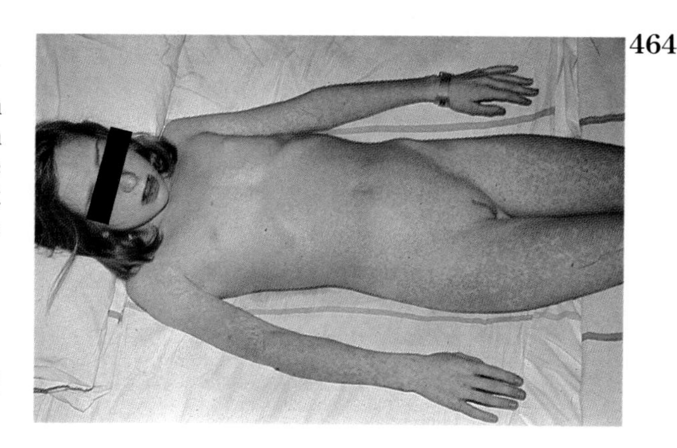

464 An erythematous rash following administration of ampicillin to a child with CMV mononucleosis.

Q fever

Q fever was first described in Queensland, Australia, but the Q stands for query. The disease is caused by the bacterium *Coxiella burnetii*. Although ticks may play a role in transmitting infection between animals, human infection usually arises by ingestion (of milk) or, more commonly, by inhalation. The incubation period lasts 2–4 weeks, with sudden onset of a high (38–40.5°C) swinging pyrexia. There may also be a dry cough or, later, endocarditis. Diagnosis is difficult (except when outbreaks occur) and usually involves serology, although the bacterium can be grown in tissue culture or in embryonated eggs. Treatment is with tetracyclines. Q fever has a low mortality (<3%) and morbidity.

Tuberculosis

Tuberculosis is a common cause of FUO, with FUO being more likely to occur with non-pulmonary tuberculosis. Patients may have active disseminated disease and a negative tuberculin test. Diagnosis requires a high index of suspicion and culture of mycobacteria from bone marrow or other biopsy specimens. Rapid cultural techniques (e.g. Bactec) or DNA detection (e.g. polymerase chain reaction) are very valuable adjuncts to diagnosis.

Typhoid

Although *Salmonella typhi* (**465**) and *S. paratyphi* A and B are the principal causes of typhoid fever, in children other salmonellae (e.g. *S. virchow, S. dublin*) may cause a typhoid-like illness or FUO. *S. typhi* is a solely human pathogen, maintained by carriers who excrete the bacterium in their faeces or, less commonly, in their urine. Transmission is by ingestion of contaminated food or water. The incubation period for *S. typhi* is up to 24 days but usually lasts 10–14 days, whereas that for *S. paratyphi* is shorter. *S. typhi* rarely produces diarrhoea, but *S. paratyphi* does so much more commonly. Following ingestion, bacteria are taken up by M cells and intestinal lymphoid tissue. They enter the lymphatics and eventually reach the bloodstream. They are then taken up by the macrophages of the reticuloendothelial system. Virulent salmonellae are well adapted to surviving within macrophages. A secondary bacteraemia results from their release from macrophages, and bacteria may lodge in Peyer's patches, producing perforation or haemorrhage. The onset of disease is insidious over a period of a week, with malaise, chills, headache and generalized aches. During this time, the temperature rises, reaching 39–40°C by the end of the week. At this point the patient may have moderate splenomegaly and may demonstrate rose spots. These spots, which are usually found on the abdomen or back, but may present at any site (**466**), consist of small (about 2 mm), pale pink macules that blanch on pressure. Diagnosis is by blood, marrow, stool and urine culture. Detection of high antibody levels to Vi and H antigens in the Widal Test can be of value in an unimmunized patient, but the test's sensitivity and specificity are not good.

Treatment is with chloramphenicol, cotrimoxazole and the newer quinolones. Untreated, the mortality is 5–15%, but treatment with antibiotics to which the organism is sensitive is usually successful. Plasmids that encode multiple drug resistance are common in *Salmonellae*.

465

465 Silver-stained smear of *S. typhi*, demonstrating the flagellae (× *1,000*).

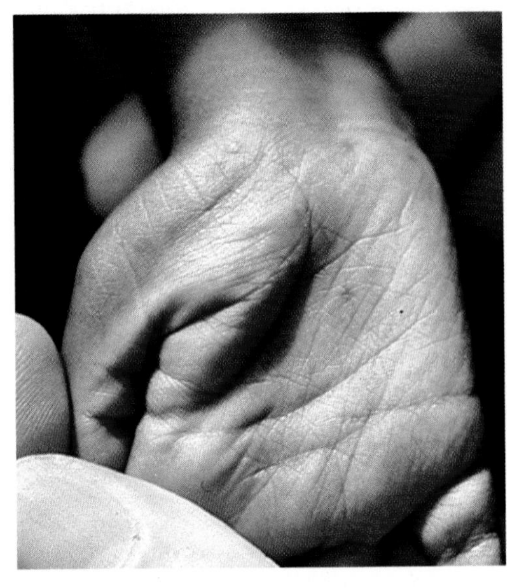

466 A rose spot on the palm of a child with typhoid.

Visceral larva migrans

Visceral larva migrans is an uncommon condition in temperate countries, where it is most often due to *Toxocara canis* or *T. cati*. The adult worm (**467**) inhabits the intestine of the dog or cat, particularly affecting puppies or kittens. Large numbers of eggs are excreted in faeces. Animal faeces often contaminate children's play areas, such as parks and sandpits. The eggs are ingested and then hatch. The second-stage larvae penetrate the intestinal wall and invade other organs, such as the liver or lungs, where granulomatous lesions occur. In the retina, such lesions may resemble retinoblastoma, and enucleation of the eye may be required (**468**). Although there may be eosinophilia, hepatosplenomegaly and fever in some children, in most cases no signs or symptoms arise. Specific diagnosis can be reached either by serology (ELISA) or by biopsy. Treatment is with diethylcarbamazine or thiabendazole. Prevention requires owners to worm their animals regularly and not to allow their pets to soil public places. The rodent whipworm *Capillaria hepatica* may cause a similar picture.

The diganosis of FUO requires a structured approach, and great care in history taking and clinical examination. The history must include questions on foreign travel, food habits and drug history.

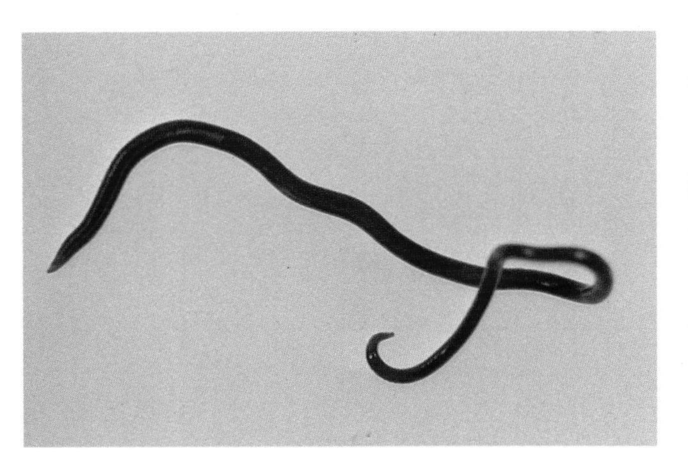

467 The adult worm of *T. canis*.

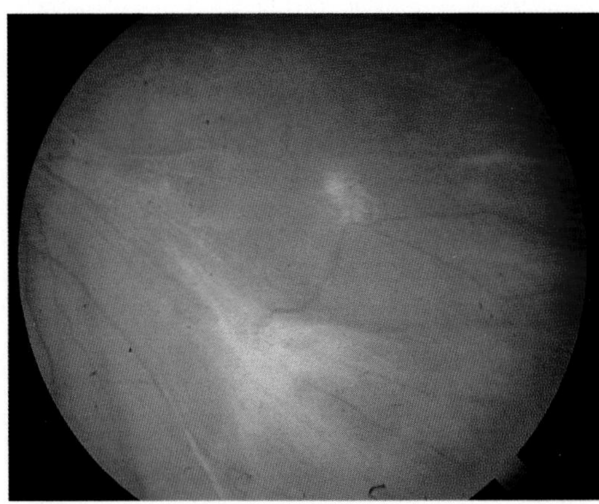

468 *T. canis* infection of the retina.

11 Infections in the immune-compromised host

The development of infection in a host is often the result of alterations in a balanced equilibrium between, on the one hand, the virulence or aggressiveness of the micro-organisms and, on the other, the integrity of the host's defences. Infection in the immune-compromised host may manifest itself in several ways (**Table 38**). In addition, the manifestation of infection will depend upon the type of immune compromise experienced. Defects may occur in both the non-specific and the specific immune systems (**Table 39**).

Table 38. Infective Manifestations of Immune Compromise.

Increased incidence of infection
Localized infection becoming generalized e.g. dissemination of shingles
Increased severity of infection
Low-grade pathogens producing disease e.g. *Pneumocystis carinii* pneumonia
Persistence of infection e.g. cryptosporidiosis
Unusual manifestations e.g. haemorrhagic chickenpox in leukaemic children
Recurrence of infection to which patient is immune
Increased frequency of recrudescence of latent infection e.g. more frequent herpes labialis
Increased frequency of reactivation of latent viruses

Table 39. Non-specific and Specific Immune Systems.

Non-specific immunity		*Specific immunity*
At body surfaces		**Antibody-mediated immunity**
Skin	Impermeability Lactic acid, fatty acids, sebaceous secretions Normal flora	Requires B cells, macrophages, T-helper and T-suppressor cells, neutrophils and complement
Respiratory mucosa	Lysozyme, lactoferrin Macrophages Mucociliary escalator	**Cell-mediated immunity** Requires T lymphocytes and macrophages
Gastrointestinal mucosa	Peristalsis Gastric acid, bile, proteolytic enzymes Lysozyme Normal flora	
Urinary tract mucosa	Urodynamics Lysozyme Tamm–Horsfall protein (false receptor)	
In tissues		
Phagocytes	Macrophages, neutrophils	
Lymphocytes	Natural killer cells	
Complement	Natural bactericidal effect of serum	
Acute-phase proteins	C-reactive protein, properidin	
Inflammatory response	Brings defence components to site of attack	
Febrile response	Limits growth of micro-organisms	

Defects in non-specific immunity

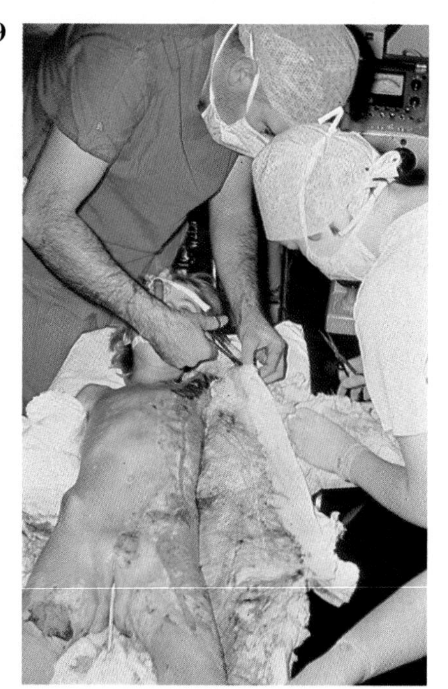

469 A child with severe burns.

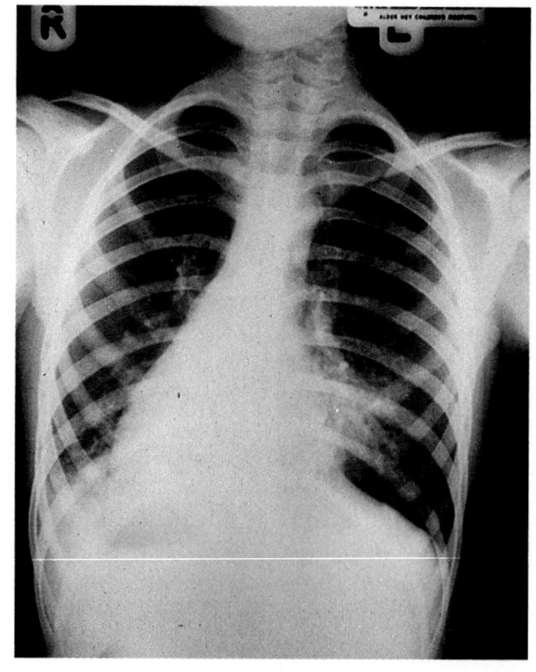

471 Chest X-ray of a child with Kartagener's syndrome, demonstrating dextrocardia.

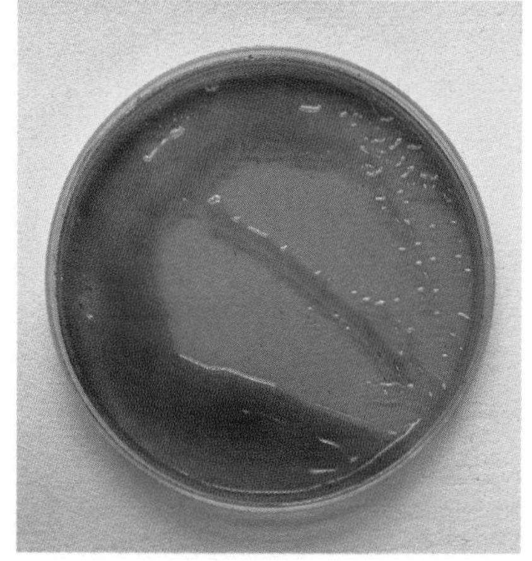

470 Mucoid *P. aeruginosa* on MacConkey agar.

In general, defects in defences at body surfaces tend to produce localized infections. For example, patients with extensive burns experience a loss of skin and produce a rich protein exudate which allows bacteria, such as *Streptococcus pyogenes* or *Staphylococcus aureus*, to multiply (**469**). Patients with cystic fibrosis have a defect in mucociliary clearance and are prone to develop colonization and chronic infection of the airways with mucoid strains of *Pseudomonas aeruginosa* (**470**). In cystic fibrosis the mucus is excessively viscid and the epithelial cilia have difficulty in propelling it upward to the larynx. In Kartagener's syndrome, in addition to dextrocardia (**471**), the dynein arms that produce the ciliary beat are defective; clearance is thus greatly impaired, leading to bronchopneumonia and bronchiectasis.

Defects in phagocytosis

The major phagocytic cells are the macrophage, which is found fixed in the reticuloendothelial system, and the polymorphonuclear neutrophil, which is found in the bloodstream. Most of the defects in phagocytosis have been described in neutrophils (**Table 40**). The defects that occur most often are due to bone marrow suppression by tumours, or to cytotoxic drugs leading to neutropenia. The number of episodes of severe

Table 40. Defects in Phagocytosis.

Congenital		Acquired	
Qualitative defects		**Qualitative defects**	
Chemotaxis	Lazy leukocyte syndrome Hyper IgE (Job's) syndrome Kartagener's syndrome LFA-1 deficiency	*Chemotaxis*	microtubule poisons e.g. vinblastine
		Phagolyzosome fusion	suramin, steroids
Adhesion	IgG deficiency Complement deficiency CD11/CD18 (receptor) deficiency	**Quantitative defects**	Most common defect encountered; due to cytotoxic drugs
Oxygen-dependent killing	Chronic granulomatous disease		
Phagolyzosome fusion	Chediak–Higachi syndrome		
Quantitative defects	Cyclic neutropenia (e.g. Schwachmann syndrome)		

infection is inversely related to the neutrophil count, with counts below 10^9/l being associated with an increased risk of infection.

However, there are also congenitally acquired defects of phagocyte function which, although rare, have greatly improved our understanding of how neutrophils kill bacteria. Recurrent infections that would cause suspicion of congenital defects of phagocytosis are shown in **Table 41**. Following invasion of tissues by micro-organisms, neutrophils in the circulation move to the site of invasion by a process known as chemotaxis. The most frequently encountered defect of chemotaxis is the hyper IgE syndrome or Job's syndrome, which is characterized by a raised serum IgE and the development of cold abscesses due to a wide variety of bacteria. **472** shows a perineal abscess

Table 41. Infections in Defective Phagocytosis.

Recurrent superficial sepsis (S. aureus, Pseudomonas spp., *Candida* spp.)	*Deep abscesses*
Paronychia	Lymphadenitis
Periodontitis	Hepatic abscess
Boils	Pneumonia, lung abscesses
Perirectal abscesses	Osteomyelitis

472

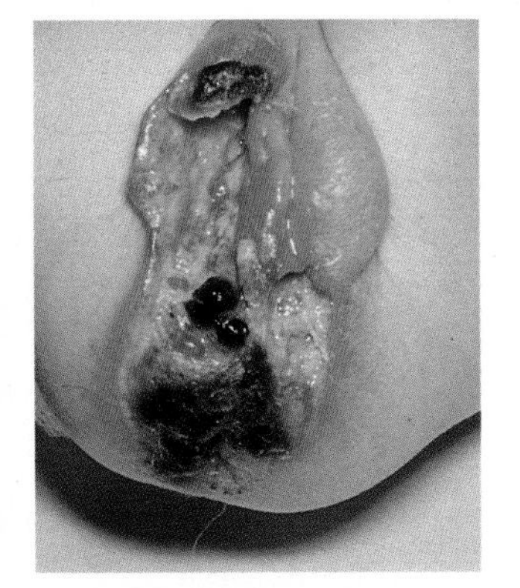

472 A large perineal abscess due to *P. aeruginosa* in a child with hyper IgE (Job's) syndrome.

473

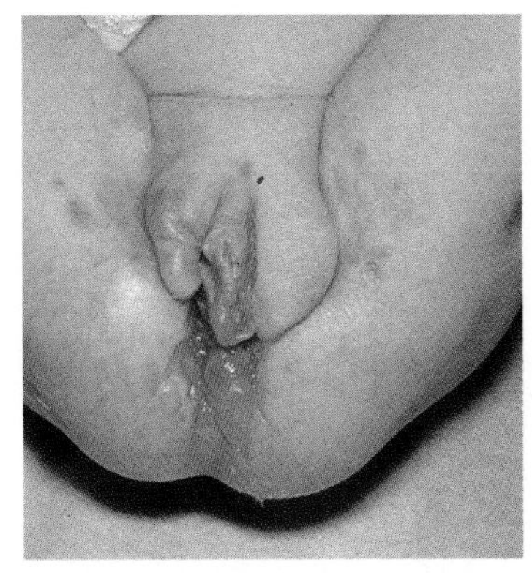

473 The same child in **472** after two weeks therapy.

474

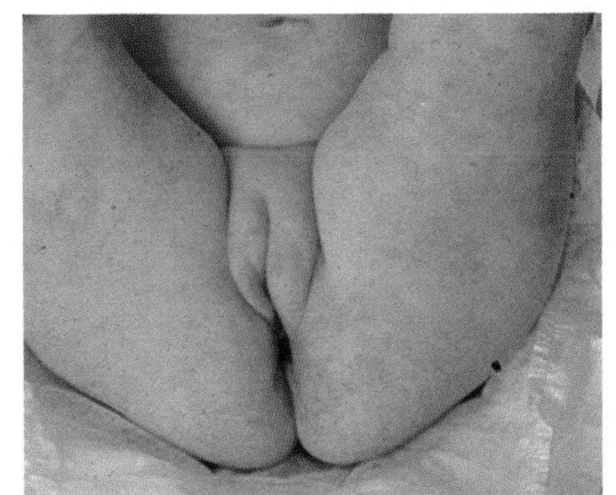

474 The same child in **472** two months later.

which contained *P. aeruginosa*. The patient had a high peripheral blood neutrophil count, but very few neutrophils were present in the pus. Her neutrophils showed a greatly diminished chemotactic response, which was reversed by exposure to cimetidine. **473** demonstrates the results of treatment with cimetidine and antibiotics after 2 weeks, and **474** illustrates the situation 2 months later.

The next stage involves adhesion of bacteria to the phagocyte surface. Problems at this stage usually result from defects in IgG production or in complement but may involve defects in receptors for IgG (CD11/CD18) or complement. As soon as bacteria adhere to the phagocyte surface, the neutrophil is activated to take in large amounts of oxygen and glucose, and an NADPH oxidase system is assembled to produce the superoxide anion (O_2^-) (**475**). The superoxide anion is a powerful oxident which can kill bacteria either in its own right or following dismutation to hydrogen peroxide. At the same time as this occurs the phagocyte throws pseudopodia around the bacterium, and lysosomal enzymes are released from granules (**476**). Myeloperoxidase, which is the major granule protein found in neutrophils, catalyses the production of hypochlorous acid (bleach) from hydrogen peroxide and Cl^- (**477**). Thus, large amounts of active oxidants are produced in close proximity to the bacterium, leading to its demise. The major defect in oxygen-dependent killing is chronic granulomatous disease (CGD). CGD usually presents as a recurrent, superficial abscess or as a deep-seated abscess, for example in the liver (**478**), brain or bone (**479**). Although infections are most often due to *S. aureus*, any catalase-positive micro-organism can be involved. Granulomata may be due to rare pathogens, such as *Aspergillus nidulans* (**480**) which in this case has produced a scalp granuloma (**481**). In CGD there is an inability to produce O_2^- and, although rare, this deficiency is the most common inherited defect of neutrophil function ($1 : 10^6$). The major form has an X-linked inheritance.

Prophylaxis can be achieved by: a rotating cycle of broad-spectrum antibiotics; long-term administration of cytokines, such as interferon, or of granulocyte colony stimulating factor; or by bone marrow transplantation.

475

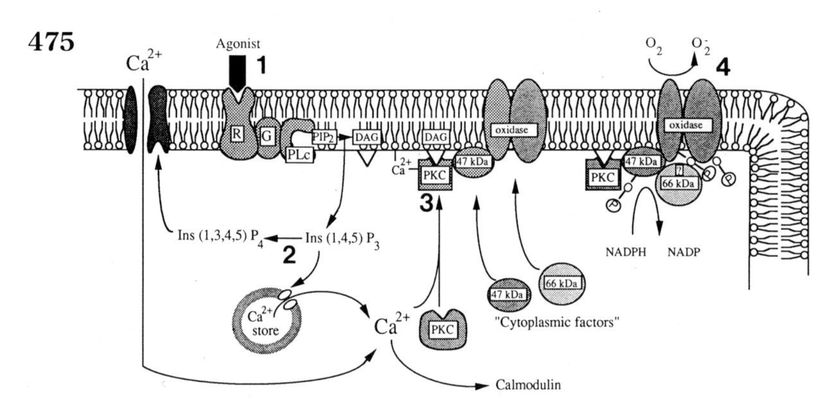

475 Activation of the neutrophil NADPH oxidase to produce superoxide anions (O_2^-). (1) Following binding of agonist (e.g. IgG) to the receptor, phospholipase C (PLc) is activated to hydrolyse phosphatidyl inositol. This yields inositol triphosphate (Ins P_3) and diacylglycerol (DAG). (2) Ins P_3 causes calcium release from calcisomes and calcium ingress. (3) Ca^{2+} and DAG activate protein kinase C (PKC), which leads to the assembly of the NADPH oxidase from membrane-associated and cytoplasmic proteins. (4) The NADPH oxidase complex catalyses the conversion of molecular oxygen to the superoxide anion, which is a potent bacteriocide.

476

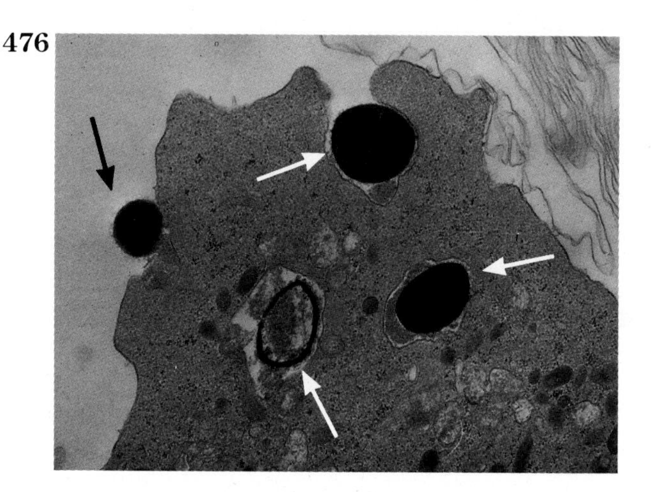

476 Thin-section electron micrograph showing the stages in the phagocytosis of *S. aureus* by a neutrophil (bacteria arrowed) (× *4,000*).

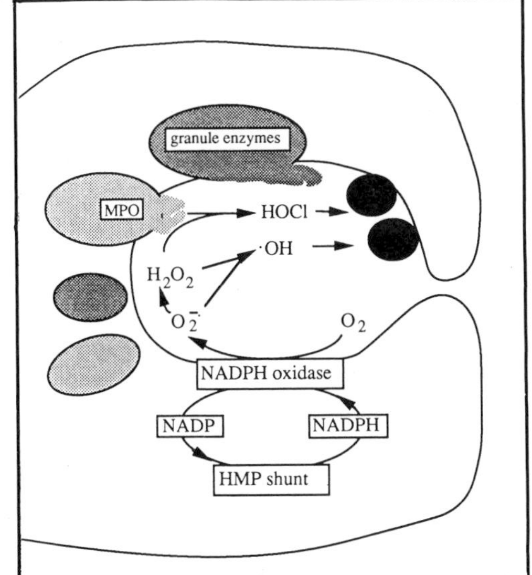

477 Diagrammatic representation of the production of active oxidants and the degranulation of myeloperoxidase.

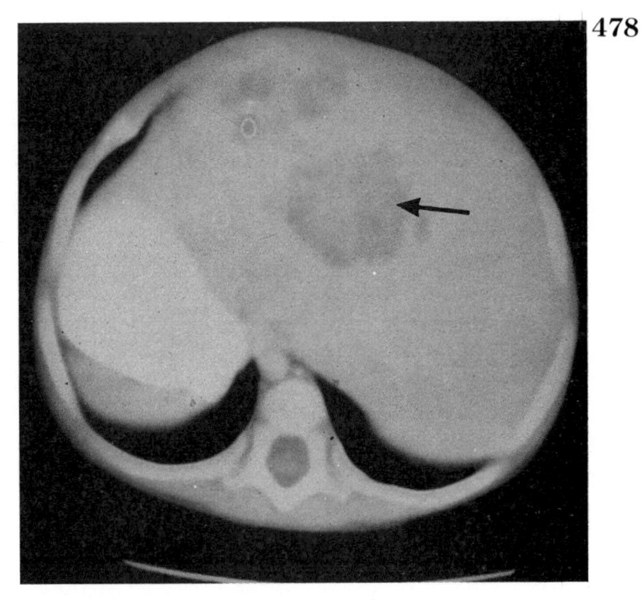

478 CT scan of a loculated liver abscess in a child with chronic granulomatous disease (CGD).

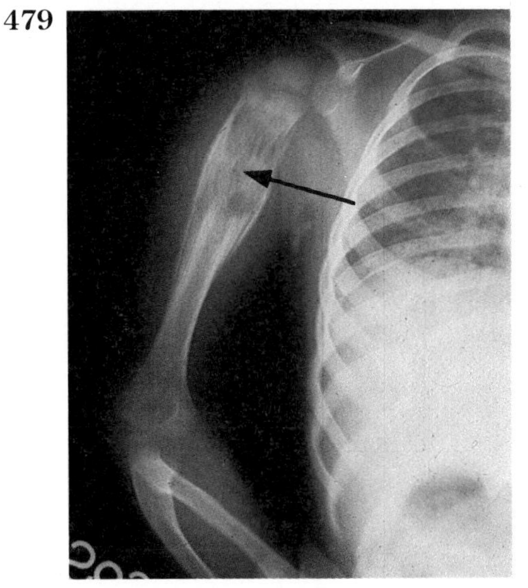

479 Multifocal osteomyelitis in a child with CGD.

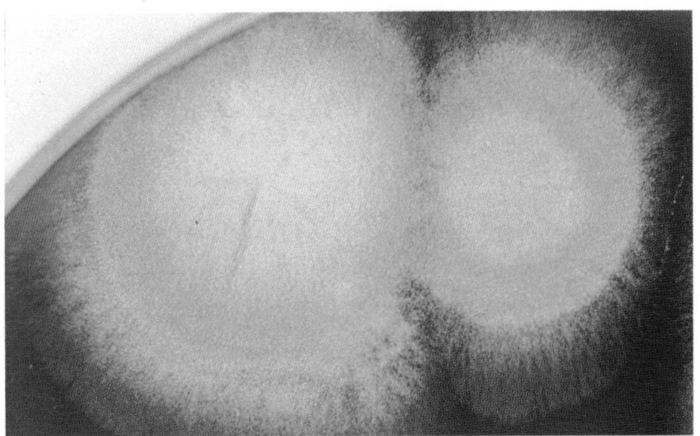

480 Two colonies of *A. nidulans* growing on blood agar.

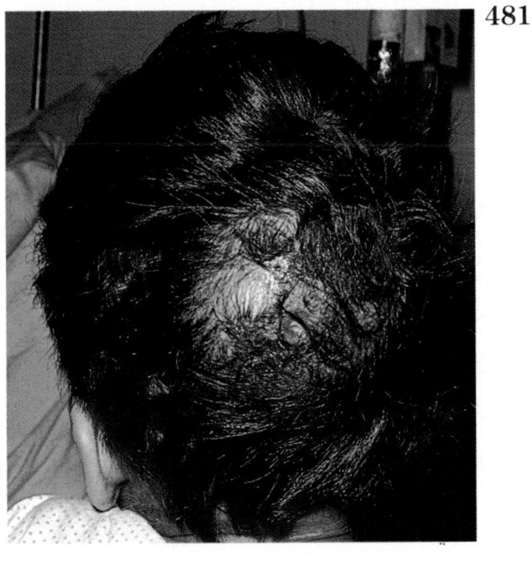

481 A large granuloma of the scalp due to *A. nidulans* in a child with CGD.

Defects in specific immunity

Defects may occur in B cell function or T cell function, or in both (**Table 42**), although all of these deficiencies are extremely rare as a rule. The most common defect in specific immunity is a selective IgA deficiency (1 : 600). The condition may be inapparent, but can be associated with atopy, recurrent pneumonia or bronchiectasis. In general, antibody deficiencies are associated with recurrent infection by capsulate bacteria such as *Streptococcus pneumoniae*, *H. influenzae* and *E. coli* K1 (**482**). Arthritis due to *Mycoplasma* spp. can also be problematic. Management involves replacement of antibodies by regular immunoglobulin infusions.

Chronic mucocutaneous candidiasis (CMC) is apparently a selective deficiency in T cell defence against *Candida* spp. In normal individuals, oral or perineal candidal infections remain localized and are self-limiting. However, in patients with CMC, infection spreads from the mouth, where it can be severe (**483**), to many other areas of the skin (**484**), and can be very disfiguring (**485**). Management consists of long-term topical treatment with nystatin.

Ataxia telangiectasia is a complex syndrome with an autosomal recessive inheritance. Cerebellar ataxia usually presents at the end of the second year and is progressive. The telangiectasia usually present by the fifth year and are normally seen on exposed areas of skin (**486**). Deficiencies in immunoglobulin classes and subclasses can be present as well as defects in T4 (helper) cell function. The disease is fatal.

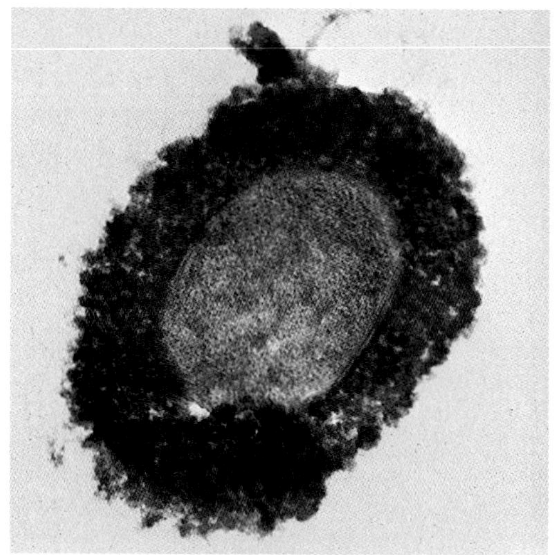

482 Thin-section electron micrograph of a capsulate strain of *E. coli*. The section has been stained with ruthenium red to demonstrate the capsule (× *8,000*).

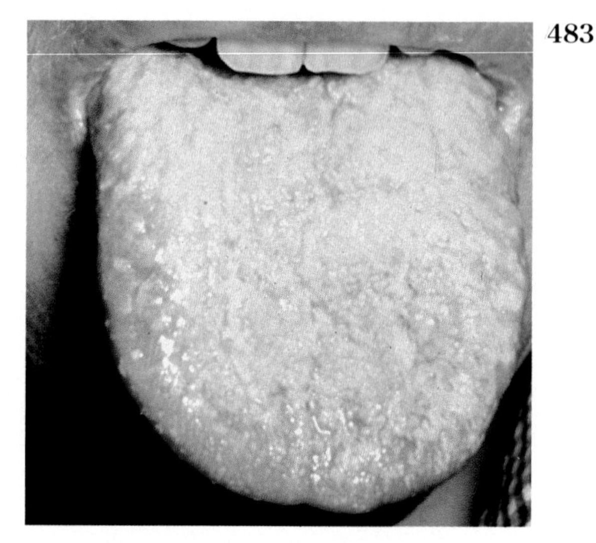

483 The tongue in chronic mucocutaneous candidiasis.

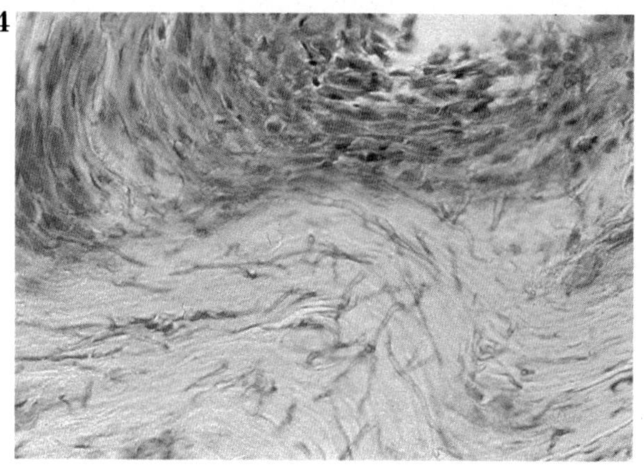

484 A histological section of skin in mucocutaneous candidiasis (× *200*).

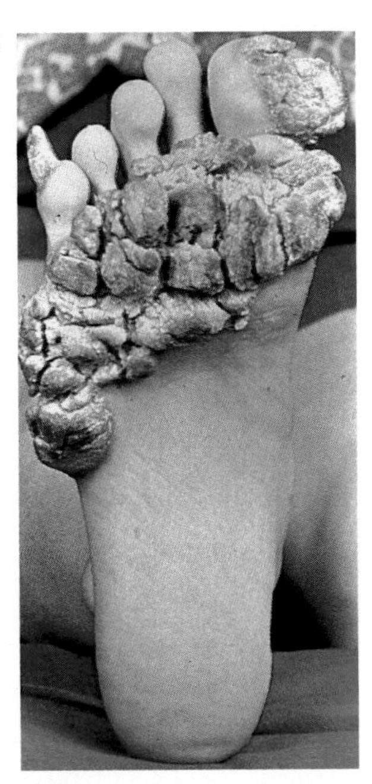

485 A large lesion on the foot of a child with mucocutaneous candidiasis.

Table 42. Defects in Specific Immunity.

B cell	Transient hypogammaglobulinaemia of infancy Selective IgA deficiency X-linked hypogammaglobulinaemia (Bruton's disease)
T cell	di George's syndrome (thymic and parathyroid aplasia) Nezelof's syndrome (thymic aplasia) Chronic mucocutaneous candidiasis
Mixed B and T cell	Severe combined immunodeficiency Adenine deaminase deficiency Purine nucleoside phosphorylase deficiency Immunodeficiency with ataxia telangiectasia Wiskott–Aldrich syndrome

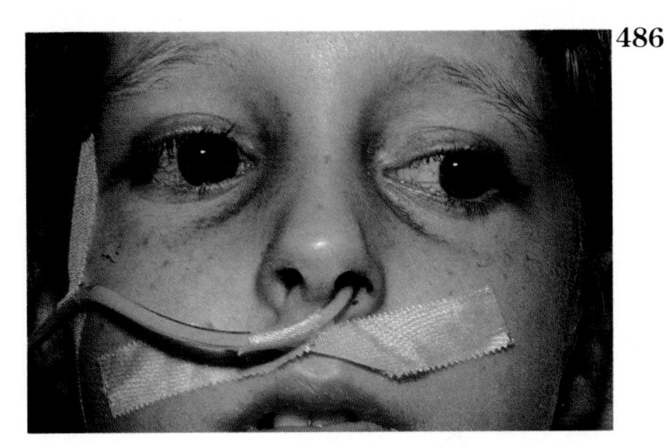

486 A girl with ataxia telangiectasia. Note the numerous telangiectasia on the cheeks.

Infections in children with leukaemia and tumours

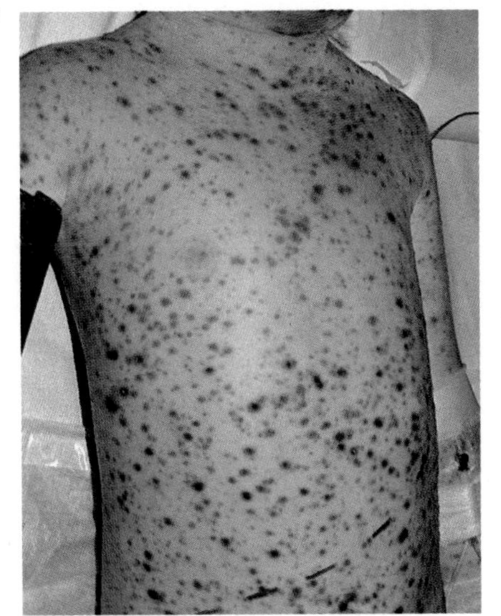

487 Haemorrhagic chickenpox in a child receiving chemotherapy for acute lymphoblastic leukaemia.

Cytotoxic drugs, steroids and radiation all seem to depress immunity by affecting T cell, B cell and neutrophil numbers. Thus, patients receiving such treatment are at risk from viral, bacterial, fungal and protozoal infections.

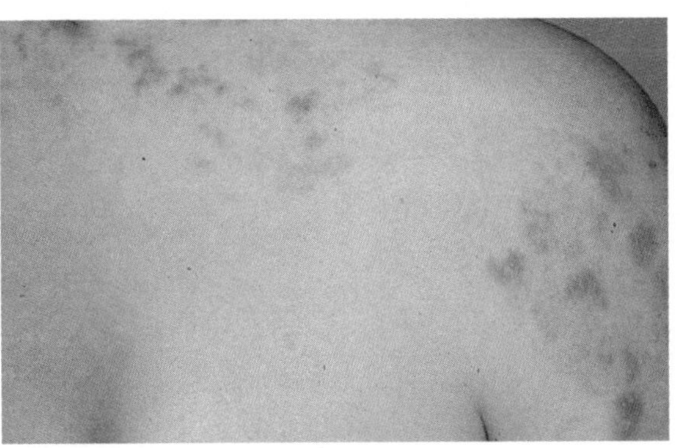

488 Shingles developing in a child receiving cytotoxic therapy.

Infection with viruses such as the herpesviruses and measles virus are particularly important. If a child develops chickenpox while receiving cytotoxic therapy, the infection can be life-threatening and often produces a haemorrhagic rash (**487**). For those previously infected with varicella–zoster virus, cytotoxic or immunosuppressive therapy can lead to the development of shingles (**488**), which may disseminate from the dermatome. CMV is another particularly important pathogen, especially in those undergoing bone marrow transplantation; instead of the innocuous infection seen in the immune-competent host, in bone marrow transplant patients CMV can produce retinitis (**489**), pneumonitis (**490**), enteritis or hepatitis. Measles can be particularly devastating in children receiving cytotoxic therapy. No rash appears, but the children develop severe life-threatening giant-cell pneumonia. **491** shows a section of lung from the first reported case (in 1955), in which it was demonstrated that measles was the cause of the giant-cell pneumonia. The fungal pathogen *Pneumocystis carinii* is an important cause of pneumonia (**492**) in such children. Treatment is either with high-dose cotrimoxazole or with nebulized pentamidine. Prophylaxis is achieved by long-term administration of cotrimoxazole.

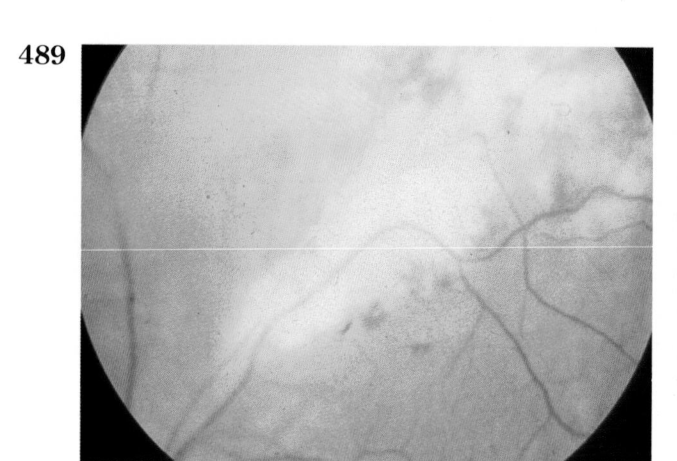

489 CMV retinitis.

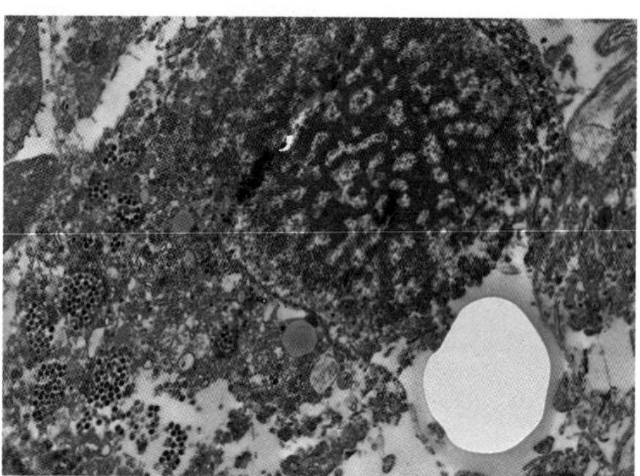

490 Thin-section electron micrograph of a lung biopsy from a child with CMV pneumonitis. Large numbers of viral particles are present in the nucleus and cytoplasm of the pneumatocyte (× *2,000*).

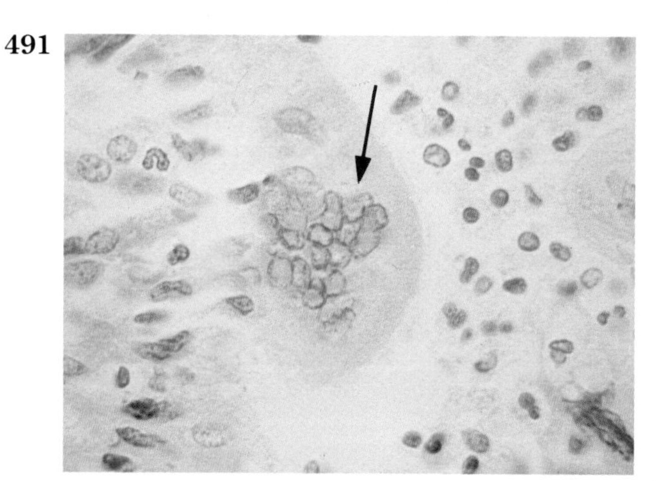

491 A section of lung from the first case in which it was shown that measles virus was responsible for giant-cell pneumonia. A large multinucleate cell is clearly visible (× *400*).

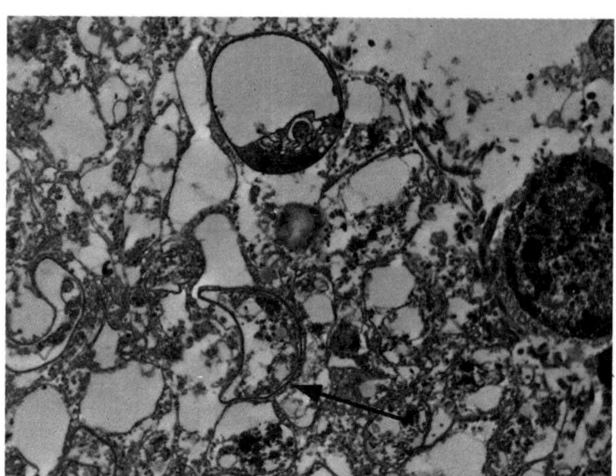

492 Thin-section electron micrograph of a lung biopsy of a patient with AIDS. Cysts of *P. carinii* are present (× *10,000*).

The acquired immunodeficiency syndrome

Acquired immunodeficiency syndrome (AIDS) is caused by the human immunodeficiency viruses (HIV-1 and HIV-2), retroviruses (**493**) that have a tropism principally for cells expressing the CD4 antigen and some neuronal cells. HIV is an enveloped RNA virus with a glycoprotein (gp 120, gp 41) fringe on its periphery (**494**). Gp 120 has an affinity for the CD4 antigen, which is present on T4-helper cells, monocytes, macrophages and some neuronal cells.

Although the initial infection is usually asymptomatic, some patients may develop a maculopapular rash, lymphadenopathy or even meningoencephalitis. During this initial period, HIV RNA genome is converted to its proviral DNA (**495**), which becomes integrated into the chromosome of the infected cells. The virus remains latent for long periods. Eventually, the virus reactivates extensively and the T-helper cells, in particular, are depleted, greatly impairing both antibody production and cell-mediated immunity. The patient is then highly susceptible both to opportunistic infection with viruses, bacteria, fungi and protozoa, and to the development of tumours, especially lymphomata.

In developed countries, HIV infection is not common in children except in certain at risk populations. It is confined to those infected perinatally and haemophiliacs who have been infected with contaminated factor VIII. Perinatal transmission occurs either *in utero*, during delivery or, rarely, by breast-feeding (there has also been one case of a neonate infecting its mother via breast-feeding). In general, perinatally acquired HIV infection has a shorter incubation period (9–18 months) than that of infection acquired in other ways (2–5 years). In addition, perinatally infected children have a much lower incidence of Kaposi's sarcoma and of infections with *Toxoplasma gondii*, *Cryptococcus neoformans* and *Histoplasma capsulatum*, but an increased incidence of lymphocytic interstitial pneumonitis and of bacterial infections.

Table 43. Clinical Features of AIDS in Perinatally Acquired HIV.

HIV-related	
Encephalopathy:	impaired head growth, failure to reach developmental milestones, progressive motor defects
Enteropathy:	failure to thrive, chronic diarrhoea
Other infections	
Candida albicans: oesophageal or bronchopulmonary	
Cryptosporidium parvum: intestinal or extraintestinal	
CMV: disseminated	
Herpes simplex virus: disseminated	
Isospora belli: chronic diarrhoea	
Mycobacterium tuberculosis: disseminated	
Atypical mycobacteria: e.g. *Mycobacterium avium/intracellulare*	
Pneumocystis carinii: pneumonia	
Recurrent bacterial infection: capsulate bacteria especially	
Mycoplasma pneumoniae: pneumonia	
Lymphocytic interstitial pneumonia: ? EBV	
Tumours	
Burkitt's lymphoma	
Other lymphomata	
Rare features	
Toxoplasma gondii: encephalitis	
Cryptococcus neoformans: extra pulmonary	
Kaposi's sarcoma: body surfaces	
Histoplasma capsulatum: disseminated	

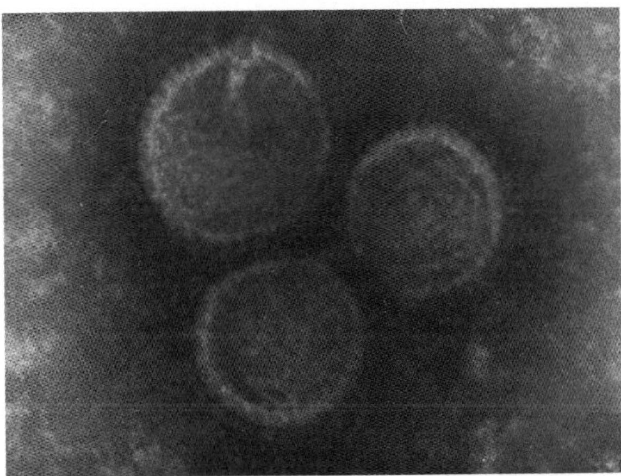

493 Negative-stain electron micrograph of the retrovirus HIV, demonstrating the fringed lipid envelope and an eccentric nucleoid (× *80,000*).

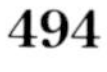

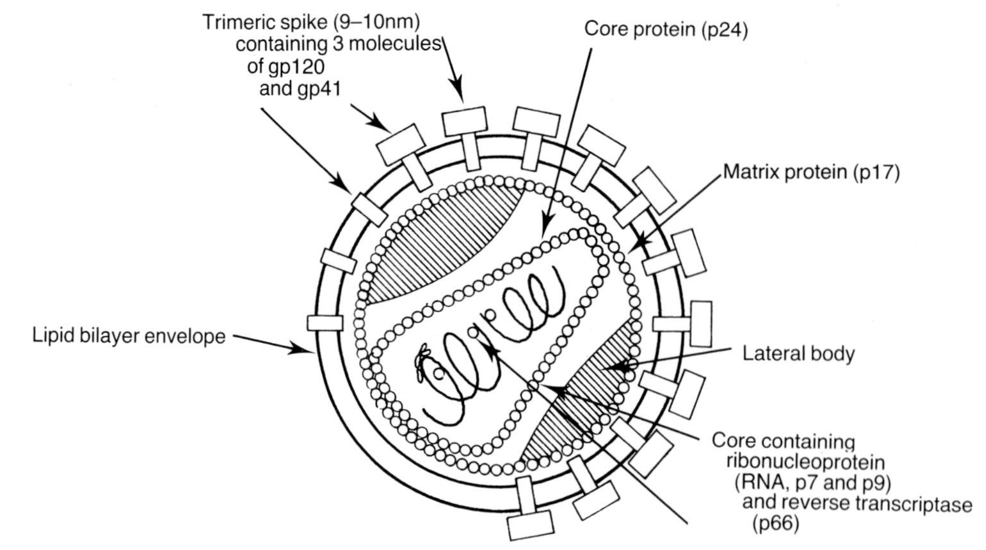

494 Diagrammatic representation of the structure of HIV.

495

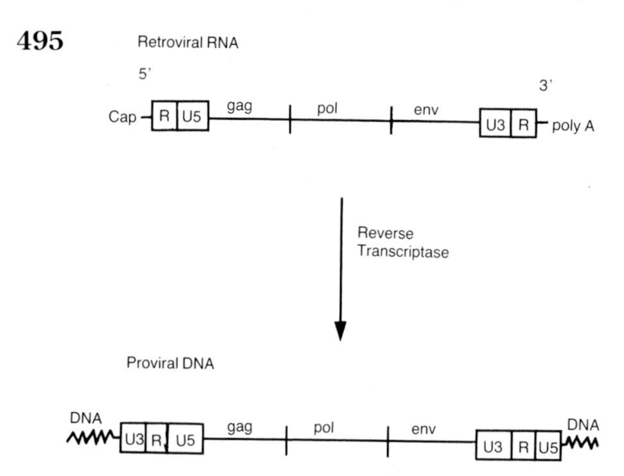

495 The conversion of the HIV RNA genome to double-stranded proviral DNA by reverse transcriptase.

The criteria for the diagnosis of AIDS in perinatally acquired HIV infection are still evolving, but they currently include the features shown in **Table 43**. (Most of the infective agents have already been covered in earlier sections). The recurrent bacterial infections present as pneumonia, arthritis, osteomyelitis, meningitis, visceral abscesses or septicaemia, all of which are due largely to capsulate bacteria such as *S. pneumoniae*, *E. coli*, *Klebsiella aerogenes* or *H. influenzae*. Although *Cryptosporidium parvum* is primarily an enteric pathogen that causes intractable diarrhoea in AIDS patients, it may spread to contiguous mucosal surfaces, such as the respiratory tract (**496**) or biliary tract. *Isospora belli* (**497**) is an uncommon cause of diarrhoea in the immunocompetent but it can cause problems in patients with AIDS.

496

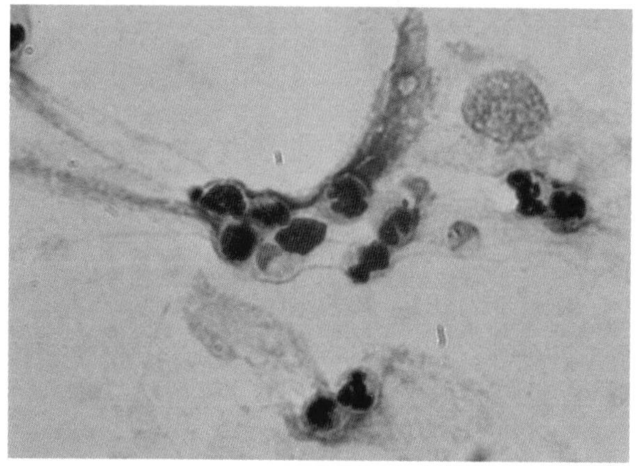

496 Smear of bronchial lavage from a child with AIDS. Safranin–methylene blue stain reveals pus cells (blue) and cryptosporidium oocysts (pink) (× *400*).

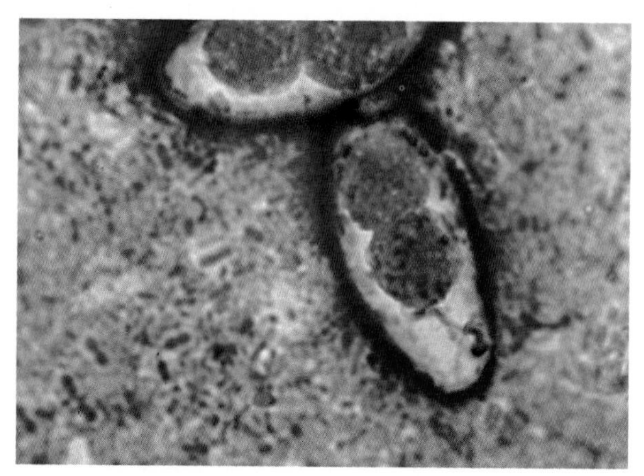

497 Faecal smear from a child with AIDS. Safranin–methylene blue stain reveals cysts (pink) of *I. belli* (× *1,000*).

12 Common tropical infections of childhood

In tropical and subtropical countries infectious diseases are responsible for the majority of deaths in childhood. The interaction of malnutrition with the consequences of impaired host resistance makes children particularly susceptible to infections. Measles and whooping cough are alone responsible for well over one million deaths per year in children because of a combination of factors including debility from malnutrition and anaemia, early and intense exposure to infection, and a poorly developed immune system.

Malaria

Malaria is responsible for many deaths in children through both direct and indirect mechanisms (**498**). In the pregnant woman malaria causes anaemia, which affects the developing fetus and produces an increase in miscarriages and stillbirths. In primigravidas an association exists between malaria and the birth of babies who are small for their gestational age. Subsequent pregnancies do not seem so badly affected. True congenital malaria does occur but it is rare. In the newborn, malarial parasites may be found but they are rapidly cleared from the circulation. Symptoms of malaria are unusual before the age of 6 months. The mother confers some short-term immunity through the passive intrauterine transfer of IgG. Moreover, erythrocytes with fetal haemoglobulin are resistant to colonization by *Plasmodium* spp. and breast-feeding is thought to inhibit the parasite by depriving it of para-aminobenzoic acid. Children with sickle-cell trait also have some resistance to malaria.

Although over 100 *Plasmodium* spp. exist, only four cause human disease: *P. falciparum*, *P. vivax*, *P. ovale* and *P. malariae*. The particular species can be distinguished by their morphology (**499** & **500**) and their effect on the red cell.

498

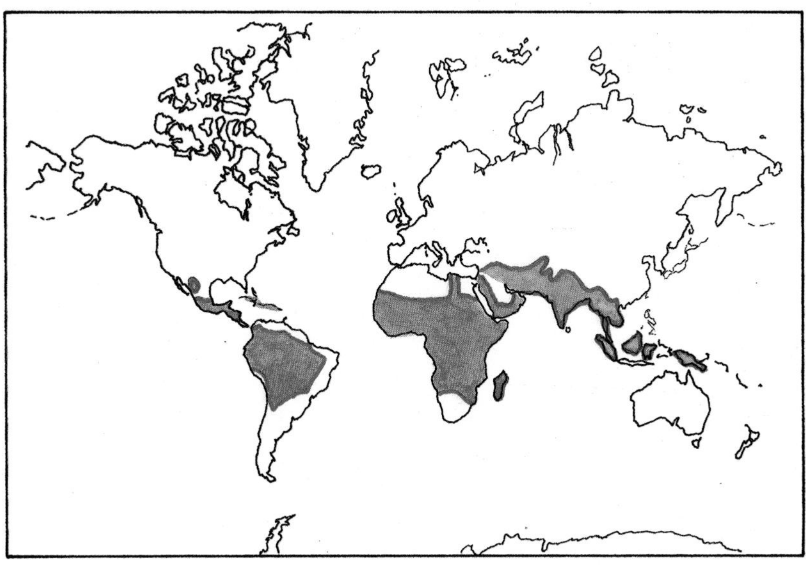

498 Areas in which malaria is endemic.

The clinical presentation of malaria can differ widely in children. In the non-immune an acute primary attack may present with non-specific symptoms of drowsiness, vomiting, refusal of feeds and loose stools. The classic features of rigor and periodicity of fever are less common in children than in adults. The temperature may rise above 39°C, precipitating a febrile convulsion in the predisposed. Physical signs often include pallor, anaemia and, later, hepatosplenomegaly. Infants in areas in which malaria is endemic develop some immunity, and symptoms of disease which include loss of appetite, fatigue, diarrhoea, anaemia and general retardation of growth may be insidious. *P. falciparum* is responsible for severe and life-threatening complications of malaria. Cerebral malaria may present suddenly with coma and convulsions. If untreated, death will almost certainly occur (**501** & **502**).

Hypoglycaemia may occur both as a result of malaria and as a complication of quinine treatment. Anaemia occurs invariably. Haemoglobin is usually below 10g/l, and the blood picture shows a normocytic or microcytic anaemia. Haemolysis may be sufficiently severe to cause jaundice. The spleen can become very large in some children, and trauma may cause rupture. Acute renal failure may develop both as a result of fluid loss from vomiting, diarrhoea and sweating, and because the parasite interferes with the microcirculation of the kidney. In children *P. malariae* is associated with a nephrotic syndrome which has a poor prognosis as it usually does not respond well to steroids (**503** & **504**).

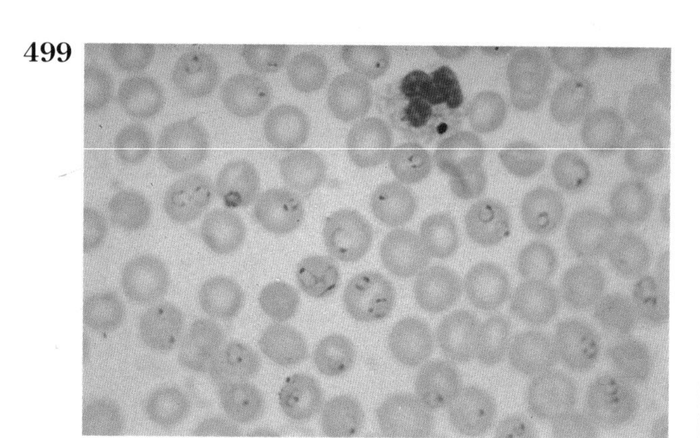

499 Leishman's stain of *P. falciparum* reveals many ring trophoizoites in erythrocytes (× *200*).

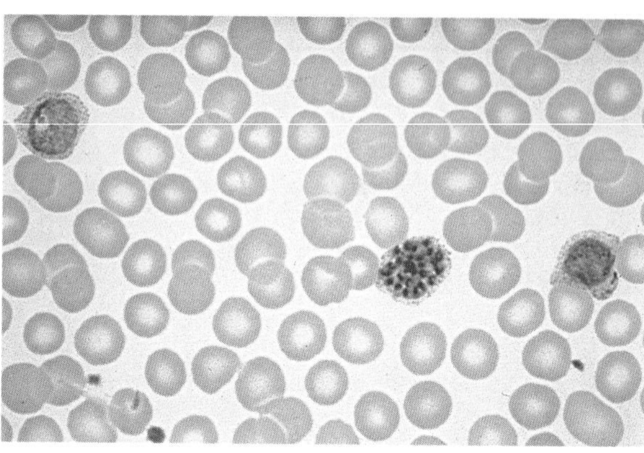

500 Leishman's stain of *P. vivax* reveals erythrocytes with merozoites (m) and two gametocytes (g) (× *200*).

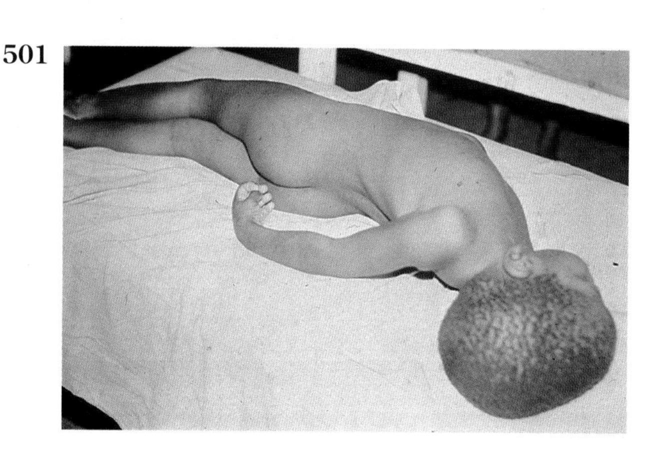

501 A child with cerebral malaria demonstrating neck retraction.

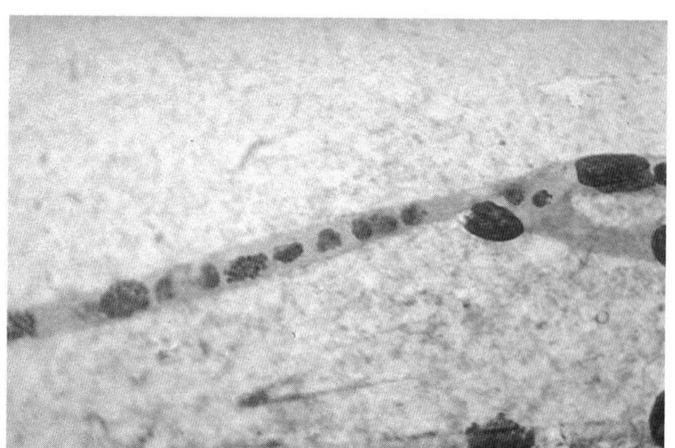

502 Brain section from a child with cerebral malaria, demonstrating capillaries packed with parasitized erythrocytes.

503

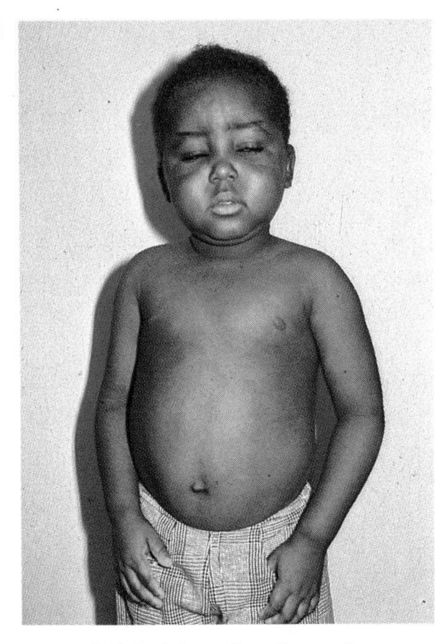

503 Child with nephrotic syndrome due to infection with *P. malariae* (quartan malaria).

504

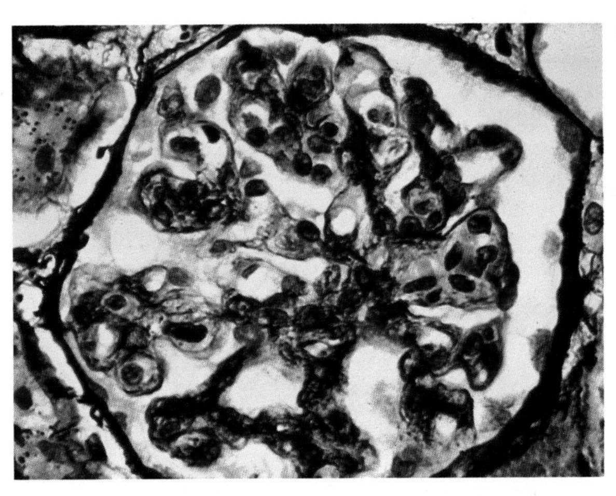

504 A glomerulus from a renal biopsy showing changes of *P. malariae* nephrotic syndrome with thickened basement membrane and virtual obliteration of capillaries (× *200*).

The diagnosis of malaria is made by taking both a thick and a thin blood film and staining them with Leishman's (**505**) or Field's stain. The species of plasmodium can then be determined by its specific morphology and its effect on the parasitized erythrocyte.

Treatment of malaria has become difficult because of the emergence of multidrug-resistant parasites. Fortunately, for the acute attack, quinine remains effective against nearly all strains of malarial parasite. Strains resistant to chloroquine, mefloquine and even to fansidar mean that prophylaxis has to be matched to up-to-date knowledge of the sensitivity of parasites in a given geographical area. Children with *P. vivax*, *P. ovale* and *P. malariae* will need a course of primaquine to eradicate the hepatic cycle of the parasite. However, children with glucose-6-phosphate dehydrogenase deficiency are at risk of developing acute haemolysis with primaquine. Prevention of malaria is currently achieved through interrupting the life cycle of the parasite, but research towards a vaccine is advancing.

505

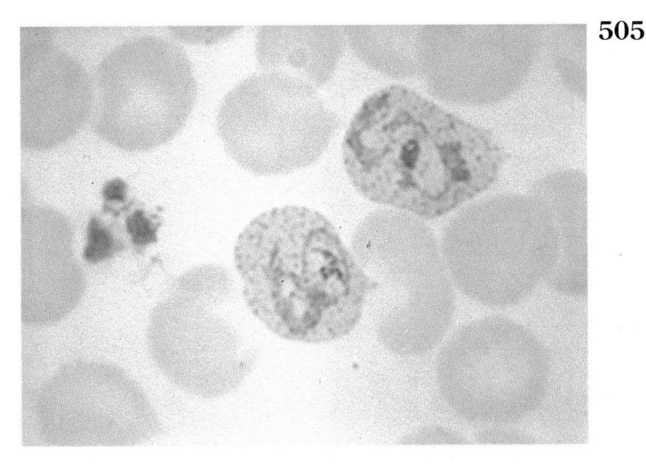

505 Leishman's stain of *P. vivax* reveals a characteristic irregular trophozoite within an enlarged erythrocyte which shows with Shuffner's dots (× *400*).

Leishmaniasis

Essentially a zoonosis, leishmaniasis is caused by a protozoan parasite *Leishmania*, of which there are several species, each with a particular geographical distribution throughout the world (**506**). The sandfly is the vector between man and reservoir hosts which include dogs, foxes and small rodents. In children, there are essentially two clinical presentations of leishmaniasis: visceral leishmaniasis and cutaneous leishmaniasis (**Table 44**).

Visceral leishmaniasis (kala-azar) is characterized by severe anaemia, diffuse lymph node enlargement, neutropenia and sometimes thrombocytopenia and massive hepatosplenomegaly (**507**). The child suffers recurrent episodes of fever and may be prone to bacterial infections due to a depressed immune response, a low white-cell count and bone marrow suppression. Diagnosis is made on a bone marrow or splenic aspiration. On examination, characteristic Leishman–Donovan bodies will be seen (**508**). Visceral leishmaniasis may need a 3-week course of treatment with a pentavalent antimonial compound.

Cutaneous leishmaniasis presents as a chronic ulcerating skin lesion, often referred to as 'oriental sore' among many other local names (**509 & 510**).

506

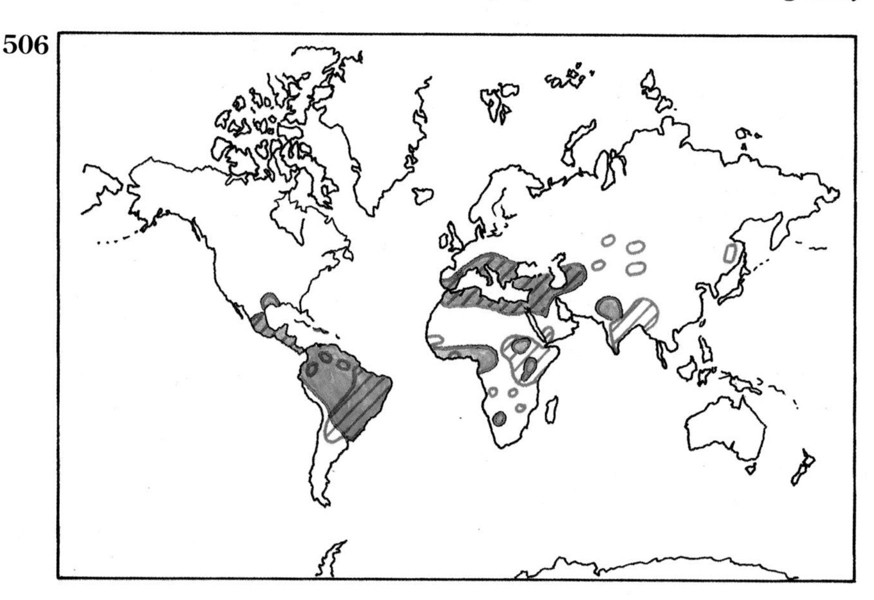

506 The geographical distribution of leishmaniasis.

Table 44. Classification of Leishmaniasis.

Type of disease	*Species*	*Host*	*Distribution*	*Infection*
Visceral leishmaniasis	*L. donovani*	Man Rodents Canines	(Old and New World) Africa, Asia, Europe South and Central America	Kala-azar Infantile leishmaniasis
Cutaneous leishmaniasis (Old World)	*L. major*	Rodents	Africa, Asia	Oriental sore (rural, deserts)
	L. tropica	Man	Africa, Mediterranean Middle East, West Asia	Oriental sore (Urban)
	L. aethiopica	Hyrax	Africa	Oriental sore Diffuse, cutaneous
Cutaneous leishmaniasis (New World)	*L. mexicana*	Rodents	South and Central America	Oriental sore Diffuse, cutaneous
Mucocutaneous leishmaniasis (New World)	*L. brasiliensis*	Canines	South America	Oriental Espundia

The lesions occur approximately 6 weeks after the initial bite of the sandfly. The parasites enter macrophages, inducing a cell-mediated response in the host. An infiltration of lymphocytes, plasma cells and large mononuclear cells occurs. The lesions usually heal themselves within 18 months, leaving a thin, depressed scar. In some children a chronic diffuse form of the disease can occur, which is thought to be due to a poor host response. The diagnosis is made by biopsy of the periphery of the ulcer, which is stained with Giemsa or with Leishman's stain. In the sandfly the promastigoate form of *Leishmania* may be found (**511**).

507

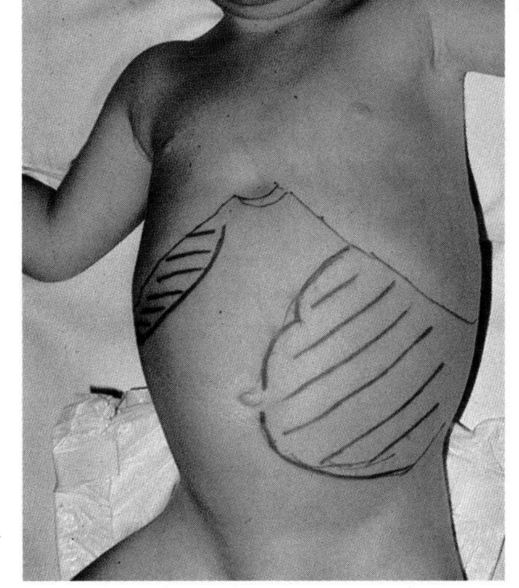

507 Visceral leishmaniasis in an 18-month-old boy, showing gross hepatosplenomegaly.

8

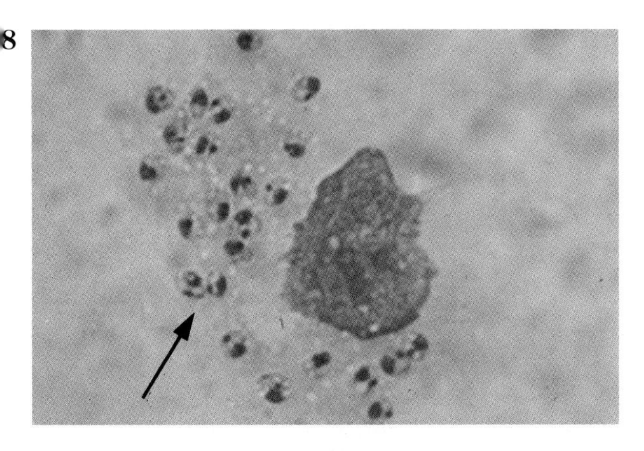

508 Bone marrow smear showing typical Leishman–Donovan bodies (amastigotes) (× *1,000*).

509

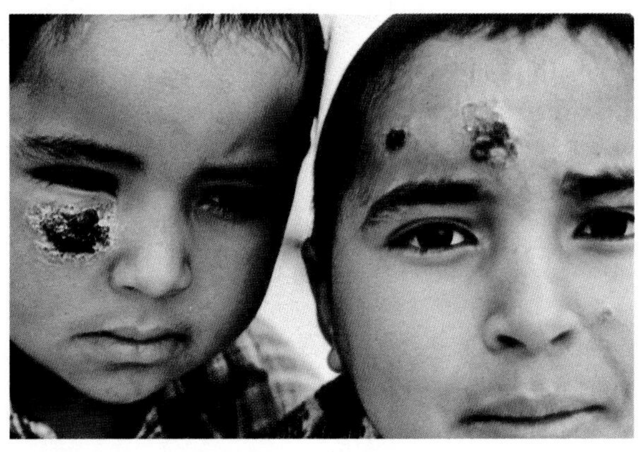

509 Cutaneous leishmaniasis on the face.

0

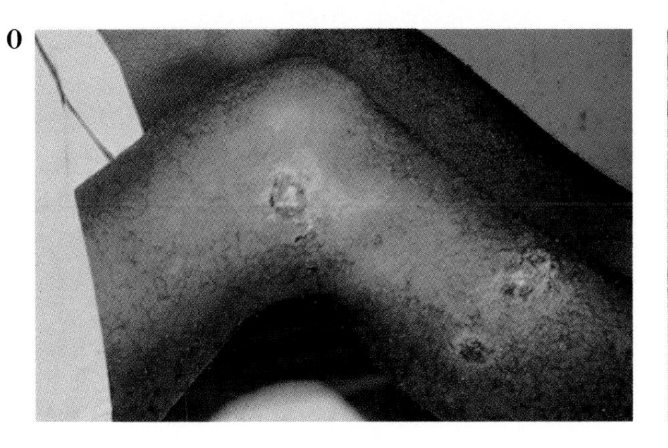

510 Cutaneous leishmaniasis on the leg.

511

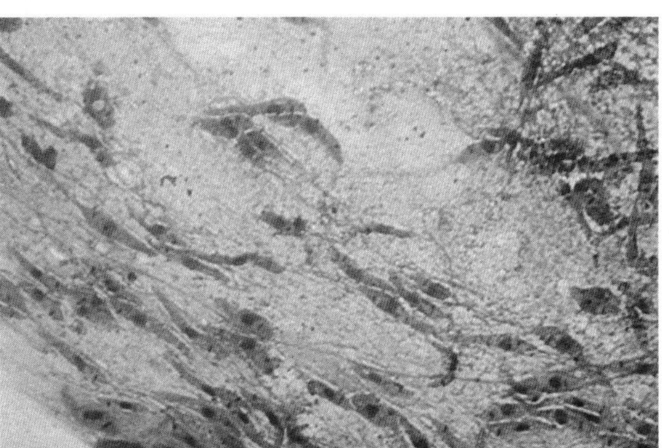

511 The promastigote form of the *Leishmania* parasite taken from the gut of the sandfly (× *1,000*).

Trypanosomiasis

Trypanosomiasis is a protozoal disease which exists in two distinct clinical forms: in Africa, *Trypanosoma gambienese* and *T. rhodesiense* cause sleeping sickness; in South America, *T. cruzi* causes Chagas' disease or American trypanosomiasis. Both types of trypanosomiasis are transmitted to man by an arthropod vector, which in Africa is the tsetse fly (*Glossina*), and in South America is a blood-sucking bug of the Reduviidae family (**512**).

African trypanosomiasis occurs after the trypanosomes are injected via the painful bite of the tsetse fly. A local chancre may result, which develops as a progressive ulcer over 7–10 days before healing (**513**). The trypanosomes multiply locally and spread via the lymph nodes into the blood stream and then into the CNS (**514**). As the trypanosomes enter the blood, they are disseminated into muscle cells and into peripheral autonomic ganglion cells. Once the brain is affected, the child will slowly deteriorate clinically in mental and motor function. The diagnosis is made from a thick blood smear or by examining the buffy layer of the blood. Serological tests are not reliable. It is often difficult to detect trypanosomes in the CSF.

Treatment for early trypanosomiasis includes suramin and pentamidine, but once the brain is affected, malarsoprol must be used. A new and less toxic drug, eflornithine, which is an ornithine carboxylase inhibitor, seems to be emerging as the treatment of choice. American trypanosomiasis is transmitted through the bite of the Reduvid bug or through the bug's faeces, which may pass through mucous membranes. If the parasite enters the body through the conjunctiva, there may be oedema (**515**) and an intense inflammatory reaction (usually involving one eye), which continues for several weeks.

Although most infections are acquired in childhood, clinical signs, which include characteristic enlargement of the viscera, in which the heart and bowel become enlarged and dilated, do not usually appear before adolescence. The disease produces a cardiomyopathy and chronic myocarditis.

512

512 The reduviid bug which transmits American trypanosomiasis through its bite or its faeces. (Copyright LSTM.)

513

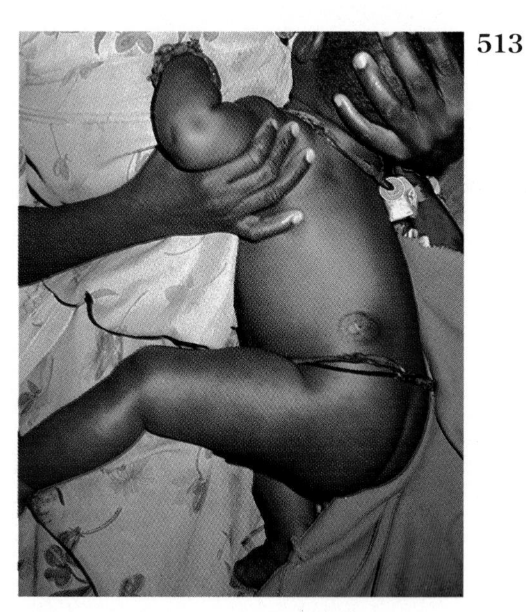

513 Chancre following the bite of the tsetse fly.

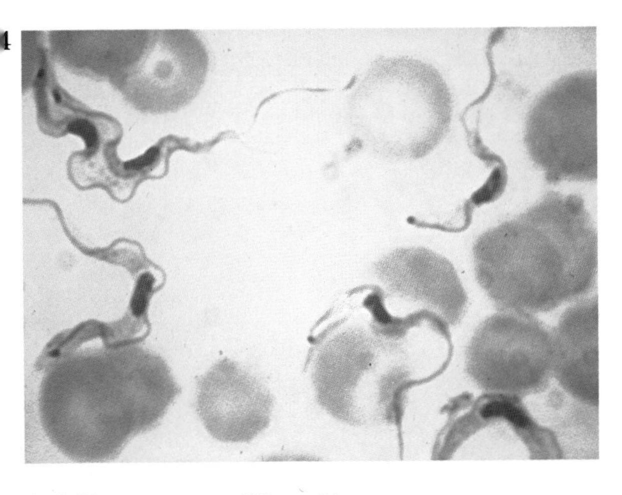

514 Trypanosomes of *T. gambiense*.

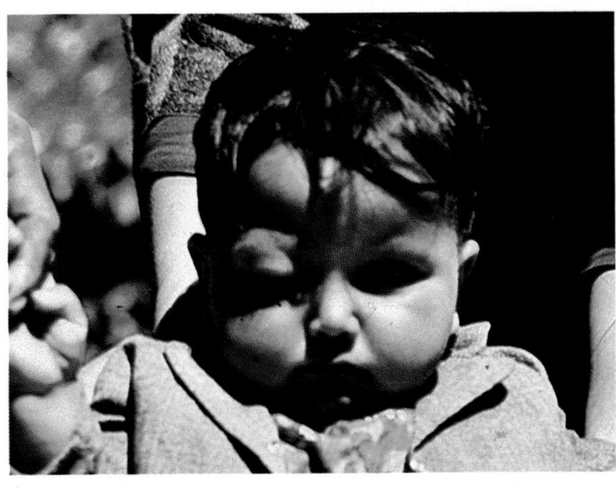

515 Oedema of the right eye (Romaña's sign) due to local inflammation caused by *T. cruzi*. (Copyright LSTM.)

Amoebiasis

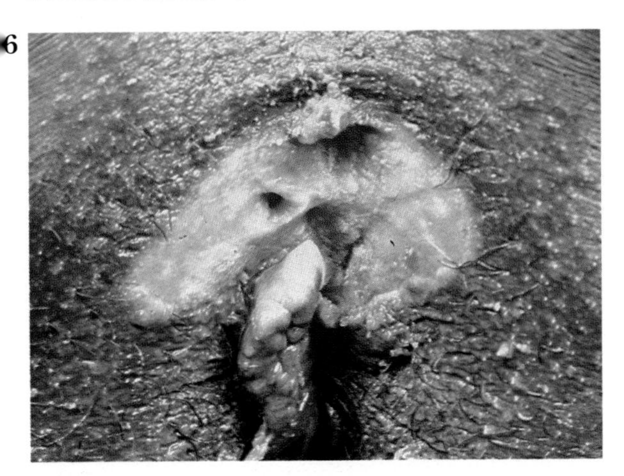

Entamoeba histolytica usually causes dysentery. However, it sometimes progresses to produce an amoebic hepatitis and liver abscesses. In some children who are seriously debilitated and who have a very heavy infection, an ulcerating lesion around the anal margin may be observed (**516**). Urgent treatment with metronidazole is essential to prevent fibrosis and permanent scarring.

516 Perianal amoebiasis.

Rickettsial disease

Rickettsial diseases are transmitted by arthropods including ticks, mites, lice and fleas. The *Rickettsiae* are gram-negative bacteria which grow only intracellularly. They are responsible for typhus and other diseases, which may be classified according to their epidemiology and the intermediate host (**Table 45**).

Rickettsiae cause symptoms and disease by being disseminated into the endothelial cells, where they cause focal perivasculitis, necrosis, and diapedisis of red cells. Any organ may be involved, and bleeding abnormalities are common. In scrub and tick typhus, a skin ulcer known as an eschar may develop at the site of the insect bite (**517**). Some children develop photophobia and neck stiffness, mimicking meningitis. Lymphadenopathy is common. Rashes, which may mimic meningococcal septicaemia, can occur in all types of typhus (**518**).

Diagnosis of rickettsial diseases can be difficult since many of the clinical features are non-specific, infection may thus present as FUO. Serology may be helpful, but false positive results are common. *Rickettsiae* are very sensitive to chloramphenicol and tetracycline.

Table 45. Classification of Rickettsial Disease.

Disease	*Organism*	*Vector*	*Mode of transmission*	*Usual host*	*Geographical distribution*
Typhus group					
Epidemic typhus	*R. prowazeki*	Body lice	Crushed louse and faeces, through skin or mucous membrane	Man	Worldwide
Brill–Zinsser disease	*R. prowazeki*	Body lice	Crushed louse and faeces, through skin or mucous membrane	Man	Worldwide
Murine typhus	*R. mooseri*	Fleas	Bites	Rodents	Worldwide
Spotted fever group					
Scrub typhus	*R. tsutsugamushi*	Chigoe or jigger fleas	Jigger bite	Rodents	Asia, Australia, Pacific
Rocky mountain spotted fever	*R. rickettsii*	Ticks	Tick bite	Small mammals	Europe, America
Boutonneuse fever	*R. conorii*	Ticks	Tick bite	Rodent, dogs	Mediterranean shores
Rickettsial pox	*R. akari*	Mite	Mouse mite bite	Mice	USA, USSR, Central Africa
Queensland tick typhus	*R. australis*	Ticks	Tick bite	Marsupials	Australia
Siberian tick typhus	*R. siberica*	Mites	Mite bite	Farm animals	USSR
Trench Fever	*R. quintana*	Lice	Crushed louse and faeces	Man	Africa, Mexico, Eastern Europe

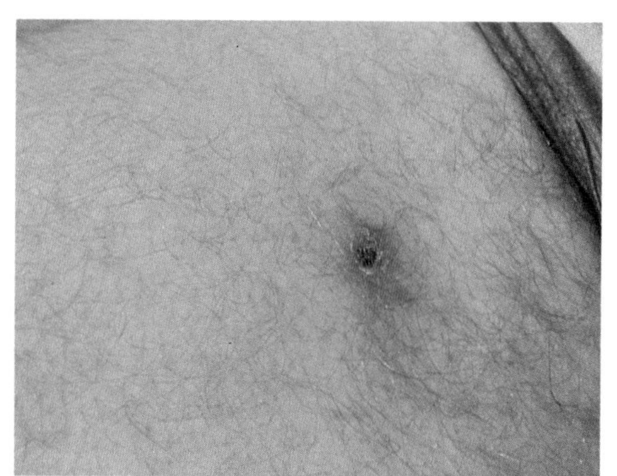

517 Eschar following the bite of a tick.

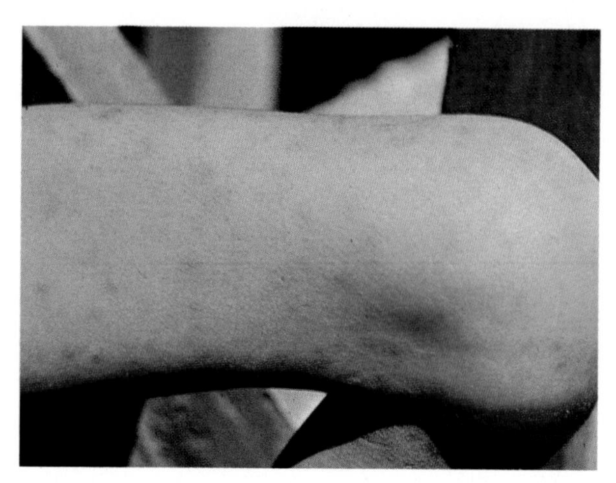

518 A rash produced by *R. tsutsugamushi* (scrub typhus). (Copyright LSTM.)

Viral haemorrhagic fevers

Viral haemorrhagic fevers comprise a group of at least 13 diseases, which share certain clinical and pathological features. These include fever, bleeding, shock and, often, liver and adrenal dysfunction. As a group they have a worldwide distribution, but principally affect tropical regions. Only Korean haemorrhagic fever and Omsk haemorrhagic fever occur exclusively in temperate zones. Most of the haemorrhagic fevers have a very limited and local distribution, for example, dengue haemorrhagic fever and yellow fever are restricted to the tropics. However, lassa fever, Argentinian haemorrhagic fever, Kyasanur Forest disease and Ebola fever may be transmitted by travellers to others via infected body fluids. They nevertheless tend to be restricted in their distribution.

The viral haemorrhagic fevers can be classified according to their mode of transmission (**Table 46**). Dengue yellow fever, chikungunya and Rift Valley fever are mosquito-borne infections. They have a great potential for wide and sudden epidemic spread.

Table 46. Classification of Viral Haemorrhagic Fevers.

Disease	*Virus*	*Arthropod vector*	*Animal host*	*Distribution*
Dengue haemorrhagic fever (togavirus)	Dengue virus (types 1–4)	Mosquitoes	Monkeys	Asia, Africa, America
Kyasanur Forest disease (togavirus)	Kyasanur Forest virus	Ticks	? Rodents and monkeys	Asia
Yellow fever (togavirus)	Yellow fever virus	Mosquitoes	Monkeys	Africa, Amercia
Chikungunya haemorrhagic fever (togavirus)	Chikungunya virus	Mosquitoes	Monkeys	Asia
Omsk haemorrhagic fever (togavirus)	Omsk haemorrhagic virus	Ticks	? Small mammals	Asia
Rift Valley fever (bunyavirus)	Rift Valley virus	Mosquitoes	Mammals	Africa
Crimean haemorrhagic fever (bunyavirus)	Crimean–Congo virus	Ticks	Small mammals	Africa, Asia
Korean haemorrhagic fever (hantavirus)	Hanta virus	–	Rodents (urine)	Asia, Africa
Lassa fever (arenavirus)	Lassa virus	–	Multimammate rats	Africa
Argentinian haemorrhagic fever (arenavirus)	Junin virus	–	Mice	South America
Bolivian haemorrhagic fever (arenavirus)	Machupo virus	–	Mice	South America
Marburg virus disease (filovirus)	Marburg virus	–	? Monkeys	Africa
Ebola virus disease (filovirus)	Ebola virus	–	? Monkeys	Africa

Dengue and dengue haemorrhagic fever

The dengue virus, which is a togavirus that exists in four serotypes, can cause two illnesses: dengue fever and dengue haemorrhagic fever. Dengue fever or 'break-bone fever' is so called because of the severe myalgia that is a main symptom. It is usually a mild self-limiting illness. In contrast, dengue haemorrhagic fever is a severe illness, especially in children. It is characterized by a bleeding tendency, shock and a high mortality. It is thought that immune mechanisms are responsible for severe disease.

Transmission of the RNA virus occurs through the mosquito *Aëdes aegypti*. Dengue is found in tropical and subtropical regions of Asia, Africa, Australasia, Central America and the Caribbean.

Classic dengue fever (break-bone fever)

Classic dengue fever occurs in epidemics which may involve thousands of adults and children. The incubation period lasts approximately 5–10 days. There is a sudden rise of fever with rigors, a transitory generalized erythematous rash, which fades after 24 hours, and a severe myalgia and arthralgia. The fever and symptoms usually last 3–5 days, after which they abate. A brief rise in temperature may follow a period of remission in biphasic manifestations of the disease. Shock, bleeding and death do not occur.

Dengue haemorrhagic fever

Dengue haemorrhagic fever is the most common haemorrhagic fever in children in South East Asia. Since 1952 it has spread throughout this area and beyond, for example, to Fiji and the Caribbean. In the period 1975–78, dengue accounted for more than 110,000 childhood hospital admissions and 3,300 deaths. It is a serious public health problem, which has the potential to spread to countries where dengue virus does not yet exist, but where the mosquito vector does exist, for example India, Latin America and tropical Africa.

If dengue is not treated energetically, the fatality rate from the accompanying shock syndrome may be as high as 15%, mainly affecting young children under 5 years of age. Autopsy findings are non-specific and include cerebral oedema, pleural effusion, ascites and enlarged liver with subcapsular haemorrhage. The main pathophysiological defect is increased vascular permeability and plasma leakage into the extravascular compartment. Children present with an abrupt onset of high fever (38–40°C), and haemorrhagic phenomena appear within 24 hours, manifested as petechiae, thrombocytopenia and hepatosplenomegaly. Circulatory failure develops in 25% of children, and is accompanied by serious bleeding (**519**). The shock syndrome occurs almost exclusively in South East Asian children, presenting between the third and sixth day of illness as the fever subsides. Abdominal pain precedes shock and is due to the plasma leakage from the vascular compartment. Severe bleeding may occur due to thrombocytopenia. Pleural effusion, which is usually right-sided and resolves spontaneously, is a common finding. The liver is enlarged and tender, but jaundice is absent. Myocarditis with abnormal ECG tracings is common. A post-dengue rash may be noted, particularly on the limbs (**520**).

519

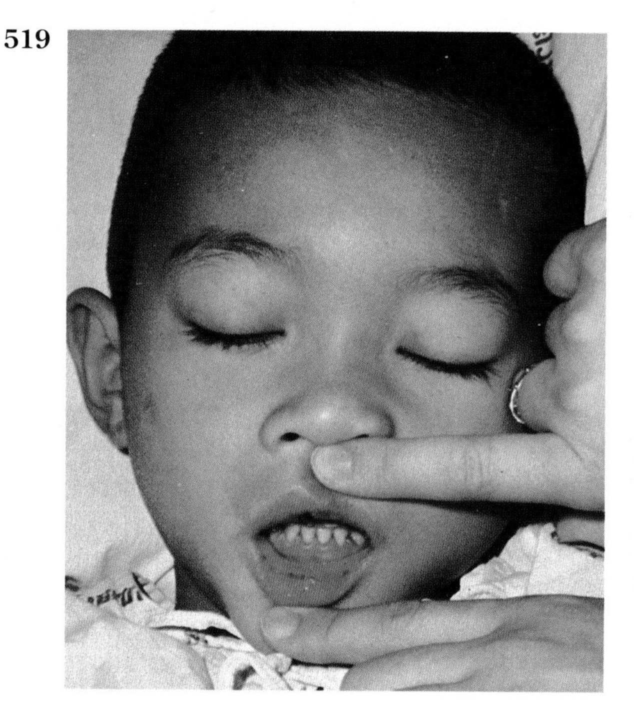

519 A Thai child with dengue haemorrhagic fever, demonstrating bleeding from the gums and mouth.

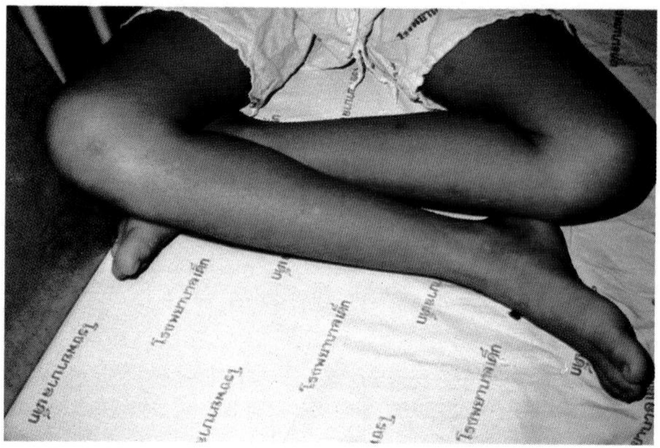

520 A post-dengue erythematous rash which blanches on pressure.

Complement fixation (CFT) and haemagglutination inhibition (HI) tests are useful in diagnosis. A positive result is indicated by a 4-fold rise in titres. Virus isolation is now routine in some parts of South East Asia.

There is no specific drug therapy for dengue haemorrhagic fever. Patients in shock must be given immediate infusions of isotonic electrolyte solution or of plasma. The rate of replacement depends upon changes in haematocrit packed-cell volume (PCV) readings, performed every 2 hours in the acute phase, and upon monitoring of vital signs. Recovery from shock occurs within 24–48 hours, with reabsorption of fluid from the extravascular compartment. Intravenous fluids should then be given with care in order to avoid overloading the circulation. If bleeding is severe, whole-blood transfusion may be necessary.

Yellow fever

Yellow fever is an acute mosquito-borne viral infection. The disease is endemic in tropical regions of South America and Africa. The yellow fever virus is a togavirus (**521**). It is enveloped with a spherical RNA nucleocapsid that is approximately 38 nm in diameter. Strains of yellow fever virus from Africa and South America are distinguishable by serological tests. The virus usually is spread by the mosquito *Aëdes aegypti* (**522**).

There are two forms of yellow fever: one is an urban type, which is transmitted from person to person by the mosquito; the other is the jungle or sylvan yellow fever, which is a zoonotic infection acquired through the bite of forest mosquito vectors that transmit the virus from monkeys to man.

The incubation period for the disease lasts 3–6 days. There can be a wide spectrum of clinical presentation, ranging from a mild febrile illness to a fulminating and fatal disease. The classic symptoms of yellow fever are probably found in only 10–20% of cases. In a mild case, there will be a sudden onset of fever and headache, which may last 48 hours or less. In other patients the fever is higher and the headache is more severe. There may be mild jaundice. In very severe infection, there is a sudden onset of high fever with headache, together with myalgia and intractable vomiting. Vomiting, haemorrhage and shock may supervene. Death occurs in 20–40% of severe cases. Treatment is supportive.

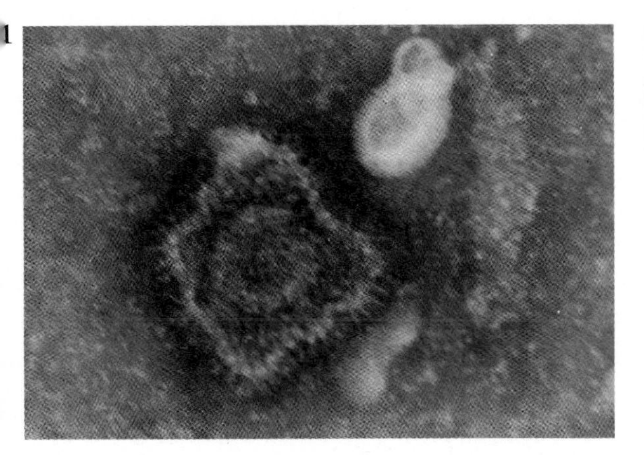

521 Negative-stain electron micrograph of a togavirus, which causes dengue and yellow fever (× *125,000*).

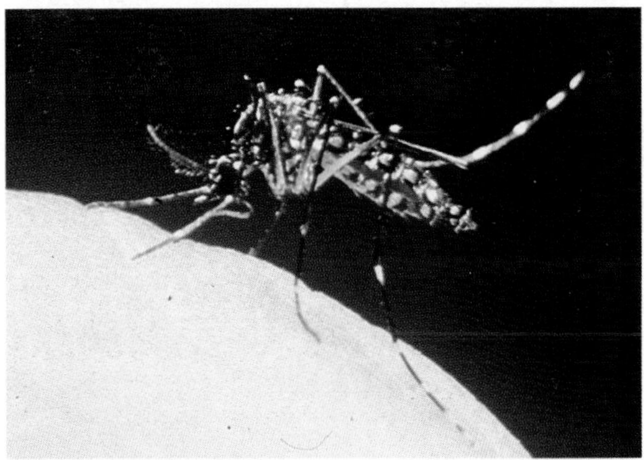

522 The *Aëdes aegypti* mosquito, the principal vector of yellow fever.

Other haemorrhagic fevers

523

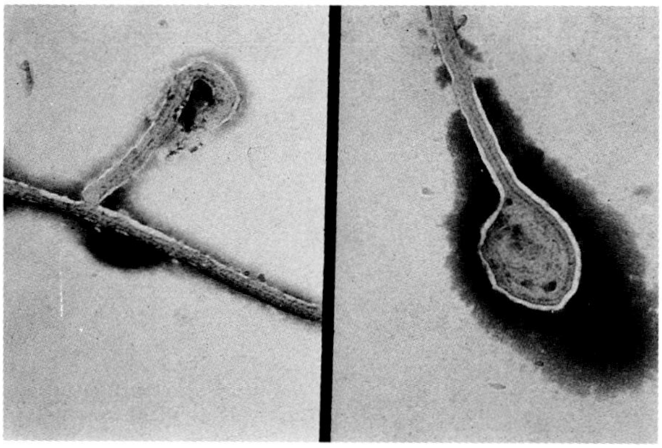

523 Negative-stain electron micrograph of filovirus which causes Ebola haemorrhagic fever (× *20,000*).

Haemorrhagic fevers caused by arenaviruses and filoviruses have in common the clinical characteristic of sudden outbreaks that, with successive transmission, become attenuated in their severity. The intermediate host is usually a small rodent or monkey. Man acquires the disease from infected blood or urine. Examples are the Ebola fever (**523**) and Marburg disease caused by filoviruses, both of which occur in East and Central Africa. The illnesses begin with flu-like symptoms which progress in severity to cause myalgia, pleurisy, respiratory symptoms and, ultimately, haemorrhage. The fatality rate is high.

Lassa fever, which is caused by an arenavirus, presents in a similar way. Children have contracted the infection by catching and playing with the reservoir host, the multimammate rat, *Mastomys natalensis*. Lassa fever is found principally in West Africa, but people have contracted the disease in Africa and then travelled abroad to infect others with their blood or body fluids.

Non-haemorrhagic arbovirus disease (arthropod-borne viruses)

524

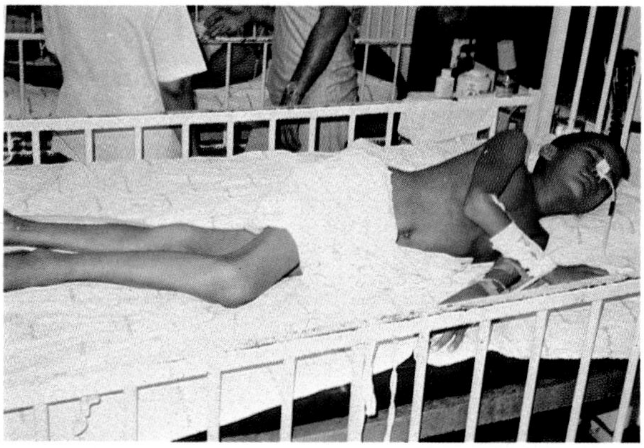

524 A Thai boy with acute Japanese encephalitis virus infection.

Arboviruses (arthropod-borne togaviruses) are transmitted by blood-sucking insects. Although there are over 400 arboviruses, only about 80 are capable of infecting man. Most of the arbovirus infections are zoonoses in which man is an incidental host. Mosquitoes are he most important vectors of disease but ticks, sandflies and *Culicoides* spp. also transmit viruses.

There is a wide spectrum of clinical presentation, ranging from a mild febrile illness to fatal encephalitis or haemorrhagic disease. Japanese encelphalitis is a severe illness with a high mortality rate in children. It is restricted to South East Asia. The intermediate hosts are pigs and some birds. Children may develop a severe encephalitis (**524**) in which the fatality rate may be as high as 60%. Those children who survive are often left with some handicap.

Management is symptomatic. Vaccines have been produced against specific viruses.

Tropical helminthic infections

There are three groups of helminths (*helmins* is Greek for worm) that infect man: annelids (segmented worms), nematodes (roundworms) and platyhelminths (flatworms or flukes). Many worms that affect man are found widely distributed throughout the world, but infestation is much more common in tropical countries because of climatic, cultural and sociological factors. Poverty, poor hygiene and overcrowding increase the risk of heavy worm infestations and children are particularly at risk.

Intestinal worm infestations are discussed in Chapter 2 (pp.46–51).

Schistosomiasis

Schistosoma is a genus of bisexual blood flukes. Man is the definitive host for three species: *S. mansoni*, *S. haematobium* and *S. japonicum*. The life cycle of these three species is similar, with man acquiring infection from cercariae, which penetrate the skin during contact with fresh infested water. The distribution of the disease can be seen in **525**.

After penetrating the skin, the cercariae are carried to the portal system, where they develop into adult worms which migrate to their final destination: *S.*

525

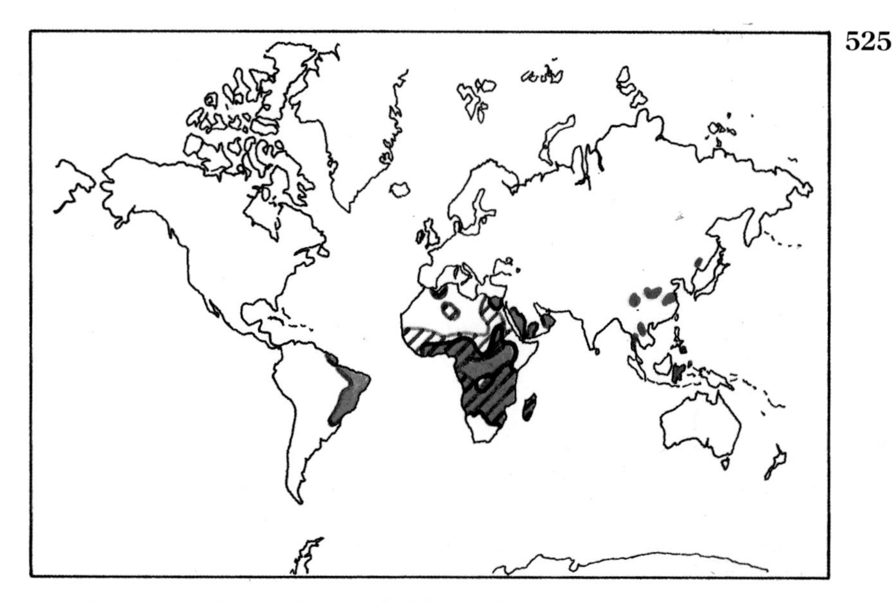

525 The geographical distribution of schistosomiasis.

526

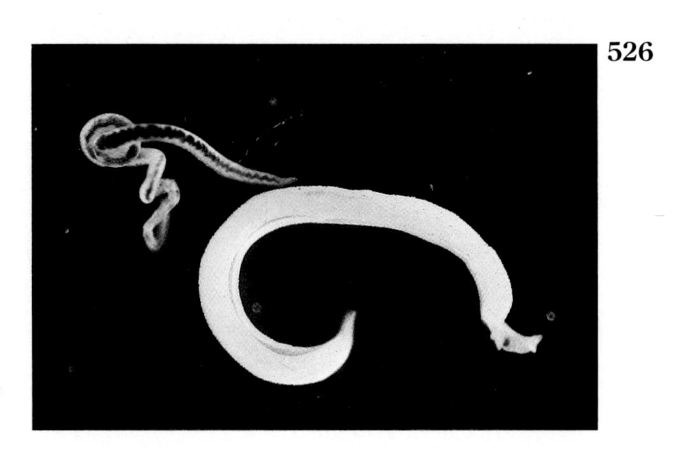

526 A small adult male worm and larger female *S. haematobium* worm. (Copyright LSTM.)

mansoni inhabits the inferior mesenteric veins, causing disease of the gastrointestinal tract; *S. haematobium* (**526**) lives mainly in the plexus of veins around the bladder, prostate and uterus, causing renal disease; and *S. japonicum* inhabits venules of the superior and inferior mesenteric veins. The female fluke lays up to 1,000 ova per day and may live up to 10 years. The pathology is caused by the ova migrating into tissue. The ova liberate histolytic enzymes which excite a granulomatous response in man. Complications arise when fibrous tissue is laid down in chronically inflamed tissue. The severity of the disease is related to the intensity of infection in a given host.

Children may acquire heavy infestations but symptoms tend to occur in late childhood. In *S. mansoni* infection the child may become anaemic from passing blood and mucus in the stools (**527**). Later, portal hypertension may develop due to intense inflammation and fibrosis of the liver (**528**). *S. haematobium* is a cause of painless haematuria. Chronic infection of the bladder may cause calcification (**529**), and stricture formation, with an obstructive uropathy. There is an association between schistosomiasis and the development of bladder cancer.

Diagnosis is made by indentification of the characteristic ova in urine in the case of *S. haematobium* (**530**), and from faeces when *S. mansoni* (**531**) and *S. japonicum* are suspected.

Fortunately, new and effective drugs have been introduced to treat all types of schistosomiasis. Praziquantel is the treatment of choice for all three types. The success rate can be as high as 80–90%, and the intensity of infection is markedly reduced. However, although the adult worms will be killed, symptoms and complications from ova may persist for many years.

527

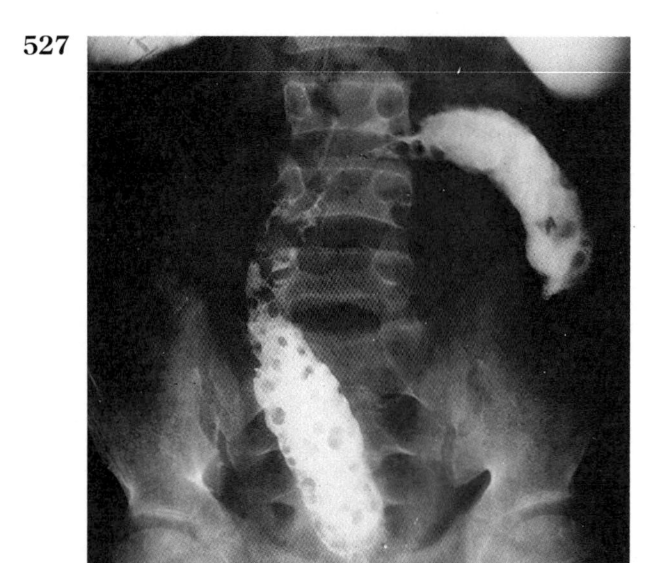

527 Barium enema reveals a cobbled appearance of the rectum and sigmoid colon due to chronic infection with *S. mansoni*.

528

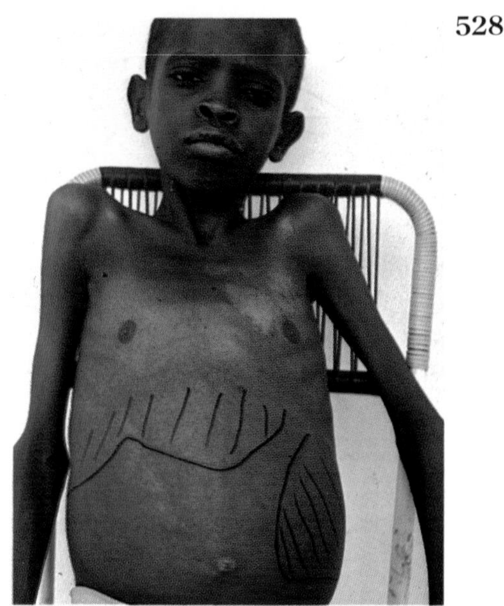

528 A Sudanese boy with portal hypertension due to *S. mansoni* infection.

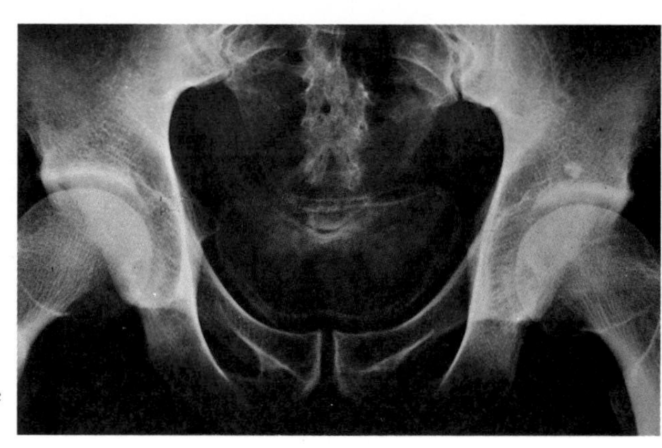

529 X-ray of the pelvis demonstrating calcification of the bladder due to chronic infection with *S. haematobium*.

0

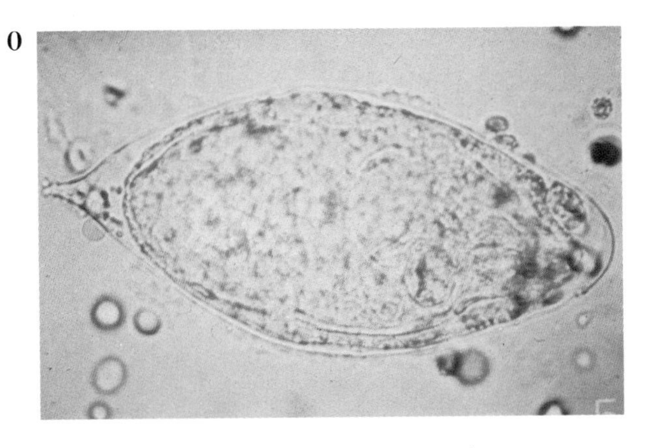

530 *S. haematobium* ova with a terminal spine.

531

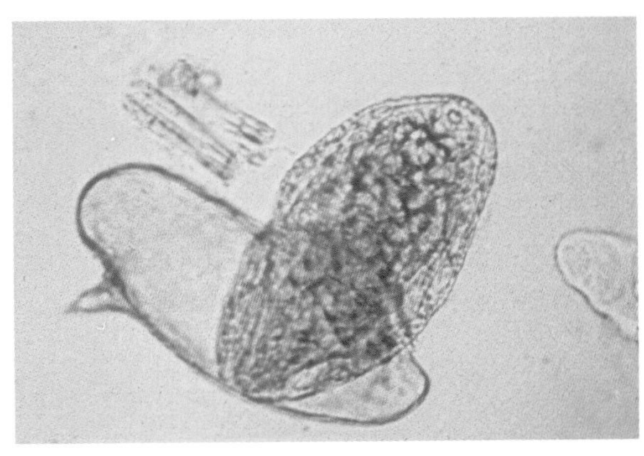

531 *S. mansoni* ova with a lateral spine.

Dracunculiasis/dracontiasis (guinea-worm infection)

Dracunculiasis or dracontiasis is caused by the nematode *Dracunculus medinensis*. Children acquire the infection by drinking water infected by the small crustacean *Cyclops* (the water flea). The larvae penetrate the bowel wall of man and invade the connective tissue. It is here that the mature worm develops, causing localized swelling. Although generalized allergic reactions may occur on initial exposure to the larvae, the first clinical sign is usually the formation of a swelling and a blister at the ankle (**532**). The blister enlarges over several days and may cause pain, which can be relieved by placing the affected limb in cold water. The female worm then extrudes part of her body and liberates the larvae (**533**).

Treatment with mebendazole or niridazole will kill the adult worm, which may then more easily be removed from the tissue. Care must be taken to extract the whole worm because secondary bacterial infection is common. Occasionally, the worm may die, subsequently becoming calcified in tissue (**534**).

532

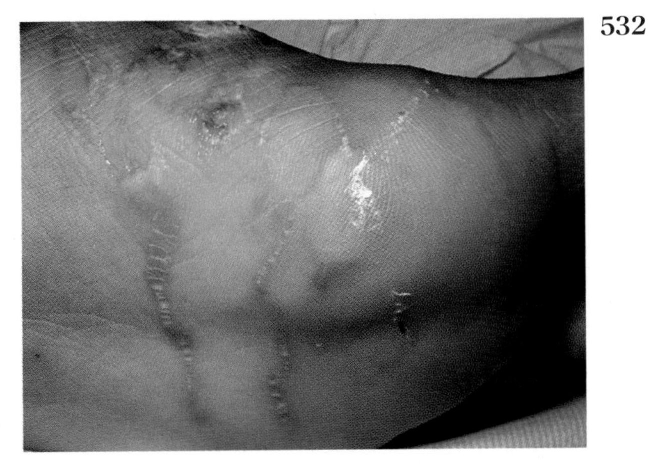

532 A blister forming on the foot prior to discharging the guinea worm larva.

33

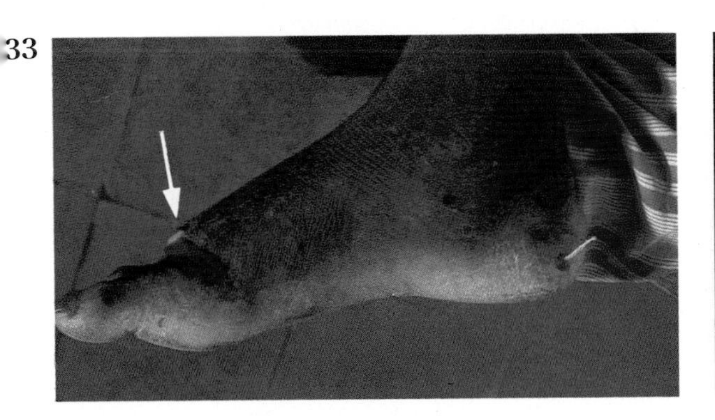

533 Guinea worm showing blister on dorsum of the foot (arrow) and the worm extruding from the heel.

534

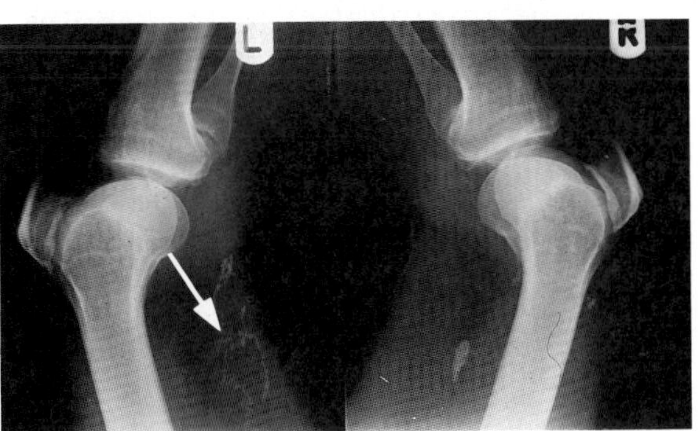

534 X-ray showing dead and calcified adult guinea worms in the popliteal space of a child.

Filariasis

Filarial parasites are nematodes, nine distinct species of which affect man (**Table 47**). Infection is acquired through the bite of blood-sucking insects. Filariasis is confined to the tropics and subtropics, the most widespread type being lymphatic filariasis, which is caused by *Wuchereria bancrofti* and *Brugia malayi*. The characteristic clinical sign of lymphoedema (**535**) or elephantiasis is rare in children. The lymphoedema is due to a lymphangitis that arises as part of the host response to the adult worm living in the lymphatic channels. The female adult worm may liberate up to 50,000 microfilarial larvae per day. These then appear in the blood and may be associated with episodes of pyrexia and chills.

The tropical pulmonary eosinophilia syndrome is caused by an aggressive host response to the larvae (**536**). The onset is usually sudden, with episodes of fever accompanied by a dry cough. There may be bronchospasm.

Table 47. Filarial Worms that Infect Man.

Nematode (Adult form)	*Geographical distribution*	*Site of microfilaria*
Wuchereria bancrofti (lymphatics)	Asia, Africa, Central and South America	Blood
Brugia malayi (lymphatics)	Asia	Blood
B. timori (lymphatics)	Indonesia	Blood
Onchocerca volvulus (skin)	Asia, Central and South America	Blood and skin
Loa loa (connective tissue)	Central Africa	Blood
Mansonella perstans (skin)	South America, Indonesia	Blood
M. streptocerca (skin)	South America, Africa	Skin
M. ozzardi (skin)	South America	Blood and skin

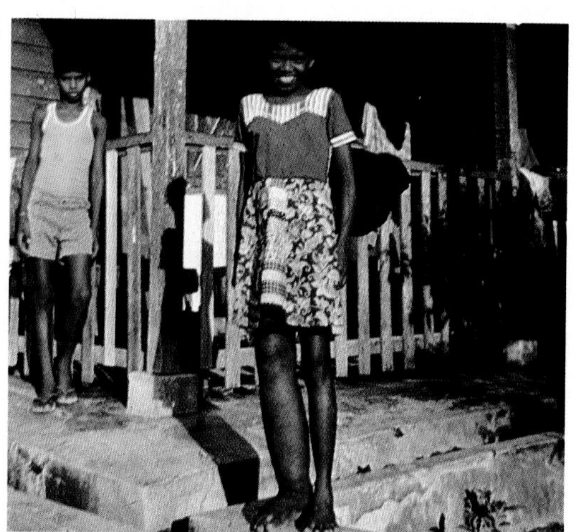

535 A girl with lymphoedema of the leg due to filariasis.

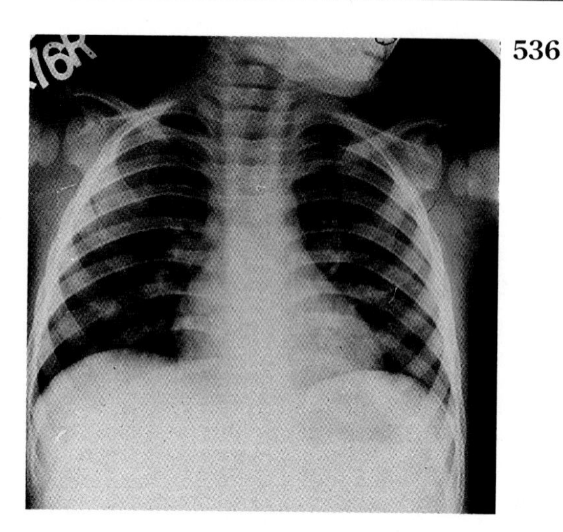

536 Chest X-ray showing bilateral soft pulmonary infiltrates in a child with pulmonary eosinophilia due to microfilaria.

Ivermectin is the treatment of choice, but diethylcarbamazine is also a well-tried and effective drug.

Onchocerciasis (river blindness) is a form of filariasis caused by *Onchocerca volvulus*, which is found in Africa, Saudi Arabia and in South America. Infection is transmitted through the bite of the blackfly (*Simulium*). Dermatitis, subcutaneous nodules and eye disease are the result of heavy infections. The most disabling complication of onchocerciasis is blindness due to microfilariae migrating through the sclera into the cornea. Dead microfilariae cause a sclerosing keratitis. The adult worms may round up into nodules, especially over bony areas (**537**). Ivermectin is the treatment of choice for onchocerciasis.

Other types of filariae include *Loa loa*, which causes tissue (kalabar) swelling, and a number of filariae that may cause a dermatitis, but give rise to few other systemic complications. An eosinophilia is usual. A cure may be effected by ivermectin or diethylcarbamazine.

537

537 A subcutaneous nodule on the chest caused by adult *O. volvulus*.

Fasciolopsiasis

Fasciolopsis buski, which is known as the giant intestinal fluke, is acquired when children eat uncooked vegetables grown in fresh water (**538**). It exists mainly in East and South East Asia. The encysted larvae are ingested and hatch in the bowel. The mature worm then attaches to the duodenum and jejunum, producing eggs. In light infections there may be a few symptoms, but children are unfortunately prone to heavy infection, and some will demonstrate oedema of the face and body. This is due partly to a toxic or allergic reaction and partly to hypoalbuminaemia secondary to protein loss or malabsorption. Treatment is effected by a single dose of praziquantel.

The liver flukes

The liver flukes include *Opisthorchis* (*Clonorchis*) and *Fasciola hepatica*. *Opisthorchis* is found in East and South East Asia, while *Fasciola* is found worldwide. In the UK, there are foci in Wales and Scotland. Children acquire infection by eating raw fish or freshwater vegetables, such as watercress, in which the larvae have encysted. The worms hatch in the gut and migrate to the bile ducts. In light infections, there are few symptoms. In heavy infections, abdominal pain, enlargement and tenderness of the liver, fever, urticaria and, occasionally, jaundice may occur. Cholangitis may be caused by secondary bacterial infection. Diagnosis can be difficult since the characteristic eggs (**539**) are only intermittently excreted with faeces. Treatment is with praziquantel.

8

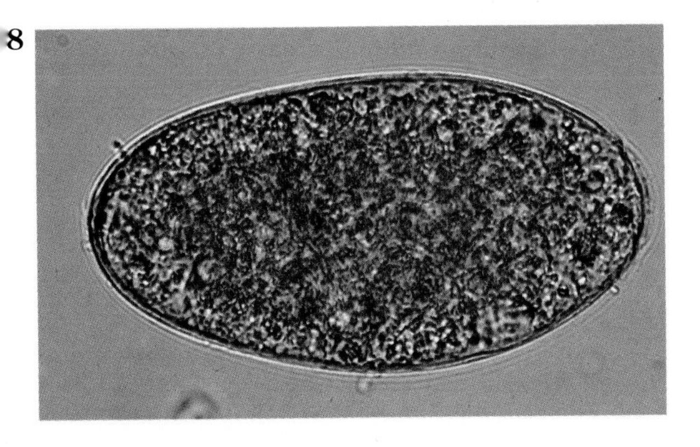

538 Ova of *F. buski*.

539

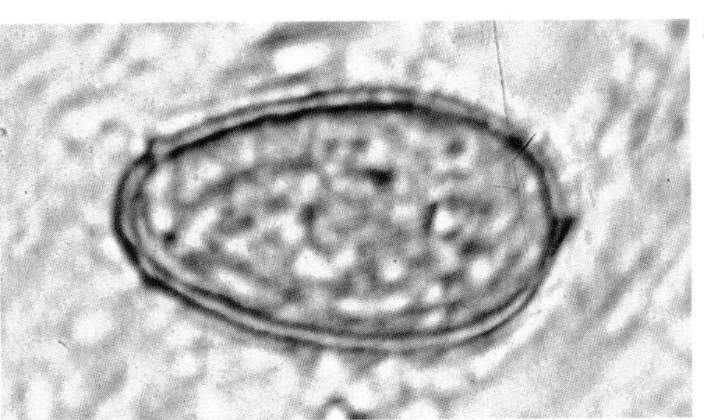

539 Ova of *O. sinensis*.

Myiasis

Myiasis is the invasion of body tissues by the larvae of certain flies. The skin, mucous membranes and the gastrointestinal tract may be involved. On the skin, the burrowing larvae may cause a painful lesion that is similar to a boil (**540**).

Creeping dermal myiasis is a form of larva migrans which arises because man is only an accidental host of animal helminths. The larvae are unable to survive in man and thus migrate in the dermis, causing severe irritation (**541**).

540

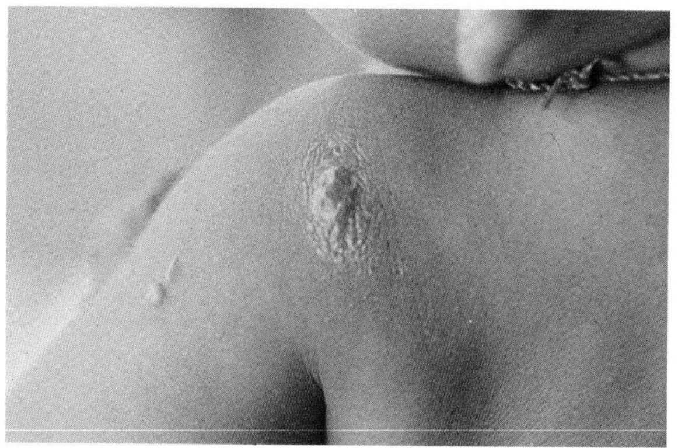

540 Myiasis showing a pustule caused by the burrowing larvae of a fly.

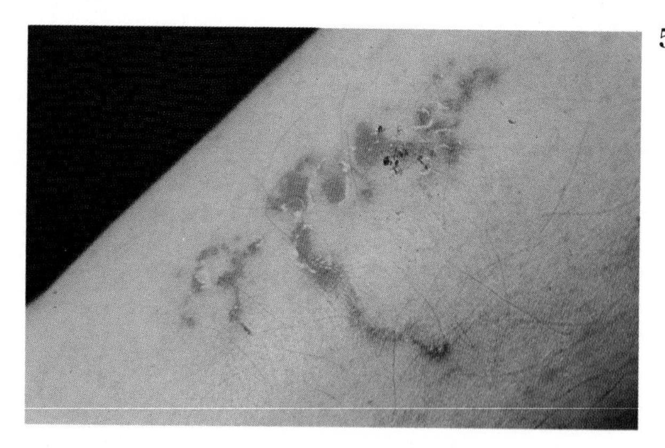

541 Cutaneous larva migrans.

Tungiasis (chigoe or jigger)

542

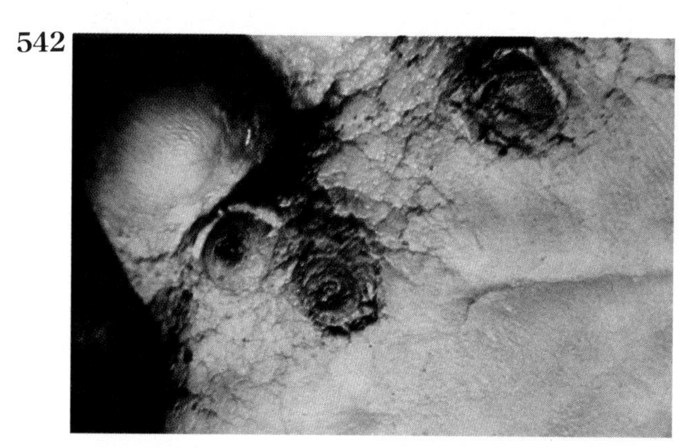

542 *T. penetrans* burrowed into the foot.

Tungiasis is caused by the chigoe or jigger flea *Tunga penetrans*, which burrows into the skin and feeds on tissue fluids. Because children are less likely to wear shoes or protective clothing, it is the feet and legs that are most often involved (**542**). The female flea enlarges with eggs, a process that can cause a very painful lesion, especially if it occurs under the nail. Children may become infected in other parts of the body when they lie on the ground near to pigs, which are the natural hosts.

Superficial and deep mycosis

The mycoses are caused by fungi. Many of the superficial dermatophyte infections such as ringworm may be found worldwide, whereas others such as Tinea imbricata (**543**) occur only in the tropics.

Superficial mycoses usually cause no serious disease. Areas of depigmentation may occur, as seen in pityriasis versicolor (**544**), which is caused by the fungus *Malassezia furfur*. However, the subcutaneous and systemic mycoses can cause serious disfigurement and life-threatening disease. Mycetoma (**545**) is a chronic subcutaneous fungal infection caused by a species of *Actinomyces* (actinomycetoma) and by some filamentous fungi (eumycetoma). The infective organism is usually introduced into the lower limb as a result of trauma and a slowly progressive soft-tissue swelling then develops. The intensity of the host reaction will determine the speed and the spread of the fungi. Sinus formation, osteitis and osteomyelitis (**546**) may arise as complications.

The systemic mycoses include a number of pathogenic fungi. These mycoses may be localized to the lung or to other organs and may also be widely disseminated throughout the body. Children and the immune-compromised are particularly vulnerable to disseminated disease (**547**). The fungi usually enter the body through the lung. Symptoms of cough and fever, and allergic reactions such as erythema nodosum, erythema multiforme, arthralgia and conjunctivitis may occur. Later, dissemination to bone, brain and other tissues takes place.

Although amphotericin B and ketoconazole will cure many children with early and localized disease, the outlook for those with meningitis and widely disseminated infection is poor.

543

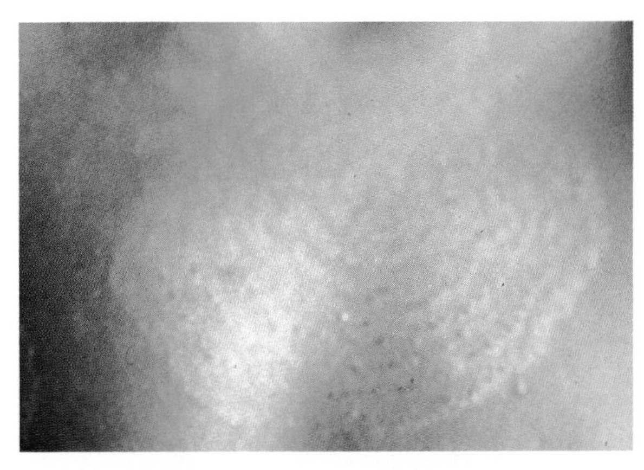

543 Tinea imbricata caused by *Trichophyton concentricum*.

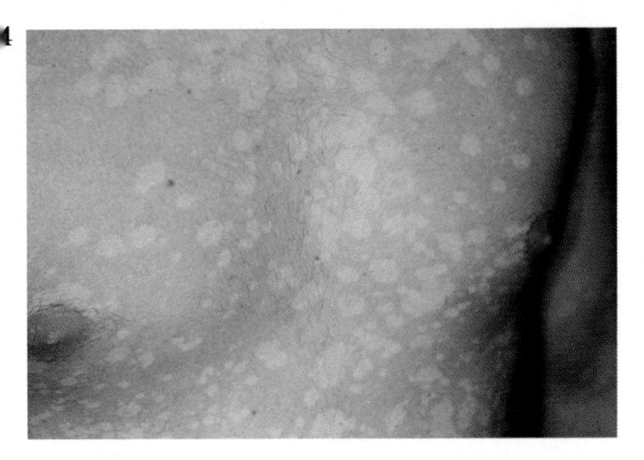

544 Pityriasis versicolor caused by *Malassezia furfur*.

545

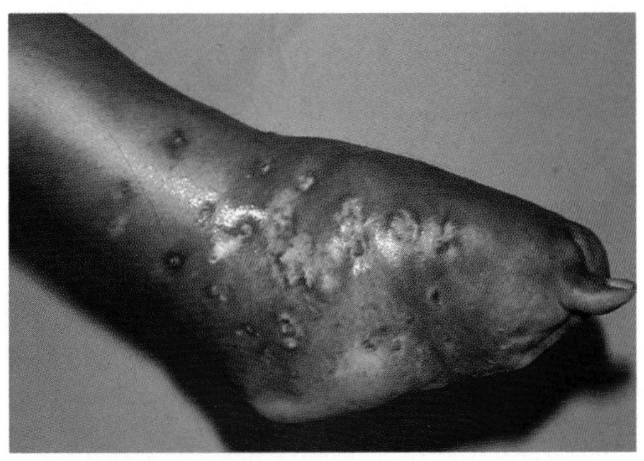

545 Mycetoma in a Sudanese boy.

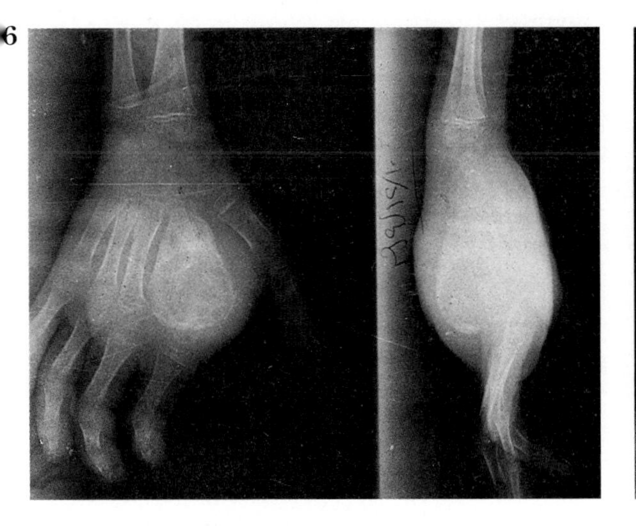

546 Mycetoma osteomyelitis.

547

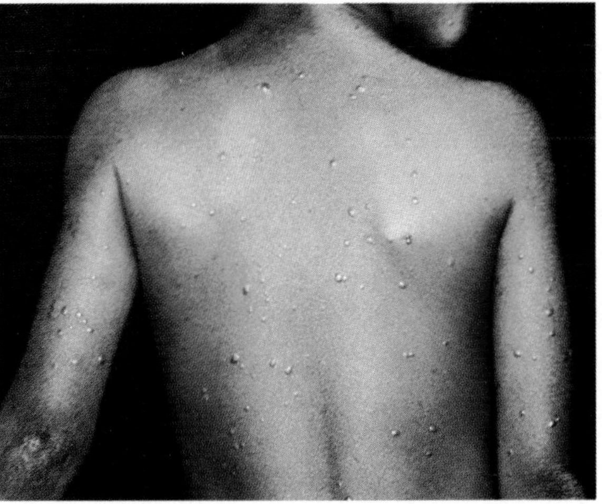

547 Scattered papular lesions in an African boy with histoplasmosis.

Yaws

Yaws is caused by the spirochaete *Treponema pertenue*, which can occur throughout the tropical world. *T. pertenue* is morphologically indistinguishable both from *T. pallidum*, which causes syphilis, and from *T. carateum*, which causes the mucocutaneous disease, pinta, and is limited to Central and South America. Yaws develops when *T. pertenue* is introduced through an abrasion of the skin. A papule then forms and progressively increases in size (**548** & **549**). There may be regional lymphadenopathy followed by secondary and tertiary lesions which can recur over many years.

T. pertenue is exquisitely sensitive to penicillin and a rapid resolution will occur with treatment.

548

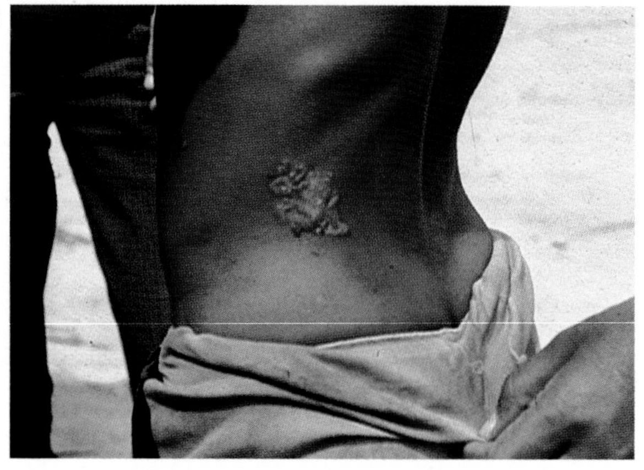

548 Yaws on the trunk.

549

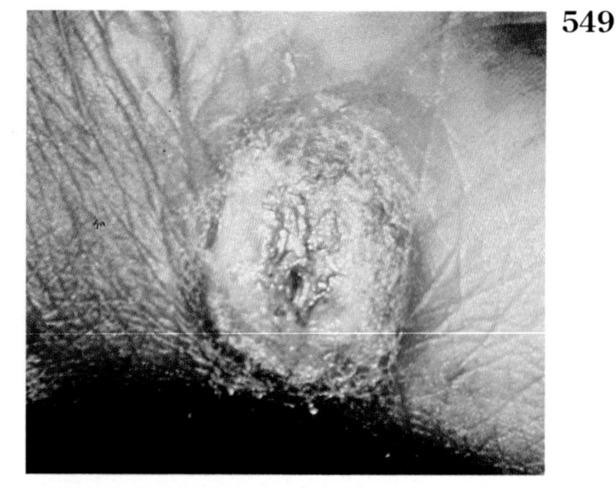

549 Yaws on the wrist.

Endemic (non-venereal) syphilis

Endemic syphilis, which is due to a treponeme that is morphologically indistinguishable from other treponemes, occurs in dry areas of North Africa and the Middle East. The initial lesion arises on the mucosa of the mouth (**550**) or nose. Secondary lesions may spread to the skin and skin folds (**551**). Treatment is with penicillin.

550

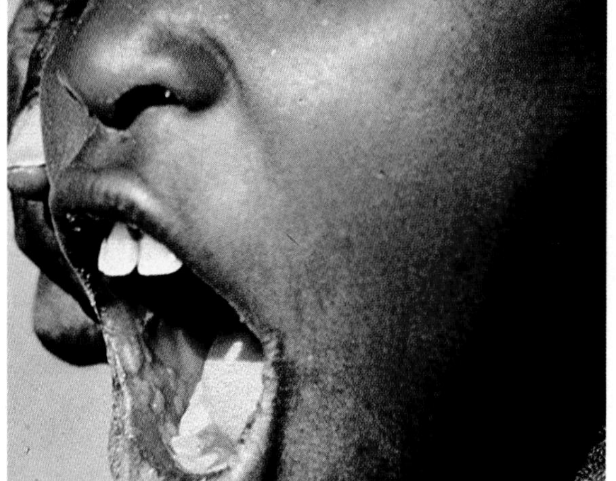

550 Endemic syphilis with a primary lesion on the mucosa of the mouth.

551

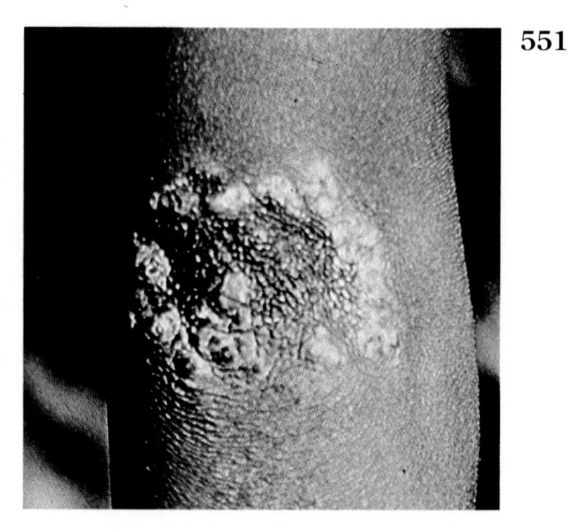

551 Endemic syphilis with a typical secondary lesion.

Atypical mycobacterial infection

Mycobacterium ulcerans (Buruli ulcer)

M. ulcerans infection, which occurs throughout the tropics, is probably transmitted to children through abraded skin. As the name suggests, the mycobacterium causes necrosis of the dermis and ulcer formation. The lesion progresses from a nodule which enlarges gradually. Some ulcers heal spontaneously, but others progress to become locally destructive, causing scarring and deformity (**552**). Other atypical mycobacteria, some of which cause chronic skin ulcers and others a lymphadenitis which may form a discharging sinus, can also infect man.

Treatment of Buruli ulcers with rifampicin may promote healing. However, with extensive lesions, local excision may be necessary.

552

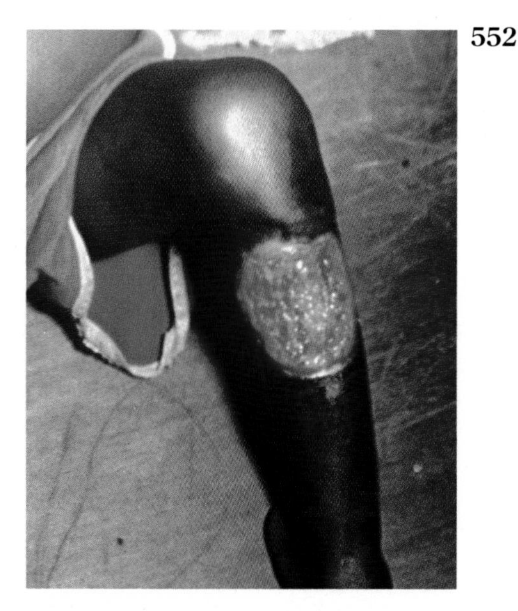

552 A destructive ulcer on the leg due to *M. ulcerans*.

Relapsing fever

Relapsing fever occurs in two forms: epidemic louse-borne relapsing fever, which is caused by *Borrelia recurrentis* (**553**); and endemic tick-borne relapsing fever, which is caused by *B. duttoni*. In both conditions the spirochaete is transmitted to man when the biting insect is crushed and its infected body fluid is rubbed into abraded skin.

Louse-borne relapsing fever occurs in epidemics in both warm and cold climates, often arising in times of social upheaval when people are herded together in refugee camps. The illness may be severe in children, and mortality may be high. Clinically, a child presents with chills, fever and malaise. Physical signs include arthritis and conjunctivitis and there may be pulmonary symptoms with meningeal signs. A rash may be present and hepatosplenomegaly is common.

Tick-borne relapsing fever may present in a clinically similar fashion. In untreated cases, each successive relapse (which lasts for 3–5 days in a 10–12 day cycle) becomes more attenuated and less severe over 6–8 cycles. Diagnosis is made by taking a peripheral blood smear at the time of fever when the spirochaete is present and staining it with Giemsa.

553

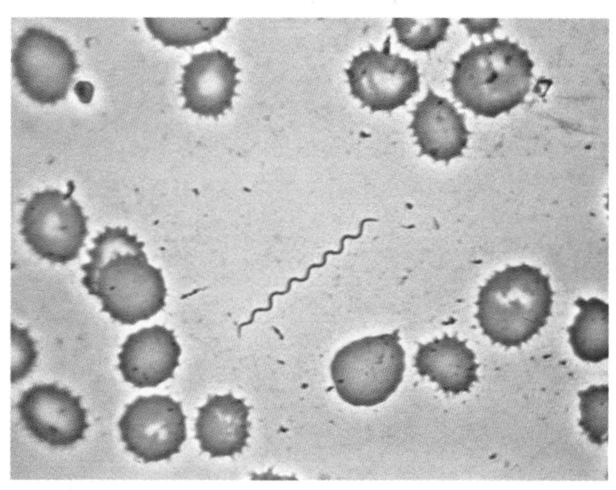

553 Blood film stained with Giemsa, demonstrating *B. recurrentis* (× *500*).

Erythromycin and tetracyline are both effective for treatment, but care must be taken where Jarisch–Herxheimer reaction occurs as this may complicate treatment.

Sickle cell disease and infection

Sickle-cell disease (**554**) predisposes children to infections, especially with *Salmonella* spp. and *Staphylococcus aureus*. Chronic osteomyelitis (**555**) and meningitis may arise as complications.

554

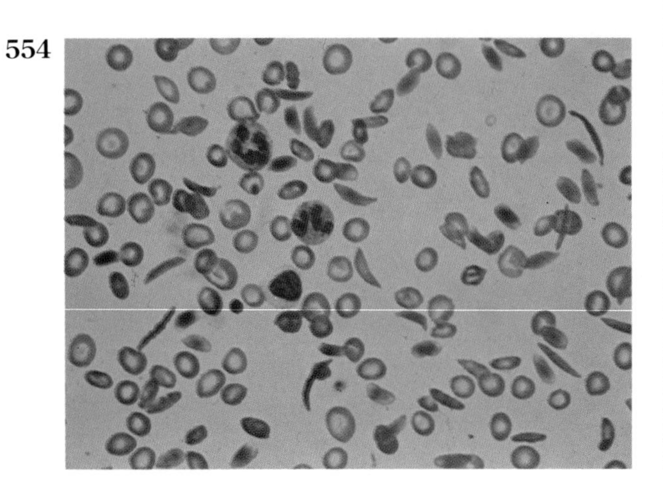

554 Blood film showing typical sickle cells (× *200*).

555

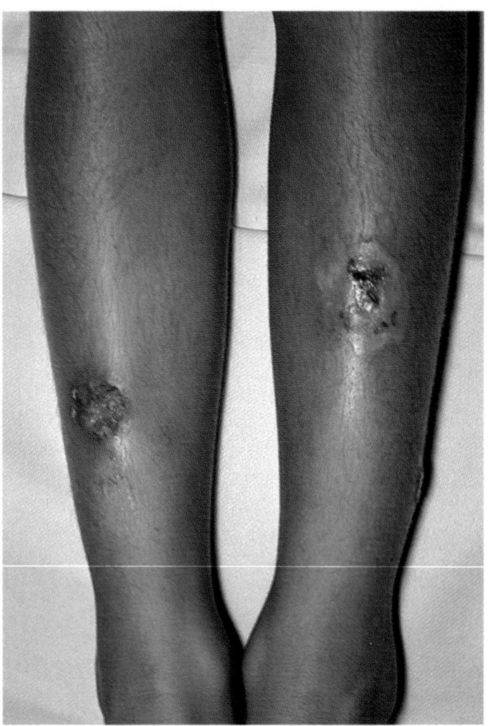

555 Osteomyelitis of both tibia due to *Salmonella* spp. infection in a boy with sickle-cell disease.

Index

Numbers in **bold** type refer to illustrations.